Improving Access to Oral Health Care for Vulnerable and Underserved Populations

Committee on Oral Health Access to Services

Board on Children, Youth, and Families

Board on Health Care Services

INSTITUTE OF MEDICINE *AND*
NATIONAL RESEARCH COUNCIL
OF THE NATIONAL ACADEMIES

THE NATIONAL ACADEMIES PRESS
Washington, D.C.
www.nap.edu

THE NATIONAL ACADEMIES PRESS 500 Fifth Street, N.W. Washington, DC 20001

NOTICE: The project that is the subject of this report was approved by the Governing Board of the National Research Council, whose members are drawn from the councils of the National Academy of Sciences, the National Academy of Engineering, and the Institute of Medicine. The members of the committee responsible for the report were chosen for their special competences and with regard for appropriate balance.

This study was supported by Contract No. HHSH25034002T between the National Academy of Sciences and the U.S. Department of Health and Human Services and Contract No. 15328 between the National Academy of Sciences and the California HealthCare Foundation. Any opinions, findings, conclusions, or recommendations expressed in this publication are those of the author(s) and do not necessarily reflect the view of the organizations or agencies that provided support for this project.

International Standard Book Number-13: 978-0-309-20946-5
International Standard Book Number-10: 0-309-20946-3

Additional copies of this report are available from the National Academies Press, 500 Fifth Street, N.W., Lockbox 285, Washington, DC 20055; (800) 624-6242 or (202) 334-3313 (in the Washington metropolitan area); Internet, http://www.nap.edu.

For more information about the Institute of Medicine, visit the IOM home page at: **www.iom.edu.**

Printed in the United States of America

The serpent has been a symbol of long life, healing, and knowledge among almost all cultures and religions since the beginning of recorded history. The serpent adopted as a logotype by the Institute of Medicine is a relief carving from ancient Greece, now held by the Staatliche Museen in Berlin.

Suggested citation: IOM (Institute of Medicine) and NRC (National Research Council). 2011. *Improving access to oral health care for vulnerable and underserved populations.* Washington, DC: The National Academies Press.

THE NATIONAL ACADEMIES

Advisers to the Nation on Science, Engineering, and Medicine

The **National Academy of Sciences** is a private, nonprofit, self-perpetuating society of distinguished scholars engaged in scientific and engineering research, dedicated to the furtherance of science and technology and to their use for the general welfare. Upon the authority of the charter granted to it by the Congress in 1863, the Academy has a mandate that requires it to advise the federal government on scientific and technical matters. Dr. Ralph J. Cicerone is president of the National Academy of Sciences.

The **National Academy of Engineering** was established in 1964, under the charter of the National Academy of Sciences, as a parallel organization of outstanding engineers. It is autonomous in its administration and in the selection of its members, sharing with the National Academy of Sciences the responsibility for advising the federal government. The National Academy of Engineering also sponsors engineering programs aimed at meeting national needs, encourages education and research, and recognizes the superior achievements of engineers. Dr. Charles M. Vest is president of the National Academy of Engineering.

The **Institute of Medicine** was established in 1970 by the National Academy of Sciences to secure the services of eminent members of appropriate professions in the examination of policy matters pertaining to the health of the public. The Institute acts under the responsibility given to the National Academy of Sciences by its congressional charter to be an adviser to the federal government and, upon its own initiative, to identify issues of medical care, research, and education. Dr. Harvey V. Fineberg is president of the Institute of Medicine.

The **National Research Council** was organized by the National Academy of Sciences in 1916 to associate the broad community of science and technology with the Academy's purposes of furthering knowledge and advising the federal government. Functioning in accordance with general policies determined by the Academy, the Council has become the principal operating agency of both the National Academy of Sciences and the National Academy of Engineering in providing services to the government, the public, and the scientific and engineering communities. The Council is administered jointly by both Academies and the Institute of Medicine. Dr. Ralph J. Cicerone and Dr. Charles M. Vest are chair and vice chair, respectively, of the National Research Council.

www.national-academies.org

COMMITTEE ON ORAL HEALTH ACCESS TO SERVICES

FREDERICK P. RIVARA (*Chair*), Seattle Children's Guild Endowed Chair in Pediatrics; Professor of Pediatrics, School of Medicine, University of Washington
PAUL C. ERWIN, Professor and Chair, Department of Public Health, University of Tennessee, Knoxville
CASWELL A. EVANS, JR., Associate Dean for Prevention and Public Health Sciences, College of Dentistry, University of Illinois, Chicago
THEODORE G. GANIATS, Professor, Department of Family and Preventive Medicine, School of Medicine, University of California, San Diego
SHELLY GEHSHAN, Director, Pew Children's Dental Campaign, Pew Center on the States
KATHY VOIGT GEURINK, Clinical Associate Professor, Department of Dental Hygiene, School of Health Professions, University of Texas Health Science Center
PAUL GLASSMAN, Professor of Dental Practice, Director of Community Oral Health, Arthur A. Dugoni School of Dentistry, University of the Pacific
DAVID M. KROL, Team Director, Senior Program Officer, Human Capital, Robert Wood Johnson Foundation
JANE PERKINS, Legal Director, National Health Law Program
MARGARET A. POTTER, Associate Dean; Director, Center for Public Health Practice; Associate Professor of Health Policy & Management, Graduate School of Public Health, University of Pittsburgh
RENEE SAMELSON, Associate Professor of Obstetrics and Gynecology, Albany Medical College
PHYLLIS W. SHARPS, Professor and Associate Dean, Community and Global Programs, School of Nursing, Johns Hopkins University
LINDA H. SOUTHWARD, Research Fellow & Research Professor, Social Science Research Center, Mississippi State University
MARIA ROSA WATSON, Research Director, Primary Care Coalition of Montgomery County
BARBARA WOLFE, Professor of Economics and Population Health Sciences; Public Affairs and Faculty Affiliate, Institute for Research on Poverty, University of Wisconsin-Madison

Study Staff

TRACY A. HARRIS, Study Director
PATTI SIMON, Senior Program Officer
MEG BARRY, Associate Program Officer
ROSEMARY CHALK, Director, Board on Children, Youth, and Families
WENDY E. KEENAN, Program Associate
AMY ASHEROFF, Senior Program Assistant

Reviewers

This report has been reviewed in draft form by individuals chosen for their diverse perspectives and technical expertise, in accordance with procedures approved by the National Research Council's Report Review Committee. The purpose of this independent review is to provide candid and critical comments that will assist the institution in making its published report as sound as possible and to ensure that the report meets institutional standards for objectivity, evidence, and responsiveness to the study charge. The review comments and draft manuscript remain confidential to protect the integrity of the deliberative process. We wish to thank the following individuals for their review of this report:

BRUCE J. BAUM, National Institute of Dental and Craniofacial Research
PAUL CASAMASSIMO, Nationwide Children's Hospital
DANIEL G. DAVIDSON, private practice
A. CONAN DAVIS, University of Alabama
R. BRUCE DONOFF, Harvard School of Dental Medicine
CHRISTINE M. FARRELL, Michigan Department of Community Health
JANE GILLETTE, Mint Dental Studio
JOHN S. GREENSPAN, University of California, San Francisco
MICHAEL J. HELGESON, Apple Tree Dental
CATHERINE HESS, National Academy for State Health Policy
CYNTHIA E. HODGE, National Dental Association Foundation
GENEVIEVE KENNEY, The Urban Institute

JULIA LEAR, The George Washington University
HUGH SILK, University of Massachusetts Medical School and Hahnemann Family Health Center
GEORGE W. TAYLOR, University of Michigan

Although the reviewers listed above have provided many constructive comments and suggestions, they were not asked to endorse the conclusions or recommendations nor did they see the final draft of the report before its release. The review of this report was overseen by **DONALD M. STEINWACHS,** Johns Hopkins University, and **GEORGES C. BENJAMIN,** American Public Health Association. Appointed by the National Research Council and the Institute of Medicine, they were responsible for making certain that an independent examination of this report was carried out in accordance with institutional procedures and that all review comments were carefully considered. Responsibility for the final content of this report rests entirely with the authoring committee and the institution.

Foreword

Oral health care is not uniformly attainable across the nation. Unfortunately, individuals who face the greatest barriers to care are often among the most vulnerable members of our society. The impact of unmet oral health care needs is magnified by the well-established connection between oral health and overall health. These problems led the Health Resources and Services Administration and the California HealthCare Foundation to ask the Institute of Medicine (IOM) to advise them on how to improve access to oral health care. The IOM committee, led by Frederick Rivara, was charged with assessing the current oral health care delivery system; exploring its strengths, limitations, and future challenges; and describing a vision for the delivery of oral health care to vulnerable and underserved populations. The committee worked in parallel with a second IOM committee that focused on the role of the U.S. Department of Health and Human Services in improving oral health. Together, they comprise an extensive examination of the status of oral health and oral health care in America.

In its examination of the evidence, the committee uncovered decades of efforts that have been insufficient in eliminating significant disparities in access to oral health care. However, this examination also revealed an array of groups committed to improving access and highlighted common goals and opportunities for collaboration and innovation. Examples appear throughout the report and inform the committee's recommendations. The committee calls for a renewed commitment and a confluence of energies directed at tackling these familiar and persistent challenges.

This report presents a vision for oral health care in the United States where everyone has access to quality oral health care throughout the life cycle. The committee acknowledges that realizing this vision will require numerous coordinated and sustained actions, with special attention to the distinct and varied needs of the nation's vulnerable and underserved populations. Achieving this goal will require flexibility and ingenuity among leaders at the federal, state, local, and community levels acting in concert with oral health and other health care professionals. We hope this report will encourage these groups to act on behalf of the nation's vulnerable and underserved populations and to take the important and necessary next steps to improve access to oral health care, reduce oral health disparities, and improve oral health.

Harvey V. Fineberg, M.D., Ph.D.
President, Institute of Medicine
July 2011

Preface

As Americans, we have become increasingly cognizant and, it is hoped, intolerant of the disparities in access to health care in this country. While our health care system has the capabilities for amazing treatment of a wide array of maladies, this care is not uniformly available to all. Disparities exist, however, not only in access to the latest in life-saving technology but also in access to the most basic of routine health care. The Patient Protection and Affordable Care Act of 2010 is intended to improve access to care for all and reduce these disparities in health care and health.

Oral health care is one of those dimensions of our health care delivery system in which striking disparities exist. More than half of the population does not visit a dentist each year. Poor and minority children are substantially less likely to have access to oral health care than are their nonpoor and nonminority peers. Americans living in rural areas have poorer oral health status and more unmet dental needs than their urban counterparts. Older adults, especially those living in long-term care facilities, have a high prevalence of oral health problems and difficulty accessing care by individuals trained in their special needs. Disabled individuals uniformly confront access barriers, regardless of their financial resources. The consequences of these disparities in access to oral health care have a strong influence not only on oral health but on overall health as well. Poor oral health can lead to malnutrition, childhood speech problems, and serious, and sometimes fatal, infections. Poor oral health is associated with diabetes, heart disease, and premature births. Oral disease in pregnant women and young mothers can be transmitted vertically to their offspring, perpetuating a cycle of disease.

In 2000, the surgeon general issued a report on oral health in this country calling for action to improve the oral health of the nation. The many efforts in both the public and private delivery systems to address these disparities have been important, but they have not been successful in eliminating them. Therefore, with support from the Health Resources and Services Administration and the California HealthCare Foundation, the National Research Council and the Institute of Medicine, through collaborative efforts between the Board on Children, Youth, and Families and the Board on Health Care Services, formed the Committee on Oral Health Access to Services. The charge was to assess current access to oral health care especially for vulnerable and underserved populations and to provide a vision of how oral health care should be addressed by public and private providers across the nation.

The committee held five meetings and one public workshop. We engaged in vigorous, thoughtful discussions regarding the causes of the current disparities in access to oral health care and the best approaches to addressing the problem both in the short and long term. We did so cognizant of the economic challenges facing the nation and individual states today, and with the awareness that oral health care is a part of our overall health care delivery system. It is our hope that the findings and recommendations of this report will help policy makers, service providers and their professional organizations, and funders and government agencies to address these access problems in new, meaningful, and innovative ways that will result in oral health for all.

The committee could not have done its work without the outstanding guidance and support provided by the NRC-IOM staff: Tracy Harris, study director; Patti Simon, senior program officer; and Meg Barry, associate program officer. Amy Asheroff provided skilled logistic support to the committee. Rosemary Chalk's guidance and counsel were invaluable throughout our deliberations. The health professionals who participated in our workshop and provided information to the committee deserve special thanks for their time and effort.

All Americans deserve to enjoy good oral health. We hope this report will help the nation achieve that vision.

Frederick P. Rivara, *Chair*
Committee on Oral Health Access to Services
July 2011

Acknowledgments

The Committee on Oral Health Access to Services benefited from the contributions of many individuals. The committee takes this opportunity to recognize those who so generously gave their time and expertise to inform its deliberations.

The committee benefited from presentations made by a number of experts outside the committee. The following individuals shared their experiences and perspectives during public meetings of the committee:

Ann Battrell, American Dental Hygienists' Association
Marcia K. Brand, Health Resources and Services Administration
Gina Capra, Health Resources and Services Administration
James Crall, American Academy of Pediatric Dentistry
Terry Dickinson, Virginia Dental Association
Bruce Dye, Centers for Disease Control and Prevention
Greg Folse
Steven Geiermann, American Dental Association
Michael Griffiths, Institutional Dental Care
David Grossman, GroupHealth Cooperative
David Halpern, Academy of General Dentistry
Lawrence Hill, CincySmiles Foundation
John McFarland, National Network for Oral Health Access
Peter Milgrom, University of Washington
Laurie Norris, Pew Children's Dental Campaign
Greg Nycz, Family Health Center of Marshfield, Inc.
Edward O'Neil, University of California, San Francisco

Jesley Ruff, American Dental Partners
Bob Russell, Iowa Department of Public Health
Mary Kate Scott, Scott & Company, Inc.
Robert Shesser, George Washington University
Mark Siegal, Ohio State Department of Health
Kristen Simmons, Willamette Dental
Woosung Sohn, University of Michigan
Ron Tankersley, American Dental Association
Jessica Van Arsdale, Humboldt State University
Louise Veselicky, West Virginia University

The committee commissioned papers to provide background information for its deliberations and to synthesize the evidence on particular issues. We thank the following individuals for their contributions to these papers:

David Armstrong, Center for Health Workforce Studies, University at Albany
Howard Bailit, University of Connecticut
John D'Adamo, University of Connecticut
Burton Edelstein, Columbia University
Margaret Langelier, Center for Health Workforce Studies, University at Albany
Jean Moore, Center for Health Workforce Studies, University at Albany

We extend special thanks to the following individuals who were essential sources of information, generously giving their time and knowledge to further the committee's efforts:

Kay Johnson, Johnson Group Consulting
Lew Lampiris, American Dental Association
Richard W. Valachovic, American Dental Education Association

Many within the Institute of Medicine were helpful to the study staff. The staff would like to thank Patrick Burke, Greta Gorman, Roger Herdman, William McLeod, Janice Mehler, Abbey Meltzer, Lauren Tobias, and Ben Wheatley for their time and support to further the committee's efforts. We also thank Mark Goodin, copyeditor.

Finally, the committee gratefully acknowledges the assistance and support of individuals instrumental in developing this project: Marcia Brand, Health Resources and Services Administration; Len Finocchio, California HealthCare Foundation; and Mark Nehring, Health Resources and Services Administration.

Contents

APPENDIXES

Summary

Vulnerable and underserved populations face persistent and systemic barriers to accessing oral health care. These barriers are numerous and complex and include social, cultural, economic, structural, and geographic factors, among others. For example:

- In 2008, 4.6 million children did not obtain needed dental care because their families could not afford it.
- In 2011, there were approximately 33.3 million unserved individuals living in dental Health Professional Shortage Areas.[1]
- In 2006, only 38 percent of retired individuals had dental coverage.

In addition, endemic low levels of oral health literacy among the public and many in the health care professions may limit their ability to understand the importance of good oral health to overall health status. Furthermore, low oral health literacy creates additional obstacles to recognizing risk for oral diseases as well as seeking and receiving needed oral health care.

Lack of access to oral health care contributes to profound and enduring oral health disparities in the United States. For example, dental caries[2]—a chronic, infectious, and largely preventable disease commonly known as tooth decay—disproportionately affects vulnerable and underserved popu-

[1] Dental Health Professional Shortage Areas are geographic areas, population groups, or facilities with shortages of dental providers.

[2] The term *dental caries* is used in the singular and refers to the disease commonly known as tooth decay (*Dorland's Illustrated Medical Dictionary*, 31st ed., s.v. "caries").

lations, groups who commonly lack access to oral health care. Vulnerable and underserved populations include but are not limited to

- Racial and ethnic minorities, including immigrants and non-English speakers;
- Children, especially those who are very young;
- Pregnant women;
- People with special needs;
- Older adults;
- Individuals living in rural and urban underserved areas;
- Uninsured and publicly insured individuals;
- Homeless individuals; and
- Populations of lower socioeconomic status.

Because good overall health requires good oral health, the unmet oral health needs of millions of American cannot be neglected.

While the majority of the U.S. population is able to routinely obtain oral health care in traditional dental practice settings, a disproportionate number of vulnerable and underserved individuals cannot. An array of providers and population-based public health programs—collectively referred to as the safety net—has emerged through uncoordinated attempts to reach these individuals. However, access to oral health care continues to elude too many Americans. Fortunately, additional opportunities exist—in both the public and private sectors—to ameliorate the situation.

STUDY CHARGE

In the fall of 2009, with support from the Health Resources and Services Administration (HRSA) and the California HealthCare Foundation, the National Research Council and the Institute of Medicine (IOM) formed the Committee on Oral Health Access to Services to assess the current oral health care system with a focus on the delivery of oral health care to vulnerable and underserved populations (see Box S-1).

The committee's vision is both aspirational and achievable (see Box S-2), but numerous coordinated and sustained actions will be needed to realize this vision.

GUIDING PRINCIPLES AND OVERALL CONCLUSIONS

To guide its deliberations, the committee began with two well-established and evidence-based principles:

1. Oral health is an integral part of overall health and, therefore, oral health care is an essential component of comprehensive health care.
2. Oral health promotion and disease prevention are essential to any strategies aimed at improving access to care.

BOX S-1
Committee Charge

The IOM-NRC Board on Children, Youth, and Families, in collaboration with the Board on Health Care Services, will undertake a study to

- Assess the current U.S. oral health system of care;
- Explore its strengths, weaknesses, and future challenges for the delivery of oral health care to vulnerable and underserved populations;
- Describe a desired vision for how oral health care for these populations should be addressed by public and private providers (including innovative programs) with a focus on safety net programs serving populations across the life cycle and Maternal and Child Health Bureau (MCHB) programs serving vulnerable women and children; and
- Recommend strategies to achieve that vision.

BOX S-2
Vision for Oral Health Care in the United States

Everyone has access to quality oral health care across the life cycle.

To be successful with underserved and vulnerable populations, an evidence-based oral health system will

1. Eliminate barriers that contribute to oral health disparities;
2. Prioritize disease prevention and health promotion;
3. Provide oral health services in a variety of settings;
4. Rely on a diverse and expanded array of providers competent, compensated, and authorized to provide evidence-based care;
5. Include collaborative and multidisciplinary teams working across the health care system; and
6. Foster continuous improvement and innovation.

These principles are woven throughout the text of this report and are fundamental to the recommendations. In addition, after reviewing the evidence, the committee came to the following overall conclusions:

1. *Improving access to oral health care is a critical and necessary first step to improving oral health outcomes and reducing disparities.*
2. *The continued separation of oral health care from overall health care contributes to limited access to oral health care for many Americans.*
3. *Sources of financing for oral health care for vulnerable and underserved populations are limited and tenuous.*
4. *Improving access to oral health care will necessarily require multiple solutions that use an array of providers in a variety of settings.*

If the current approaches to oral health education, financing, and regulation continue unchanged, equitable access to oral health care cannot be achieved. This report, however, should not be perceived as simply a call for more spending. Investing additional money in a delivery system that is poorly designed to meet the oral health care needs of the nation's underserved and vulnerable populations would produce limited results. Rather, the report calls for transformation through targeted investments in programs and policies that are most likely to yield the greatest impact. Therefore, the committee makes recommendations in key areas, suggests actions that various stakeholders can take, and identifies the relevant policy levers that are most likely to produce both short-term and long-term change.

RECOMMENDATIONS

Integrating Oral Health Care into Overall Health Care

Nondental health care professionals need to take a role in oral health care.[3] Young children, for example, visit pediatricians and family physicians earlier and more frequently than they visit dentists. Similarly, for older adults living in institutions, nurses and nursing assistants often provide personal oral health care. With proper training, these and other primary care providers are well situated to educate individuals about how to prevent oral

[3] In this report, the committee uses the term *dental professionals* to refer to dentists, dental hygienists, dental assistants, and dental laboratory technicians. The term *nondental health care professionals* includes all other types of health care professionals (e.g., nurses, pharmacists, physician assistants, physicians). Together, they are referred to as *oral health care professionals.*

diseases, to assess risk and screen for oral diseases, and to deliver preventive services (e.g., fluoride varnish).

Several nondental health care professions have made great strides in improving the oral health education and training of their students through development of oral health curricula and requirements for training in oral health care. The available evidence indicates that these efforts have been effective at increasing knowledge about oral health and integrating oral health care into primary care practices. However, these types of initiatives have not spread widely through the health professions.

Defining a core set of oral health competencies would describe essential skills that nondental health care professionals need in order to provide quality oral health care. Instead of having each profession develop their own set of competencies, one strategy is to develop a core set of competencies that would be broad and applicable to many nondental health professions. Once developed, this core set would need to be adopted by health professional schools and incorporated into the curricula. The committee concludes that the best way to encourage adoption is for professional accreditation and certification bodies to require these competencies for accreditation and maintenance of certification. Therefore, the committee recommends

> **RECOMMENDATION 1a: The Healthcare Resources and Services Administration (HRSA) should convene key stakeholders from both the public and private sectors to develop a core set of oral health competencies for nondental health care professionals.**

> **RECOMMENDATION 1b: Following the development of a core set of oral health competencies**
> - **Accrediting bodies for undergraduate and graduate-level nondental health professional education programs should integrate these core competencies into their requirements for accreditation; and**
> - **All certification and maintenance of certification for health care professionals should include demonstration of competence in oral health care as a criterion.**

The minimum core competencies will need to prepare graduates to

- Recognize risk for oral disease through competent oral examinations,
- Provide basic oral health information,
- Integrate oral health information with diet and lifestyle counseling, and
- Make and track referrals to dental professionals.

The committee suggests the following strategies:

- HRSA can require that Title VII–funded programs include interprofessional education on oral health.
- HRSA can support curriculum development and dissemination efforts for nondental health professional education programs.

Creating Optimal Laws and Regulations

A variety of regulations and policies determine *how* and *by whom* oral health care is provided. In spite of the existence of national accreditation standards on education and training of health care professionals, regulations defining supervision levels and scopes of practice vary widely from state to state and even by procedure. Some states have altered their scope-of-practice and supervision regulations to allow a broader range of competent oral health care professionals to treat patients, or for existing oral health care professionals to perform a wider range of procedures under various levels of supervision.

When expansions to existing scopes of practice are proposed, concerns inevitably arise about the quality of care provided when patients are treated by individuals with less training.[4] However, many have called for state practice acts to be expanded in alignment with professional competence. Moreover, the Federal Trade Commission suggests that lawmakers consider whether overly restrictive regulations preclude a countervailing benefit, such as through increased access to care. Therefore, the committee recommends

RECOMMENDATION 2: State legislatures should amend existing state laws, including practice acts, to maximize access to oral health care.

At minimum, state dental practice acts should

- **Allow allied dental professionals to practice to the full extent of their education and training,**
- **Allow allied dental professionals to work in a variety of settings under evidence-supported supervision levels, and**
- **Allow technology-supported remote collaboration and supervision.**

This recommendation will enable members of a stratified workforce of professionals to work in community settings, change supervision require-

[4] The IOM defines *quality* as being safe, timely, effective, efficient, equitable, and patient-centered.

ments to levels supported by evidence, and allow the appropriate use of telehealth technologies to reach underserved populations.

States can be supported in these efforts with strong evidence and clear guidance. This committee, therefore, proposes the following strategies:

- The Centers for Medicare and Medicaid Services (CMS) can disseminate rules and policies that promote Medicaid and Children's Health Insurance Program (CHIP) beneficiaries' access to appropriate care, and ensure that these rules and policies reflect the practice abilities of current and new types of licensed professionals.
- The Office of the Assistant Secretary for Planning and Evaluation can examine and report on the impact of state practice acts on oral health care delivery to vulnerable and underserved populations. These reports would need to be conducted and published periodically to support sustained attention.
- Foundations, professional organizations, and public policy organizations can conduct and disseminate an initial review of state practice acts with a focus on access to services.
- Foundations, professional organizations, and public policy organizations can issue "best practices" briefs to highlight what each state is doing and what impact it is having on access.

Improving Dental Education and Training

An improved and responsive dental education system is needed to ensure that current and future generations of dental professionals can deliver quality care to diverse populations, in a variety of settings, using a variety of service-delivery mechanisms, and across the life cycle. Diversity in the health care workforce is associated with expanded access to care for racial and ethnic minority patients, greater patient choice and satisfaction, better patient–provider communication, and better educational experiences for all students. Furthermore, all dental professionals need to develop the necessary skills to work in a variety of community-based settings and with vulnerable and underserved populations, such as the ability to work in interprofessional teams with general health, education, and social service professionals; the ability to work in dental professional teams; and the ability to use new service-delivery mechanisms such as telehealth technologies for supervision, consultation, and collaboration.

Evidence points to limited training of dental students in community-based settings, thereby limiting their exposure to and practical experience with the broad range of patients cared for in these settings. This creates missed opportunities to improve cultural competence and to reinforce the professional and ethical role of caring for the vulnerable and underserved populations. Providing students with clinical experiences in community-based settings helps them acquire skills that cannot be learned in academic settings, improves their comfort level with caring for vulnerable and underserved populations, and increases the likelihood that students may return to such settings in their future careers. Finally, schools will require more faculty members with experience and expertise in caring for vulnerable and underserved populations to adequately prepare students in this manner. Therefore, the committee recommends

RECOMMENDATION 3: Dental professional education programs should

- **Increase recruitment and support for enrollment of students from underrepresented minority, lower-income, and rural populations;**
- **Require all students to participate in community-based education rotations with opportunities to work with interprofessional teams; and**
- **Recruit and retain faculty with experience and expertise in caring for underserved and vulnerable populations.**

To support Recommendation 3, the committee further recommends

RECOMMENDATION 4: HRSA should dedicate Title VII funding to

- **Support the development, implementation, and maintenance of substantial community-based education rotations, and**
- **Increase funding for recruitment and scholarships for underrepresented minority, lower-income, and rural populations to attend dental professional schools.**

Continuation of proven strategies will help prepare—and ultimately promote—a greater desire among dental professionals to provide care to underserved and vulnerable populations. The committee suggests that private foundations and professional organizations can strengthen efforts of dental professional education programs to

- Increase enrollment of students from underrepresented minority, lower-income, and rural populations by funding bridge programs.
- Develop and evaluate innovative educational models to prepare students to work in diverse settings and with new delivery mechanisms.

Upon completion of dental school, students may have had limited opportunities to integrate their skills and knowledge with practical hands-on experience and may not feel adequately prepared for dental practice. In the

1995 IOM report *Dental Education at the Crossroads* (*Crossroads*) the committee noted:

> A year of postgraduate or advanced education in general dentistry would allow students to gain speed and confidence in procedures, broaden their patient management skills to cover more complex problems, and mature in the nontechnical aspects of patient care.

Dentists who have completed general dentistry residency programs report feeling more comfortable caring for underserved patients and patients with complex health care needs, and tend to care for those patients more often, even after completing residency. Dental residencies are also a source of care for underserved and vulnerable populations, and some evidence shows that, with appropriate funding, requiring a year of residency training can expand the capacity of these programs to care for more individuals. Therefore, the committee recommends

RECOMMENDATION 5: HRSA should dedicate Title VII funding to support and expand opportunities for dental residencies in community-based settings.

- **Subsequently, state legislatures should require a minimum of one year of dental residency before a dentist can be licensed to practice.**

To be optimally effective, dental residency programs especially need to include clinical experiences with young children, individuals with special health care needs, and older adults. For this reason, these residency programs need to be located in settings where services to these and other vulnerable and underserved populations are most needed.

In alignment with the *Crossroads* report, this committee recommends increased opportunities rather than requirements for residencies as a short-term goal.

Since funding of residency programs has been tenuous, the committee recommends a continuous source of existing funding—Title VII of the Public Health Services Act—be directed to support dental residencies. This will require that Title VII receives priority within current and future funding levels. In the long term, the committee recommends that states should ultimately *require* a minimum of 1 year of dental residency before a dentist can be licensed to practice. This will involve, among other actions, the need for each state to revise its statutes and the need to increase the capacity of dental residency programs.

The committee suggests the following as potential strategies:

- HRSA can support care for underserved and vulnerable populations where they live, work, and learn by designating the types of clinical experiences and settings that would qualify for dental residencies.
- The public and private sectors can help identify and address barriers to having all states make postgraduate education a requirement for licensure.
- Hospitals and dental schools can increase the number of formal relationships with community-based care settings (e.g., Federally Qualified Health Centers [FQHCs], nursing homes, state and local health departments, and prisons) for dental residency programs.

Reducing Financial and Administrative Barriers

Dental coverage is a major determinant of access to and utilization of oral health care. In addition, a parent's insurance status and utilization of oral health care is associated with whether his or her children receive oral health care. All states are required to provide comprehensive dental benefits for all children enrolled in Medicaid or CHIP. In contrast, states are not required to provide Medicaid benefits for adults. Among states that offer dental coverage for adult Medicaid recipients, the benefits are often limited to emergency coverage.

Recognizing that publicly funded programs are the primary source of coverage for underserved and vulnerable populations, the committee concludes that Medicaid cannot properly address access to oral health services if it excludes oral health benefits. However, in the absence of a comprehensive cost-benefit analysis and in a climate of significantly limited resources, the committee lacks the necessary evidence base and appropriate fiscal conditions to recommend that all states be required to cover essential dental benefits for all Medicaid beneficiaries. Nevertheless, the committee firmly concludes that including dental benefits for all Medicaid beneficiaries is a critical and necessary goal. Toward this end, the committee recommends

RECOMMENDATION 6: CMS should fund and evaluate state-based demonstration projects that cover essential oral health benefits for Medicaid beneficiaries.

State-based demonstration projects will help establish a basis for sound policy and fiscal decision making both for participating states and for future federal and state actions. Recognizing the different challenges faced by individual states, the committee suggests that CMS build in flexibility and encourage innovation in the demonstrations. For example, states may choose to focus on providing oral health benefits to specific populations (e.g., "high-risk" enrollees) or to examine the effects of providing benefits to all enrolled populations. The committee suggests the following strategies:

- CMS can ensure that Medicaid beneficiaries receive the appropriate level of care by appointing and convening a committee of key stakeholders to establish an essential dental benefits package for Medicaid.
- CMS can provide technical assistance and oversight to state-based demonstration projects including guidance on program design elements that address the specialized needs of targeted beneficiaries and consultation on program evaluation and monitoring systems.
- CMS can develop a report at the culmination of the demonstration projects to review, translate, and disseminate evidence and guidance to all states.
- Private foundations can partner with CMS and participating states to support outreach for state-based demonstration projects including campaigns to raise awareness of changes in state oral health benefits available and to promote the use of newly covered services.

Financing also influences providers' practice patterns. For example, low reimbursement by public programs is often cited as a disincentive to provider participation. Increases in reimbursement rates have shown promise in increasing dentists' participation in these programs. However, increasing reimbursement rates alone is not sufficient. To that end, many states have taken measures to reduce the administrative burdens of publicly funded programs. These actions, in conjunction with rate increases and other supportive strategies (e.g., increased education and outreach to beneficiaries) can have a greater impact on increasing provider participation and patient utilization rates. Therefore, the committee recommends

RECOMMENDATION 7: To increase provider participation in publicly funded programs, states should

- **Set Medicaid and CHIP reimbursement rates so that beneficiaries have equitable access to essential oral health services, as required by law;**
- **Provide case-management services; and**
- **Streamline administrative processes.**

In a climate of limited resources and perennial demands on tight state budgets, states will need additional support in these efforts. Therefore, the committee suggests the following as strategies:

- Congress can provide enhanced federal matching funds to help offset the additional expense to the states. To be most effective, Congress can require that an enhanced match be tied to efforts of states to streamline administrative procedures related to provider participation and patient utilization in Medicaid.
- CMS can ensure that Medicaid beneficiaries have equitable access to essential oral health services by appointing and convening a committee of key stakeholders to establish an essential dental benefits package for Medicaid.

As noted above, simply increasing reimbursement rates, in the absence of other actions, will not be sufficient in improving access to care. Therefore, the committee proposes the following strategies:

- CMS can issue guidance to state Medicaid officers on strategies to reduce administrative burdens associated with provider participation in Medicaid.
- States can use Maternal and Child Health Services Block Grant (Title V) funds to evaluate and assess their case-management services to determine the most effective strategies to expand access to oral health care.
- Professional organizations and patient advocacy organizations can work with their constituencies to help identify populations in need of case management and the specific administrative barriers serving these populations.

Promoting Research

Over the course of this study, the committee encountered considerable gaps in the evidence base. For example, little is known about the best ways to care for the distinct segments of the American public that are not well served by the traditional oral health care system. To this end, there are a number of programs currently under way designed to deliver oral health care through innovations in the workforce and in delivery of care in nontraditional settings.

First, as discussed earlier, research is needed on how to best include nondental health care professionals in oral health care. Further, several new models seek to develop new types of dental professionals or expand the role of existing dental professionals. For example, while limited, evaluations of the dental health aide therapist program in Alaska to date point to the quality and acceptability of dental therapists, but more research is needed to determine the broader impact and implementation of these types of programs. Similar research is also needed on the provision of oral health care in nontraditional settings (e.g., school-based health centers, mobile equipment) and through innovative technologies (e.g., telehealth).

Quality assessment and improvement efforts in oral health are hampered by a deficiency in the collection, analysis, and use of data related to important aspects of oral health. Because of the limited infrastructure and the current paucity of measures in use to assess the technical competence, practice procedures, and quality of care and outcomes of care provided by *any* dental professionals, making comparisons of care rendered by different types of professionals is even more challenging.

Finally, little has been done to investigate better methods of financing and regulation that might lead to improvements in dental coverage, access to oral health care, and, again, improvements in oral health status.

Therefore, the committee recommends

RECOMMENDATION 8: Congress, the Department of Health and Human Services, federal agencies, and private foundations should fund oral health research and evaluation related to underserved and vulnerable populations, including

- **New methods and technologies (e.g., nontraditional settings, nondental professionals, new types of dental professionals, and telehealth);**
- **Measures of access, quality, and outcomes; and**
- **Payment and regulatory systems.**

Given the need for further research, the committee concludes that a variety of stakeholders will need to take additional actions to support this recommendation, including

- Federal agencies can increase funding for programs that successfully provide education and preventive and treatment services to vulnerable and underserved populations such as Head Start; the Women, Infants, and Children program; and school-based health centers.
- HRSA can provide new funding toward demonstration projects that promote innovations in oral health care delivery, such as new workforce models, nontraditional settings of care, and new ways to finance oral health care.

Expanding Capacity

State oral health programs are essential to direct resources and monitor the impact of oral health efforts. One important aspect of state oral health programs is their ability to monitor and analyze the burden of oral health disease, conditions, and personal behaviors over time. Other functions of state oral health programs (e.g., community water fluoridation, dental sealant programs, fluoride varnish programs, dental screening programs, and oral health programs specifically for pregnant women) also have a positive impact on oral health. According to the Association of State and Territorial Dental Directors,

> with expanded infrastructure and capacity, state oral health programs are better able to monitor oral health status, address high-risk populations, increase population-based prevention activities, and extend resources to local health agencies and communities in order to implement oral health strategies.

In spite of this impact, funding for state and local dental public health services continues to be limited and often insufficient. In FY 2010, the Centers for Disease Control and Prevention (CDC) provided $6.8 million to 19 state oral health programs to support evidence-based prevention programs, surveillance of oral disease burden, and to develop plans to improve oral health and address disparities.

Recognizing the critical role of state-based programs, the committee recommends

RECOMMENDATION 9: The Centers for Disease Control and Prevention (CDC) and the Maternal and Child Health Bureau (MCHB) should collaborate with states to ensure that each state has the infrastructure and support necessary to perform core dental public health functions (e.g., assessment, policy development, and assurance).

The committee proposes the following strategies:

- The CDC can continue to increase the number of states that receive cooperative agreement funding for dental public health programs.
- The MCHB can support an oral health component under Title V through block grants (formulary grants to states), discretionary funds, and/or "set asides" (a percentage of funds) for oral health.
- Congress can fund the *Oral Healthcare Prevention Education Campaign* authorized by the Patient Protection and Affordable Care Act (ACA) [Public Law 111-148, Title IV, Sec. 4102] which calls for a national public education campaign focused on oral health and disease prevention targeted toward vulnerable and underserved populations.
- Private foundations can partner with public agencies to develop, implement, and evaluate public education and oral health literacy campaigns.

Expanding the capacity of FQHCs to deliver oral health care is also important to meet the needs of vulnerable and underserved populations. FQHCs are required to provide certain oral health services—including preventive, but not comprehensive, dental services—either in the clinic or by referral. In 2009, HRSA funded 1,131 FQHCs in all 50 states, the District of Columbia, and Puerto Rico. The American Recovery and Rehabilitation Act included $2 billion for FQHCs, and the ACA included $11 billion for a Community Health Centers Trust Fund that will allow FQHCs to expand access and make capital improvements, and also appropriated $1.5 billion to a new National Health Service Corps Trust Fund.

In 2009, over 3.4 million patients used dental services in the health center system. Still, this is only a small fraction of the underserved population. The committee concludes that with adequate support, FQHCs are well positioned to significantly expand the delivery of oral health care to vulnerable and underserved populations.

The committee, therefore, recommends

RECOMMENDATION 10: To expand the capacity of FQHCs to deliver essential oral health services, HRSA should

- **Support the use of a variety of oral health care professionals;**
- **Enhance financial incentives to attract and retain more oral health care professionals;**
- **Provide guidance to implement best practices in management, operation, and efficiency; and**
- **Assist FQHCs in all states to operate programs outside their physical facilities and take advantage of new systems to improve the oral health of the population they serve.**

Each of the specific actions outlined for FQHCs in this recommendation build upon the committee's previous recommendations and the evidence that supports them.

The committee proposes the following strategies:

- Public–private partnerships can supplement educational loan repayment programs for oral health care professionals who are willing to serve a designated amount of time in medically underserved areas.
- HRSA can support dissemination and implementation of this recommendation by identifying FQHC "best practices" to highlight what states or individual clinics are doing and what impact these efforts are having on access.
- HRSA can support the demonstration and dissemination of models that extend the reach of FQHCs by operating programs out-

side their physical facilities and that use new delivery models and techniques.

- Other nonprofit community health centers can take the steps outlined in this recommendation to increase the delivery of essential oral health services to greater numbers of vulnerable and underserved individuals.

CONCLUSION

The release of this report coincides with a transformative moment in the nation's health care system. As the nation struggles to address the larger systemic issues of access to health care, greater effort will be needed to ensure that oral health is included in this conversation.

The recommendations presented in this report are directed to national, state, and local governments; all types of health care professions; licensing and accreditation bodies; educational institutions; health care researchers; and philanthropic and advocacy organizations. Together, these groups have the power to transform the delivery of oral health care to vulnerable and underserved populations. This report envisions an integrated delivery system that provides quality oral health care to vulnerable and underserved people where they live, work, and learn through changes in the education, financing, and regulation of oral health care. The recommendations support the creation of a diverse workforce that is competent, compensated, and authorized to serve vulnerable and underserved populations across the life cycle. Implementation of these recommendations will be a critical next step in increasing access to oral health care, reducing persistent oral health disparities, and improving oral health outcomes among vulnerable and underserved populations.

1

Introduction

Access to oral health care is essential to promoting and maintaining overall health and well-being. When individuals are able to access oral health care, they are more likely to receive basic preventive services and education on personal behaviors. They are also more likely to have oral diseases detected in the earlier stages and obtain restorative care as needed. In contrast, lack of access to oral health care can result in delayed diagnosis, untreated oral diseases and conditions, compromised health status, and, occasionally, even death. Unfortunately, access to oral health care eludes many Americans.

A significant portion of the U.S. population is not adequately served by the current oral health care system, and millions of Americans have unmet oral health needs (Bloom et al., 2010; Brown, 2005; HHS, 2000). This is especially true for the nation's vulnerable and underserved populations. Commonly studied populations include but are not limited to

- Racial and ethnic minorities, including immigrants and non–English speakers (Bloom et al., 2010; Cruz et al., 2004; Edelstein and Chinn, 2009; Pleis et al., 2010);
- Children, especially those who are very young (Dye et al., 2010; Edelstein and Chinn, 2009; GAO, 2008);
- Pregnant women (Silk et al., 2008; Steinberg et al., 2008);
- People with special health care needs (Anders and Davis, 2010; Armour et al., 2008; Havercamp et al., 2004; Owens et al., 2006);
- Older adults (Dye et al., 2007; Manski et al., 2004, 2010);

- Individuals living in rural and urban underserved areas (Maserejian et al., 2008; Vargas et al., 2002, 2003a,b,c);
- Uninsured and publicly insured individuals (GAO, 2008; Liu et al., 2007);
- Homeless individuals (Conte et al., 2006; Gibson et al., 2003); and
- Populations of lower socioeconomic status (Bloom et al., 2010; GAO, 2000; Vargas et al., 1998).

For example, in 2009, 4.6 million children did not obtain needed dental care because their families stated that they could not afford it (Bloom et al., 2009), and people with disabilities are less likely to have seen a dentist in the past year than people without disabilities (Armour et al., 2008).

Although other health conditions frequently draw attention in health policy and health services discussions, oral health issues seldom rise to the top of the national health and health policy agenda. As a result, oral health concerns have persisted as a major, largely preventable, health problem across the life span.

BARRIERS TO ORAL HEALTH CARE ACCESS

The factors that contribute to problems with access to oral health care are numerous and complex. These include social, cultural, economic, structural, and geographic factors, among others. A thorough review of these factors is included in the chapters that follow. For example, *dental coverage* (discussed in Chapter 5) is correlated to access to and utilization of oral health care (AHRQ, 2010; Decker, 2011; Sohn et al., 2007). One recent report found that individuals who lacked dental insurance were about two-thirds less likely than people with private insurance to have had a dental visit within the last year (16.1 percent compared with 50.9 percent) (AHRQ, 2010). In addition, poor *oral health literacy* of both individuals and all types of health care professionals (discussed in Chapter 2) contributes to poor access because individuals may not understand the importance of oral health care or their options for accessing such care (Caspary et al., 2008; Gussy et al., 2008; Jones et al., 2007; Kutner et al., 2006; Sakai et al., 2008).

Likewise, the *geographic distribution* of oral health professionals in relation to the general public (discussed in Chapter 3) has a considerable impact on access to oral health care (HHS, 2000; IOM, 2009b). For example, as of March 2011, there were 4,639 dental Health Professional Shortage Areas (HPSAs) (a geographic area, population group, or facility with a shortage of dental professionals) (HRSA, 2011). An estimated 9,642 additional dentists would be required to meet the need of unserved populations in these areas (based on a 3,000:1 population-to-practitioner ratio). It should be noted that making estimates of underservice and unmet need are complicated and that shortcomings in the current criteria and methodologies used to make HPSA designations have been identified (GAO, 2006). For example, the dental HPSA criteria have not recently been updated and may not adequately capture broader issues of access to care, including a greater focus on indicators of need as opposed to simple population to provider ratios (Orlans et al., 2002). However, population-to-provider data are continuously collected and will likely serve as the basis for estimates of underservice and unmet need until improved methodologies and criteria are developed.

THE CONSEQUENCES OF POOR ORAL HEALTH

The consequences of insufficient access to oral health care and resultant poor oral health—at both the individual and population levels—are far reaching. Nontreatment of dental caries,[1] for example, may be associated with inappropriate use of emergency departments (Cohen et al., 2011; Davis et al., 2010). Moreover, strong evidence documents the clear linkages between oral health and respiratory disease (Scannapieco and Ho, 2001), cardiovascular disease (Blaizot et al., 2009; Offenbacher et al., 2009; Scannapieco et al., 2003; Slavkin and Baum, 2000), and diabetes (Chávarry et al., 2009; Löe, 1993; Taylor, 2001; Teeuw et al., 2010).

Lack of access to oral health care also contributes to the profound and persistent oral health disparities that exist in the United States. For example, dental caries—a chronic, infectious, and largely preventable disease—disproportionately affects racial/ethnic minority groups (Flores and Tomany-Korman, 2008; HHS, 2000; Nash and Nagel, 2005), rural populations (Skillman et al., 2010; Vargas et al., 2003a,b,c), children (Dye et al., 2010), individuals with special health care needs (Owens et al., 2006), and low-income populations (Vargas and Ronzio, 2006), among others. A recent analysis of the National Survey of Children with Special Health Care Needs found that 8.9 percent of children with special health care needs were unable to obtain needed dental care (Lewis, 2009).

EFFORTS TO IMPROVE ACCESS TO ORAL HEALTH CARE

Multiple agencies within the Department of Health and Human Services (HHS) and other federal departments have sought to develop resources and strategies to improve access to and quality of oral health care for vulnerable populations. Programs administered by the Health Resources and Services

[1] The term *dental caries* is used in the singular and refers to the disease commonly known as tooth decay (*Dorland's Illustrated Medical Dictionary*, 31st ed., s.v. "caries").

Administration (HRSA), the Centers for Disease Control and Prevention (CDC), the Food and Drug Administration, the Indian Health Service (IHS), the National Institute of Dental and Craniofacial Research, and other agencies have focused on multiple dimensions of the service system: building the supply of dental professionals; strengthening state capacity and dental public health infrastructure; providing direct oral health care to selected populations (including veterans, military personnel and their families, incarcerated individuals in federal prisons, Native Americans and Alaska Natives, migrant and homeless populations, pregnant women, low-income children and adolescents, and others); and developing population-based services such as fluoridation of drinking water. In addition, federal agencies provide technical assistance on oral health issues to state and local health departments, support national surveys and examinations to assess the status of children's oral health, sponsor basic and applied research, sponsor public education materials and programs, and develop consumer protection services such as regulation of devices and pharmaceuticals used in dentistry. In other areas, federal funds finance the provision of oral health services by public and private dental professionals through health insurance programs such as Medicaid and the Children's Health Insurance Program (CHIP).

In addition to the federal-level strategies described above, stakeholders across the country have been encouraged to increase the resources available to meet the oral health needs of the public and take action to address the poor oral health status of vulnerable and underserved populations. For example, the private sector has sponsored several types of voluntary programs to care for these populations. The Missions of Mercy projects are short-term, temporary clinics, staffed by volunteer dental professionals that are set up in easily accessible locations to provide oral health care to underserved populations on a first-come, first-served basis. Another example is the American Dental Association's (ADA's) *Give Kids A Smile Day*. This annual program includes regional one-day events that provide education, screening, preventive, and clinical (e.g., restorative) services to underserved children. Donated Dental Services, a program of the National Foundation of Dentistry for the Handicapped, assists volunteer dentists and laboratories in providing care to older adults and individuals with special health care needs. Collectively, these and other efforts have temporarily mitigated some of the burden related to inadequate access to oral health care, but they have been insufficient in fully addressing existing challenges and underlying problems. What is lacking at present is a systems-level approach that can establish priorities among multiple and fragmented efforts and focus public resources on priority areas of need in the areas of service delivery, system capacity, and public health infrastructure.

Within the context of these previous efforts and the persistent challenges to achieving good oral health and reducing oral health disparities, there is a clear need to reexamine the way oral health care is delivered to vulnerable and underserved populations, and to design strategic policies that support the health care professionals and programs that serve these populations. This report examines these needs, highlights the successes that have been achieved, and makes recommendations for the work that remains to be done.

STUDY CHARGE, SCOPE, AND APPROACH

The 2000 surgeon general's report *Oral Health in America* raised the profile of oral health issues nationally; it continues to be cited frequently, and it is viewed as a benchmark for oral health system reform. However, there is also a growing recognition among policy makers and other stakeholders that little has changed in the intervening years. Access to oral health coverage and oral health care remains disparate and inadequate to meet the need; oral health status among many population groups remains poor; avoidable oral health complications continue to occur with great frequency; the worlds of dentistry and medicine remain substantially divided; and oral health continues to be marginalized in many crucial respects.

Study Charge

In light of these issues, in the fall of 2009, with support from HRSA and the California HealthCare Foundation, the National Research Council (NRC) and the Institute of Medicine (IOM), through collaborative efforts between the Board on Children, Youth, and Families and the Board on Health Care Services, formed the Committee on Oral Health Access to Services to assess the current oral health care system with a focus on the delivery of oral health care to vulnerable and underserved populations. Further, the committee was asked to provide a vision of how oral health care for these populations should be addressed by public and private providers (see Box 1-1).

Scope

This committee was tasked with describing a delivery system better able to provide access to oral health care to vulnerable and underserved populations. The committee recognizes that, while access to care is one critical component needed to improve oral health outcomes and reduce oral health disparities, it is not an end in and of itself. Improving access will, however, help provide needed services to the millions of Americans for whom oral health care is currently out of reach. The committee was not asked to make recommendations to improve oral health outcomes and reduce oral health

BOX 1-1
The Committee on Oral Health Access to Services Statement of Task

The IOM-NRC Board on Children, Youth, and Families, in collaboration with the Board on Health Care Services, will undertake a study to

- Assess the current U.S. oral health system of care;
- Explore its strengths, weaknesses, and future challenges for the delivery of oral health care to vulnerable and underserved populations;
- Describe a desired vision for how oral health care for these populations should be addressed by public and private providers (including innovative programs) with a focus on safety net programs serving populations across the life cycle and Maternal and Child Health Bureau (MCHB) programs serving vulnerable women and children; and
- Recommend strategies to achieve that vision.

disparities among vulnerable and underserved populations. Recommendations of this nature are beyond the scope of this study. Moreover, the focus of this study is directed specifically on those populations that are not served by the current system. The committee was not asked to examine or make recommendations on how the overall oral health care system might be improved. This, too, goes beyond the scope of this study. Therefore, the committee limited its examination to those issues directly related to improving access to oral health care and has sought, through the careful and thorough examination of available evidence, the best and most realistic paths to pursue.

The committee does not suggest that the findings, conclusions, and recommendations within this report will resolve all problems related to access to oral health care in this country. Nor is this report intended to supplant effective and innovative initiatives currently under way at the community, state, and national levels (a number of which are highlighted in the chapters that follow). Instead, this report is intended to complement those efforts as a part of a larger solution that will require efforts from a variety of stakeholders.

As directed by the statement of task, the committee sought opportunities to improve access to oral health care through both public- and private-sector actions. While a number of the recommendations are geared toward state and federal agencies, the recommendations require action and support from the private sector to be successful. Some of the recommendations designate priority areas within current funding levels; others call for new or increased state and federal investments. Recognizing the vital role that the private sector will play in improving access to oral health care, the committee has identified areas where private investments and support from the private sector are needed. These actions and investments are included as suggested strategies for implementation following each recommendation.

It is also important to note that this study was conducted at the same time that the IOM's Committee on an Oral Health Initiative study was under way. While the two studies have related statements of task, the two projects had separate committees, meetings, and report review processes. The two committees were not made aware of the other's conclusions or recommendations. *Advancing Oral Health in America*, the report from the Committee on an Oral Health Initiative, was released in April 2011. A brief summary of the report's key findings, conclusions, and recommendations is included in Appendix D.

Study Approach

The study committee included 15 members with expertise in dentistry and dental hygiene, dental public health, pediatric dentistry, pediatrics, family medicine, obstetrics/gynecology, health law, health policy, nursing, prenatal care, neonatal and infant health, public health, health disparities, and health finance. (See Appendix E for biographies of the committee members.)

A variety of sources informed the committee's work. The committee met in person five times and during two of those meetings held public workshops to obtain vital input from a broad range of relevant stakeholders including parents and patients; oral health care professionals; public and private insurers; local, state, and federal agencies; and research experts. In addition, the committee commissioned four papers on various topics (see Appendix B). The committee conducted a review of the literature to identify issues that affect underserved populations who are most vulnerable to oral disease and the role of the safety net providers, both public and private, who serve them, with a specific focus on the provision of oral health care to women and children.

The committee made every effort to include the most up-to-date research published in peer-reviewed journals. However, strong evidence was sometimes found in older studies; as these studies had not been replicated in recent years, they were the only available sources of data. In other cases, large-scale studies have not been done, and so the committee looked to available data from smaller-scale studies, such as case reports. Finally, in some instances, the committee cited secondary sources such as reports. In such cases, the committee referred back to the original citations to assess the quality of the evidence.

In addition, the committee was limited by what was available in the published literature. For example, the committee found that there were areas of research (e.g., oral health financing, quality measures) that were considerably less developed than other areas (e.g., preventive care). Through its review of evidence, the committee also became aware of the existence of newer data in several key areas that have not yet been fully analyzed. The committee was not equipped to or charged with conducting data analysis, and so the most current published data analyses are included in the report. The evidence included in the report is almost exclusively focused on the United States. However, in cases in which the committee determined that it was important to include relevant international research, this research is cited. In the chapters that follow, the committee evaluates available relevant data, identifies specific gaps in the literature, and addresses the need for additional research in its recommendations in Chapter 6.

In approaching its charge, the committee sought to gain an understanding of the full spectrum of influences, challenges, and opportunities facing the delivery of oral health care services to vulnerable and underserved populations. This chapter describes why such efforts are necessary and provides an overview of key issues related to the committee's charge, each of which is expanded upon, in greater detail, in the chapters that follow. In addition, one of the committee's early tasks was to establish guiding principles, reach consensus on how to define several key terms, and to determine how to approach the task of assessing the current oral health system of care in the United States.

GUIDING PRINCIPLES

To guide its deliberations on improving access to oral health care among vulnerable and underserved populations, the committee began with two well-established and evidence-based principles:

1. Oral health is an integral part of overall health and, therefore, oral health care is an essential component of comprehensive health care.
2. Oral health promotion and disease prevention are essential to any strategies aimed at improving access to care.

These principles are woven throughout the text of this report and are fundamental to the recommendations. The committee strongly believes that these two principles need to be better understood by the general public and policy makers and emphasized to improve access to oral health care with the ultimate goal of improving oral health outcomes for vulnerable and underserved populations.

DEFINITIONS OF KEY TERMS

This section provides definitions of several key terms that are relevant to this report.

Access

Many other reports have examined issues related to access to health care. The current challenges to understanding and measuring access to oral health care in the United States are similar to those that apply to access to all health care services. Therefore, the committee chose to focus on previous definitions of access to health care.

An earlier NRC-IOM committee developed an enduring definition of access, as set forth in the report *Access to Health Care in America*: "the timely use of personal health services to achieve the best possible health outcomes" (IOM, 1993). Other work has broadened this definition to underscore issues specific to health care disparities (AHRQ, 2010; Bierman et al., 1998). For example, the 2009 Agency for Healthcare Research and Quality (AHRQ) *National Healthcare Disparities Report* includes concepts such as an individual's ability to gain entry to the health care system and appropriate sites of care to receive needed services. The report also stated that having access to providers who meet the needs of individual patients was an essential component of access to care (AHRQ, 2010).

This committee endorses a broad definition of access as applied to oral health care. Moreover, the committee finds that in order to promote and maintain overall health individuals require access to quality *oral disease preventive services at regular intervals* and *treatment services when needed.* Because access is seldom as straightforward as adequate availability of services and providers, this report thoroughly examines the various barriers to care that inhibit timely receipt of services. In addition, the committee contends that the implicit goal in improving access is improving access to *quality* oral health care—care that is safe, timely, effective, efficient, equitable, and patient centered (IOM, 2001). This concept of quality should be applied wherever the term *access* is used in the pages that follow. Finally, the broad definition of access described above underscores both the *availability* and *use* of care. The committee concludes that these are essential components of access. Therefore, strategies to improve access are necessarily broader than simply improving an individual's or population's ability to "get in the door." This concept is echoed throughout the report.

Oral Health

The Surgeon General's report *Oral Health in America* firmly established that oral health care encompasses more than dental care, and that a healthy mouth is more than just healthy teeth (HHS, 2000). The World Health Organization captures this broader definition of oral health in the following way: "Oral health is a state of being free from chronic mouth and facial pain, oral and throat cancer, oral sores, birth defects such as cleft lip and palate, periodontal (gum) disease, tooth decay and tooth loss, and other diseases and disorders that affect the oral cavity" (WHO, 2010). To ensure that the recommendations of this report are applied to their fullest extent, the committee has chosen to endorse a broad definition of oral health that aligns with the definitions above. Moreover, as described earlier, oral health is fundamental to overall health. Therefore, the committee encourages readers of this report to keep this underlying premise in mind whenever they encounter the term *oral health* in the pages that follow.

Oral Health Care Workforce

This report considers the oral health care workforce broadly—that is, to be inclusive of all the members of the health care workforce who are, or could be, involved in oral health care. Traditionally, a combination of dentists, dental hygienists, dental assistants, and others (*dental professionals*) contribute to oral health care. As oral health has become increasingly recognized as part of overall health, *nondental health care professionals* (e.g., nurses, pharmacists, physician assistants, physicians) have become involved in the prevention, diagnosis, and treatment of oral diseases. In addition, in efforts to expand oral health access, new types of dental professionals (e.g., dental therapists) have evolved, and expanded scopes of practice have been explored for existing professionals. Together, all of these professionals are recognized in this report as *oral health care professionals*.

Vulnerable and Underserved

The committee's charge specifically refers to improving access for vulnerable and underserved populations. These are individuals and populations that are systematically excluded from obtaining oral health care. However, there are no universally accepted definitions for these two groups. Vulnerability, for example, may be temporal in nature. That is, an individual or a community may experience pervasive and lasting vulnerability (e.g., persistent poverty or chronic illness) or may become vulnerable for a discreet period of time (e.g., during pregnancy or following a catastrophic event). Likewise, whether an individual or a community is considered underserved may change over time. For example, individuals residing in a designated HPSA are considered to be underserved. If a health care professional moves to the area, it may lose its HPSA designation, and its residents will no longer be considered underserved. The reverse situation, of course, would also be true.

Given the complex and variable nature of these designations, the committee determined early in the study process it would consider *vulnerable* and *underserved* populations in terms of a general set of characteristics. These groups would include those who are made vulnerable by or underserved due to

- Financial circumstances,
- Insurance status,
- Place of residence,
- Health status,
- Age,
- Personal characteristics,
- Functional or developmental status,
- Ability to communicate effectively, and
- Presence of chronic illness or disability (IOM, 2000a; President's Advisory Commission on Consumer Protection and Quality in the Health Care Industry, 1998).

This list is not meant to be exhaustive. Similarly, the vulnerable and underserved populations discussed in the chapters that follow should not be viewed as comprehensive. They have been included as examples based on the amount of data and evidence available in the literature. Additional factors and characteristics that contribute to whether individuals and populations are underserved such as the supply of trained professionals available to provide care are also examined in this report.

NOTABLE PAST WORK

The committee drew important lessons from the collection of efforts aimed at improving access to oral health care. The following review of notable past work highlights the breadth of efforts over time and calls attention to the range of engaged stakeholders.

The Institute of Medicine

Over 30 years have passed since the IOM's first significant look at oral health issues, *Public Policy Options for Better Dental Health* (IOM, 1980), in which the committee was charged to consider the inclusion of dental services under national health insurance plans. At that time, the IOM found a substantial unmet need for dental care in the United States and that the methods to prevent and reduce dental disease were well known. The IOM explicitly recognized the lack of a national plan for the prevention of dental disease, the significant financial barriers that prevented access for many Americans, and the omission of oral health from larger public policy discussions. The IOM recommended the inclusion of dental services in any national health insurance plan, the delivery of preventive services (at a minimum) to children in school-based settings, the use of dental hygienists and assistants (with appropriate training) to provide preventive care in school-based settings, the development of a system for quality and utilization review of dental services, and the institution of a population-based information system.

Over 15 years ago, the IOM focused on dental education issues in *Dental Education at the Crossroads* (IOM, 1995). In that report, the committee envisioned a future in which dentistry is more integrated in the overall health care system (e.g., education, research, and patient care); dental students have more diverse, hands-on clinical experiences; dental schools demonstrate their contributions to the larger health care community (e.g., research, technology transfer, service to community); dental leaders cooperate to reform accreditation and licensing; and dental professionals continue to test alternative models of education, practice, and performance assessment. The committee laid out four broad objectives: to improve knowledge of what works; to encourage prevention at both the individual and community level; to reduce disparities; and to promote attention to oral health by those outside of the dental fields.

In early 2009, the IOM convened a workshop to address one dimension of these issues: the oral health workforce. The workshop summary, *The U.S. Oral Health Workforce in the Coming Decade,* highlighted the connection between oral health and overall health and well-being, current oral health needs and the status of access to care, the demographics and future trends of the oral health workforce, the structure and characteristics of current delivery systems, and challenges in the current workforce and delivery systems (IOM, 2009b). The workshop speakers also reviewed workforce strategies for improving access, with a particular focus on improving children's access to oral health services, as well as opportunities to reframe the oral health delivery system with special attention to the roles of federal and state health agencies, dental educators and policy leaders, advocates, and the media.

Many other IOM studies that did not focus solely on oral health have highlighted particular oral health issues (e.g., the needs of adolescent populations, rural populations, and older adults) and made recommendations related to oral health (IOM, 1992, 2000b, 2005b, 2008, 2009a,b). Among two of its most recent reports, the IOM found that the training of most members of the health care workforce (specifically including dentists and dental hygienists) in the care of older adults is inadequate (IOM, 2008) and that existing oral health services are generally insufficient to meet the needs of many adolescents (IOM, 2009a). Another recent IOM report that examined the impact of health insurance status in the United States found that children's access to dental care and use of dental services improved significantly for children with health insurance (IOM, 2009c).

Previous IOM reports include recommendations such as that the National Institute of Dental and Craniofacial Research should implement programs to increase dental school applicants interested in careers in oral health research, should require that loan forgiveness recipients spend a significant amount of time on research, and should fund required years of the D.D.S./Ph.D. program (IOM, 2005a), and that the National Institutes of Health should expand medical and dentist scientist training programs "specifically for training investigators in the skills of performing patient-oriented clinical research" (IOM, 1994). Certainly the many reports in IOM's history related to primary care, health literacy, access to care, diversity, nutrition, and improving public health have direct implications for all oral health professionals (IOM, 1993, 1996, 1997, 2002, 2004a,b, 2005b).

Professional Organizations

Oral health professional organizations have made improving access to oral health care a major focus of their research efforts and their national agendas. For example, the ADA has convened three recent meetings focused on increasing access to oral health care: an American Indian/Alaska Native (AI/AN) Oral Health Access Summit, a Medicaid Provider Symposium, and an Access to Dental Care Summit (ADA, 2007, 2008, 2009). Each of these meetings brought together diverse groups of stakeholders from the public and private sectors to discuss the dental profession's role in improving the oral health of underserved and vulnerable populations and to identify innovative approaches. The AI/AN Oral Health Access Summit focused on the role of allied dental professionals; multidisciplinary approaches to oral health promotion and disease prevention; and the resources needed to address oral health issues among AI/AN populations (e.g., recruitment and retention of oral health professionals). The Medicaid Provider Symposium focused on the challenges to providing care to Medicaid patients and discussed promising strategies to integrate Medicaid patients into private practice settings. Finally, the overall goal of the Access to Dental Care Summit was to develop a shared vision among diverse stakeholders for improving access to oral health care. The findings from each of these meetings have been used to develop and implement the ADA's work on access.

Other health professional organizations have also made improving access to oral health care a priority in their outreach, research efforts, and their strategic plans. Notably, the American Academy of Pediatrics (AAP) identified oral health as one of its four strategic priority areas of which access to care is a major component. In 2008, the AAP convened a National Summit on Children's Oral Health to examine strategies to overcome barriers to children's access to oral health care services in the United States (AAP, 2011b). The meeting was attended by an array of stakeholders from medical, dental, and other health organizations; advocacy organizations; and federal agencies. The findings from this meeting were published as a collection in a special issue of *Academic Pediatrics* on children's oral health and have helped inform the work of AAP's broader Oral Health Initiative (AAP, 2011a). The Society of Teachers of Family Medicine (STFM) has supported the role of primary care providers in oral health promotion and disease prevention. In 2005, the STFM Group on Oral Health developed *Smiles for Life*, a comprehensive oral health curriculum for primary care providers including physicians, physician assistants, and nurse practitioners (Douglass et al., 2010). This curriculum was developed with guidance from dentists, physicians, and educators through a series of regional consortia. It addresses oral health education across the life cycle and includes online training modules on the needs of underserved and vulnerable populations among other topics (Douglass et al., 2010).

Foundations

A number of philanthropic organizations have also made access to oral health care a significant part of their work. The following are examples of several recent foundation-led initiatives.

The Pew Charitable Trusts established the Pew Children's Dental Campaign to raise awareness and promote policies that ensure children have access to oral health care. In 2010, the campaign released a report, *The Cost of Delay: State Dental Policies Fail One in Five Children*, that underscored the issue of inadequate access to oral health care for low-income children (Pew Center on the States, 2010). *The Cost of Delay* found that two-thirds of states were doing an inadequate job of ensuring that children have access to basic, preventive dental care. A follow-up study in 2011, *The State of Children's Dental Health: Making Coverage Matter,* found that "while many states improved their performance on one or more of the Pew's policy benchmarks, too many still fall short" (Pew Center on the States, 2011).

The Robert Wood Johnson Foundation (RWJF), in collaboration with the California Endowment and the W.K. Kellogg Foundation, created the *Pipeline, Profession, and Practice: Community-Based Dental Education*[2]

[2] For information on participating schools, funding levels, activities, accomplishments, and community partners, see the RWJF project website at http://www.dentalpipeline.org.

initiative to increase the time that senior dental students spend in community settings providing care to underserved populations; and to increase enrollment of low-income and underrepresented minority students in dental school (Bailit and Formicola, 2010). Evaluations of the dental pipeline program found that among pipeline schools, there were increases in first-year enrollment of underrepresented minority students (up 54 percent) (Andersen et al., 2009), increases in the number of days senior students spent in community sites (Formicola et al., 2010), and substantial numbers of services provided through extramural rotations (Atchison et al., 2009).

The W.K. Kellogg Foundation recently announced plans to invest over $16 million in the *Dental Therapist Project*, in Kansas, New Mexico, Ohio, Vermont, and Washington, to improve oral health access in underserved communities (W.K. Kellogg Foundation, 2010). This announcement followed on the heels of a recently released evaluation of the Alaska Native Tribal Health Consortium's Alaska Dental Health Aide Initiative (sponsored by the W.K. Kellogg Foundation, the Rasmuson Foundation, and the Bethel Community Services Foundation). The evaluation (self-described as an "in-depth case study") assessed the performance of dental health aide therapists practicing in remote Alaskan villages. The evaluation found that "the therapists are performing well and operating safely within their scope of practice" (under the general supervision of dentists) (Wetterhall et al., 2010).

DentaQuest Foundation supports the National Interprofessional Initiative on Oral Health which focuses on the education and training of health care providers from primary care disciplines (e.g., family medicine, pediatrics, nursing, physician assisting, obstetrics and gynecology, and internal medicine). And, in Massachusetts, DentaQuest helped lead a statewide coalition of stakeholders to create a state plan for oral health that addresses barriers to care, oral health disparities, and community-based prevention.

The U.S. Department of Health and Human Services

HHS supports a broad array of oral health activities focused on improving the nation's oral health, including

- Oral health financing,
- Research,
- Workforce development,
- Public health action,
- Quality initiatives, and
- Technology (HHS, 2010).

BOX 1-2
Examples of Current HHS Efforts to Improve Access to Oral Health Care

The Administration for Children and Families (ACF)
Oral health activities in the ACF center on its Head Start program, which is operated through the Office of Head Start. For example, ACF requires Head Start programs to determine whether a child has received age-appropriate preventive dental care within 90 days of the child entering the Head Start program.[a]

The Agency for Healthcare Research and Quality (AHRQ)
AHRQ contributes to oral health research by collecting data, funding both intramural and external research, and disseminating innovations in health care delivery. AHRQ collects information on oral health care needs, access, and expenditures through the Medical Expenditure Panel Survey.

The Centers for Disease Control and Prevention (CDC) and the National Institutes of Health (NIH)
The CDC and the NIH are developing a comprehensive Oral Health Surveillance Plan that will allow HHS to create a "report card" for oral health in the United States (HHS, 2010). In addition, the CDC provided $6.8 million in FY 2010 to 19 state oral health programs to support evidence-based prevention programs (e.g., community water fluoridation and school-based sealant programs), surveillance of oral disease burden, and to develop plans to improve oral health and address disparities.

The CDC/National Center for Health Statistics (NCHS)
NCHS contributes to oral health research by collecting, analyzing, and disseminating data. NCHS collects information on oral health status and access to services through the National Health Interview Survey and the National Health and Nutrition Examination Survey.

The Centers for Medicare and Medicaid Services (CMS)
CMS is reviewing state Medicaid dental programs for innovative practices that have increased access to dental care among children and will be sharing the information about those practices with other states (HHS, 2010). CMS has also set goals to increase the rate of children who are enrolled in Medicaid or CHIP and to increase the percentage of these children who receive dental sealants (CMS, 2010). CMS plays an important role in financing oral health care, particularly for low-income children (described in Chapter 5).

The Health Resources and Services Administration (HRSA)
Bureau of Primary Health Care (BPHC)
The BPHC allocates capital and operating funds to federally funded community health centers that receive grants under §330 of the Public Health Service Act (HRSA, 2010a). These health centers provide oral

health care services to low-income individuals both directly and through referrals to private professionals.[b] BPHC also manages the Service Expansion in Oral Health grants that provided additional funding to Fully Qualified Health Centers to expand oral health care services (Anderson, 2010).

Bureau of Clinician Recruitment and Service
The Bureau of Clinician Recruitment and Service manages the National Health Service Corps, which provides scholarships and loan repayment to clinicians, including dentists and dental hygienists, who agree to serve for 2–4 years in Health Professional Shortage Areas (HRSA, 2010b).

The HIV/AIDS Bureau
The HIV/AIDS Bureau sponsors several activities to improve the oral health care of persons with HIV/AIDS through both education of students and residents, as well as grant funding to increase opportunities for provision of oral health care to this population. For example, the Ryan White Special Projects of National Significance Oral Health Initiative funds 15 demonstration sites for up to 5 years to support organizations using innovative models of care to provide oral health care to HIV-positive, underserved populations in both urban and nonurban settings (Anderson, 2010).

Maternal and Child Health Bureau (MCHB)
The MCHB sponsors two centers focused on oral health: the National Maternal and Child Oral Health Resource Center (OHRC) and the National Oral Health Policy Center (OHPC). Specific activities include the OHPC Children's Dental Health Project that provides information and support to federal, state, and local programs and policy makers to promote policies that address disparities in children's oral health (National Maternal and Child Oral Health Policy Center, 2010). The MCHB also funds a number of oral health activities through Title V Block/Formula Grants, Special Projects of Regional and National Significance (SPRANS) grants, and Community Integrated Service Systems (CISS) discretionary grants.

Indian Health Service (IHS)
The IHS is working with community partners such as Head Start; the Special Supplemental Nutrition Program for Women, Infants, and Children (WIC) Program; nurses; doctors; and community health representatives to reduce the prevalence of early childhood caries in American Indian/Alaska Native children.

SOURCE: HHS, 2010.

[a] *Code of Federal Regulations,* Office of Human Development Services, Department of Health and Human Services, title 45, sec. 1304.20 (2009).
[b] 42 U.S.C. §254b.

A review of past and present HHS oral health activities was addressed by the previously mentioned concurrent study by the IOM Committee on an Oral Health Initiative. Box 1-2 provides an overview of several current efforts within HHS, by agency, that are directly related to improving access to oral health care.

ORGANIZATION OF THE REPORT

This report reviews the literature on the oral health status and the delivery of oral health care to vulnerable and underserved populations; presents the committee's findings; and offers recommendations to both public and private entities for investing in, strengthening, and improving the delivery of care to individuals who are currently unable to access oral health services.

The report has six chapters. Chapter 2 provides an overview of oral health status and its connection to overall health. It also provides a closer examination of oral health status by specific subpopulations and establishes the extent of unmet oral health care needs among these populations. Finally, the chapter describes factors that differentially influence oral health status and utilization of oral health care services in the United States.

Chapters 3, 4, and 5 frame the challenges and types of solutions that are typically used to improve access for vulnerable and underserved populations within the context of the resources that are currently available. To that end, Chapter 3 focuses on the characteristics of the oral health care workforce that may help improve access to oral health care; Chapter 4 describes the variety of settings in which oral health care is, or could be, provided; and Chapter 5 provides an overview of the various sources and mechanisms of financing for oral health care in the United States and describes the impact these expenditures have on access to care. Each of these chapters also includes examples of innovative strategies designed to increase access to oral health care.

Finally, Chapter 6 provides a vision of access to quality oral health care across the lifespan that addresses the multitude of needs and barriers to care described in the preceding chapters. The chapter also presents the committee's recommendations for specific actions that should be taken to achieve this vision and additional strategies that will be needed in the near term and over time with an eye toward what can be achieved and sustained during periods of transformation (e.g., health care reform) and in a climate of significantly limited resources.

The report includes several appendixes. Appendix A provides a list of acronyms used throughout the report, and Appendix B contains the authors and titles of the papers commissioned by this committee. Appendix C lists the agendas for the March and July committee workshops. A brief summary of *Advancing Oral Health in America*, the report from the Committee on an Oral Health Initiative, is included in Appendix D. Finally, Appendix E contains biographical sketches of the committee members and IOM project staff.

REFERENCES

AAP (American Academy of Pediatrics). 2011a. *Oral health initiative*. http://www.aap.org/oralhealth/ (accessed March 16, 2011).

AAP. 2011b. *Results of the AAP national summit on children's oral health and* Academic Pediatrics' *special issue on children's oral health*. http://www.aap.org/oralhealth/summit/ (accessed March 16, 2011).

ADA (American Dental Association). 2007. *American Indian and Alaska Native Oral Health Access Summit: Summary report*. Santa Ana Pueblo, NM: American Dental Association.

ADA. 2008. *Report on the June 23, 2008, Medicaid Provider Symposium*. Chicago, IL: American Dental Association.

ADA. 2009. *Proceedings of the March 23–25, 2009, Access to Dental Care Summit*. Chicago, IL: American Dental Association.

AHRQ (Agency for Healthcare Research and Quality). 2010. *2009 National healthcare disparities report*. Rockville, MD: U.S. Department of Health and Human Services.

Anders, P. L., and E. L. Davis. 2010. Oral health of patients with intellectual disabilities: A systematic review. *Special Care in Dentistry* 30(3):110-117.

Andersen, R. M., P. L. Davidson, K. A. Atchison, J. J. Crall, J.-A. Friedman, E. R. Hewlett, and A. Thind. 2009. Summary and implications of the dental pipeline program evaluation. *Journal of Dental Education* 73(Supp. 2):S319-S330.

Anderson, J. R. 2010. *HRSA oral health programs*. Paper presented at 2010 Dental Management Coalition, June 27, Annapolis, MD.

Armour, B. S., M. Swanson, H. B. Waldman, and S. P. Perlman. 2008. A profile of state-level differences in the oral health of people with and without disabilities, in the U.S., in 2004. *Public Health Reports* 123(1):67-75.

Atchison, K. A., A. Thind, T. T. Nakazono, D. Wong, J. J. Gutierrez, D. C. Carreon, and R. M. Andersen. 2009. Community-based clinical dental education: Effects of the pipeline program. *Journal of Dental Education* 73(Supp. 2):S269-S282.

Bailit, H., and A. Formicola. 2010. Preface: About the dental pipeline program. *Journal of Dental Education* 7(10):S5-S6.

Bierman, A. S., E. S. Magari, A. M. Jette, M. Splaine, and J. H. Wasson. 1998. Assessing access as a first step toward improving the quality of care for very old adults. *Journal of Ambulatory Care Management* 21(3):17-26.

Blaizot, A., J. N. Vergnes, S. Nuwwareh, J. Amar, and M. Sixou. 2009. Periodontal diseases and cardiovascular events: Meta-analysis of observational studies. *International Dental Journal* 59(4):197-209.

Bloom, B., R. Cohen, et al. 2009. *Summary health statistics for U.S. children: National Health Interview Survey, 2008*. Hyattsville, MD: National Center for Health Statistics.

Bloom, B., R. Cohen, and G. Freeman. 2010. *Summary health statistics for U.S. children: National Health Interview Survey, 2009*. Hyattsville, MD: National Center for Health Statistics.

Brown, L. J. 2005. *Adequacy of current and future dental workforce: Theory and analysis*. Chicago, IL: American Dental Association.

Caspary, G., D. M. Krol, S. Boulter, M. A. Keels, and G. Romano-Clarke. 2008. Perceptions of oral health training and attitudes toward performing oral health screenings among graduating pediatric residents. *Pediatrics* 122(2):e465-e471.

Chávarry, N., M. V. Vettore, et al. 2009. The relationship between diabetes mellitus and destructive periodontal disease: A meta-analysis. *Oral health & preventive dentistry* 7(2):107-127.

CMS (Centers for Medicare and Medicaid Services). 2010. *Written testimony of CMS to the Committee on an Oral Health Initiative.* Available in Committee on Oral Health Access to Services' public access file.

Cohen, L. A., A. J. Bonito, C. Eicheldinger, R. J. Manski, M. D. Macek, R. R. Edwards, and N. Khanna. 2011. Comparison of patient visits to emergency departments, physician offices, and dental offices for dental problems and injuries. *Journal of Public Health Dentistry* 71(1):13-22.

Conte, M., H. L. Broder, G. Jenkins, R. Reed, and M. N. Janal. 2006. Oral health, related behaviors and oral health impacts among homeless adults. *Journal of Public Health Dentistry* 66(4):276-278.

Cruz, G. D., R. Shore, et al. 2004. Effect of acculturation on objective measures of oral health in Haitian immigrants in New York City. *Journal of Dental Research* 83(2):180-184.

Davis, E. E., A. S. Deinard, and E. W. H. Maïga. 2010. Doctor, my tooth hurts: The costs of incomplete dental care in the emergency room. *Journal of Public Health Dentistry* 70(3):205-210.

Decker, S. L. 2011. Medicaid payment levels to dentists and access to dental care among children and adolescents. *Journal of the American Medical Association* 306(2): 187-193.

Douglass, A. B., R. Maier, et al. 2010. *Smiles for Life: A National Oral Health Curriculum.* 3rd Edition. Retrieved April 26, 2011, from www.smilesforlifeoralhealth.com.

Dye, B. A., S. Tan, V. Smith, B. G. Lewis, L. K. Barker, G. Thornton-Evans, P. I. Eke, E. D. Beltran-Aguilar, A. M. Horowitz, and L. Chien-Hsun. 2007. *Trends in oral health status: United States, 1988-1994 and 1999-2004.* Hyattsville, MD: National Center for Health Statistics.

Dye, B. A., O. Arevalo, and C. M. Vargas. 2010. Trends in paediatric dental caries by poverty status in the United States, 1988-1994 and 1999-2004. *International Journal of Paediatric Dentistry* 20(2):132-143.

Edelstein, B. L., and C. H. Chinn. 2009. Update on disparities in oral health and access to dental care for America's children. *Academic Pediatrics* 9(6):415-419.

Flores, G., and S. C. Tomany-Korman. 2008. The language spoken at home and disparities in medical and dental health, access to care, and use of services in U.S. children. *Pediatrics* 121(6):e1703-e1714.

Formicola, A. J., K. C. D'Abreu, and L. A. Tedesco. 2010. Underrepresented minority dental student recruitment and enrollment programs: An overview from the dental pipeline program. *Journal of Dental Education* 74(Supp. 10):S67-S73.

GAO (Government Accountability Office). 2000. *Dental disease is a chronic problem among low-income populations.* Washington, DC: U.S. General Acccounting Office.

GAO. 2006. *Health professional shortage areas: Problems remain with primary care shortage area designation system.* Washington, DC: U.S. General Accounting Office.

GAO. 2008. *Extent of dental disease in children has not decreased, and millions are estimated to have untreated tooth decay.* Washington, DC: U.S. Government Accountability Office.

Gibson, G., R. Rosenheck, J. Tullner, R. Grimes, C. Seibyl, A. Rivera-Torres, H. Goodman, and M. Nunn. 2003. A national survey of the oral health status of homeless veterans. *Journal of Public Health Dentistry* 63(1):30-37.

Gussy, M. G., E. B. Waters, E. M. Riggs, S. K. Lo, and N. M. Kilpatrick. 2008. Parental knowledge, beliefs and behaviours for oral health of toddlers residing in rural Victoria. *Australian Dental Journal* 53(1):52-60.

Havercamp, S. M., D. Scandlin, and M. Roth. 2004. Health disparities among adults with developmental disabilities, adults with other disabilities, and adults not reporting disability in North Carolina. *Public Health Reports* 119(4):418-426.

HHS (U.S. Department of Health and Human Services). 2000. *Oral health in America: A report of the surgeon general.* Rockville, MD: U.S. Department of Health and Human Services.

HHS. 2010. *HHS Oral Health Initiative 2010.* http://www.hrsa.gov/publichealth/clinical/oralhealth/hhsinitiative.pdf (accessed August 19, 2010).

HRSA (Health Resources and Services Administration). 2010a. *Bureau of Primary Health Care.* http://www.hrsa.gov/about/organization/bureaus/bphc/ (accessed December 22, 2010).

HRSA. 2010b. *NHSC loan repayment.* http://nhsc.hrsa.gov/loanrepayment/ (accessed December 22, 2010).

HRSA. 2011. *Designated health professional shortage areas (HPSA) statistics.* http://ersrs.hrsa.gov/ReportServer?/HGDW_Reports/BCD_HPSA/BCD_HPSA_SCR50_Smry&rs:Format=HTML3.2 (accessed March 14, 2011).

IOM (Institute of Medicine). 1980. *Public policy options for better dental health.* Washington, DC: National Academy Press.

IOM. 1992. *The second fifty years: Promoting health and preventing disability.* Washington, DC: National Academy Press.

IOM. 1993. *Access to health care in America.* Washington, DC: National Academy Press.

IOM. 1994. *Careers in clinical research: Obstacles and opportunities.* Washington, DC: National Academy Press.

IOM. 1995. *Dental education at the crossroads: Challenges and change.* Washington, DC: National Academy Press.

IOM. 1996. *Primary care: America's health in a new era.* Washington, DC: National Academy Press.

IOM. 1997. *Dietary reference intakes.* Washington, DC: National Academy Press.

IOM. 2000a. *America's health care safety net: Intact but endangered* Washington, DC: National Academy Press.

IOM. 2000b. *Extending Medicare coverage for preventive and other services.* Washington, DC: National Academy Press.

IOM. 2001. *Crossing the quality chasm: A new health system for the 21st century.* Washington, DC: National Academy Press.

IOM. 2002. *The future of the public's health in the 21st century.* Washington, DC: The National Academies Press.

IOM. 2004a. *Health literacy: A prescription to end confusion.* Washington, DC: The National Academies Press.

IOM. 2004b. *In the nation's compelling interest: Ensuring diversity in the health-care workforce.* Washington, DC: The National Academies Press.

IOM. 2005a. *Advancing the nation's health needs: NIH research training programs.* Washington, DC: The National Acadmies Press.

IOM. 2005b. *Quality through collaboration: The future of rural health care.* Washington, DC: The National Academies Press.

IOM. 2008. *Retooling for an aging America: Building the health care workforce.* Washington, DC: The National Academies Press.

IOM. 2009a. *Adolescent health services: Missing opportunities.* Washington, DC: The National Academies Press.

IOM. 2009b. *The U.S. oral health workforce in the coming decade: Workshop summary.* Washington, DC: The National Academies Press.

IOM. 2009c. *America's uninsured crisis: Consequences for health and health care*. Washington, DC: The National Academies Press.

Jones, M., J. Y. Lee, and R. G. Rozier. 2007. Oral health literacy among adult patients seeking dental care. *Journal of the American Dental Association* 138(9):1199-1208.

Kutner, M., E. Greenberg, Y. Jin, and C. Paulsen. 2006. *The health literacy of America's adults: Results from the 2003 National Assessment of Adult Literacy*. Washington, DC: National Center for Health Statistics.

Lewis, C. W. 2009. Dental care and children with special health care needs: A population-based perspective. *Academic Pediatrics* 9(6):420-426.

Liu, J., J. C. Probst, A. B. Martin, J.-Y. Wang, and C. F. Salinas. 2007. Disparities in dental insurance coverage and dental care among U.S. children: The National Survey of Children's Health. *Pediatrics* 119(Supp. 1):S12-S21.

Löe, H. 1993. Periodontal disease. The sixth complication of diabetes mellitus. *Diabetes Care* 16(1):329-334.

Manski, R. J., H. S. Goodman, et al. 2004. Dental insurance visits and expenditures among older adults. *American Journal of Public Health* 94(5):759-764.

Manski, R. J., J. Moeller, et al. 2010. Dental care expenditures and retirement. *Journal of Public Health Dentistry* 70(2):148-155.

Maserejian, N. N., M. A. Tavares, C. Hayes, J. A. Soncini, and F. L. Trachtenberg. 2008. Rural and urban disparities in caries prevalence in children with unmet dental needs: The New England children's amalgam trial. *Journal of Public Health Dentistry* 68(1):7-13.

Nash, D. A., and R. J. Nagel. 2005. Confronting oral health disparities among American Indian/Alaska Native children: The pediatric oral health therapist. *American Journal of Public Health* 95(8):1325-1329.

National Maternal and Child Oral Health Policy Center. 2010. *About us*. http://nmcohpc.net/?page_id=2 (accessed December 22, 2010).

Offenbacher, S., J. D. Beck, et al. 2009. Results from the Periodontitis and Vascular Events (PAVE) Study: A pilot multicentered, randomized, controlled trial to study effects of periodontal therapy in a secondary prevention model of cardiovascular disease. *Journal of Periodontology* 80(2):190-201.

Orlans, J., E. Mertz, and K. Grumbach. 2002. *Dental health professional shortage area methodology: A critical review*. San Francisco, CA: UCSF Center for the Health Professions.

Owens, P. L., B. D. Kerker, E. Zigler, and S. M. Horwitz. 2006. Vision and oral health needs of individuals with intellectual disability. *Mental Retardation and Developmental Disabilities Research Reviews* 12(1):28-40.

Pew Center on the States. 2010. *The cost of delay: State dental policies fail one in five children*. Washington, DC: Pew Center on the States.

Pew Center on the States. 2011. *The state of children's dental health: Making coverage matter*. Washington, DC: Pew Center on the States.

Pleis, J. R., B. W. Ward, and J. W. Lucas. 2010. *Summary health statistics for U.S. adults: National Health Interview Survey, 2009*. Hyattsville, MD: Department of Health and Human Services.

President's Advisory Commission on Consumer Protection and Quality in the Health Care Industry. 1998. *Quality first: Better health care for all Americans*. Final Report to the President of the United States. Washington, DC: The President's Advisory Commission on Consumer Protection and Quality in the Health Care Industry.

Sakai, V. T., T. M. Oliveira, T. C. Silva, A. B. S. Moretti, D. Geller-Palti, V. A. Biella, and M. A. A. M. Machado. 2008. Knowledge and attitude of parents or caretakers regarding transmissibility of caries disease. *Journal of Applied Oral Science* 16(2):150-154.

Scannapieco, F. A., and A. W. Ho. 2001. Potential associations between chronic respiratory disease and periodontal disease: Analysis of National Health and Nutrition Examination Survey III. *Journal of Periodontology* 72(1):50-56.

Scannapieco, F. A., R. B. Bush, et al. 2003. Associations between periodontal disease and risk for atherosclerosis, cardiovascular disease, and stroke. A systematic review. *Annals of Periodontology* 8(1):38-53.

Silk, H., A. B. Douglass, J. M. Douglass, and L. Silk. 2008. Oral health during pregnancy. *American Family Physician* 77(8):1139-1144.

Skillman, S. M., M. P. Doescher, W. E. Mouradian, and D. K. Brunson. 2010. The challenge to delivering oral health services in rural America. *Journal of Public Health Dentistry* 70(Supp. 1):S49-S57.

Slavkin, H. C. and B. J. Baum 2000. Relationship of dental and oral pathology to systemic illness. *Journal of the American Medical Association* 284(10):1215-1217.

Sohn, W., A. Ismail, A. Amaya, and J. Lepkowski. 2007. Determinants of dental care visits among low-income African-American children. *Journal of the American Dental Association* 138(3):309-318.

Steinberg, B. J., L. Minsk, J. I. Gluch, and S. K. Giorgio. 2008. Women's oral health issues. In *Women's health in clinical practice*. Totowa, NJ: Humana Press. Pp. 273-293.

Taylor, G. W. 2001. Bidirectional interrelationships between diabetes and periodontal diseases: An epidemiologic perspective. *Annals of Periodontology* 6(1):99-112.

Teeuw, W. J., V. E. A. Gerdes, et al. 2010. Effect of periodontal treatment on glycemic control of diabetic patients: A systematic review and meta-analysis. *Diabetes Care* 33(2): 421-427.

Vargas, C. M., and C. R. Ronzio. 2006. Disparities in early childhood caries. *BMC Oral Health* 6(Supp. 1):S3-S7.

Vargas, C., J. Crall, and D. Schneider. 1998. Sociodemographic distribution of pediatric dental caries: NHANES III, 1988-1994. *Journal of the American Dental Association* 129(9):1229.

Vargas, C. M., B. A. Dye, et al. 2002. Oral health status of rural adults in the United States. *Journal of the American Dental Association* 133(12):1672-1681.

Vargas, C. M., B. A. Dye, and K. L. Hayes. 2003a. Oral health care utilization by U.S. rural residents, National Health Interview Survey 1999. *Journal of Public Health Dentistry* 63(3):150-157.

Vargas, C. M., C. R. Ronzio, and K. L. Hayes. 2003b. Oral health status of children and adolescents by rural residence, United States. *Journal of Rural Health* 19(3):260-268.

Vargas, C. M., J. A. Yellowitz, and K. L. Hayes. 2003c. Oral health status of older rural adults in the United States. *Journal of the American Dental Association* 134(4):479-486.

Wetterhall, S., J. D. Bader, B. B. Burrus, J. Y. Lee, and D. A. Shugars. 2010. *Evaluation of the dental health aide therapist workforce model in Alaska*. Research Triangle Park, NC: W.K. Kellogg Foundation, Rasmuson Foundation, Bethel Community Services Foundation.

WHO (World Health Organization). 2010. *Oral health*. http://www.who.int/topics/oral_health/en/ (accessed December 3, 2010).

W.K. Kellogg Foundation. 2010. *W.K. Kellogg Foundation supports community-led efforts in five states to increase oral health care access by adding dental therapist to the dental team*. http://www.wkkf.org/news/Articles/2010/11/WK-Kellogg-Foundation-Supports-Community-Led-Efforts.aspx (accessed March 16, 2011).

2

Oral Health Status and Utilization

Many of the country's most vulnerable populations face the greatest oral health needs and the largest barriers to accessing oral health care. Because oral health is inextricably linked to overall health, the effects of poor oral health are felt far beyond the mouth. Oral health providers, policy makers, and other stakeholders need to coalesce around a common ground of basic preventive strategies, health literacy, and quality of care principles to improve the oral health of the entire U.S. population.

This chapter begins with a discussion of the connection between oral health and overall health. Next, the chapter gives a brief overview of the oral health status and access to oral health care for the nation as a whole. The specific oral health needs and access issues for individual vulnerable and underserved populations follows. Finally, the chapter considers several barriers to improving access to oral health care (and ultimately, oral health status) including poor oral health literacy, inadequate use of preventive services, and relative lack of oral health quality measures. These barriers are briefly considered here, as a fuller discussion of literacy, prevention, and quality measures can be found in the IOM report *Advancing Oral Health in America* (IOM, 2011).

THE CONNECTION BETWEEN ORAL HEALTH AND OVERALL HEALTH

For people suffering from dental, oral, or craniofacial diseases, the link between oral health and general health and well-being is beyond dispute. However, for policy makers, payers, and health care professionals, a chasm

BOX 2-1
Dental, Oral, and Craniofacial

The word *oral* refers to the mouth. The mouth includes not only the teeth and the gums (gingiva) and their supporting tissues, but also the hard and soft palate, the mucosal lining of the mouth and throat, the tongue, the lips, the salivary glands, the chewing muscles, and the upper and lower jaws. Equally important are the branches of the nervous, immune, and vascular systems that animate, protect, and nourish the oral tissues, as well as provide connections to the brain and the rest of the body. The genetic patterning of development in utero further reveals the intimate relationship of the oral tissues to the developing brain and to the tissues of the face and head that surround the mouth, structures whose location is captured in the word *craniofacial*.

SOURCE: HHS, 2000b.

has divided them. Dental coverage is provided and paid for separately from general health insurance (see Chapter 5), dentists are trained separately from physicians (see Chapter 3), and legislators often fail to consider oral health in health care policy decisions. In effect, the oral health care field has remained separated from general health care. Recently, however, researchers and others have placed a greater emphasis on establishing and clarifying the oral-systemic linkages.

The surgeon general's report *Oral Health in America* emphasized that oral health care is broader than dental care, and that a healthy mouth is more than just healthy teeth (see Box 2-1). The report described the mouth as a mirror of health or disease occurring in the rest of the body in part because a thorough oral examination can detect signs of numerous general health problems, such as nutritional deficiencies and systemic diseases, including microbial infections, immune disorders, injuries, and some cancers (HHS, 2000b). For example, oral lesions are often the first manifestation of HIV infection, and may be used to predict progression from HIV to AIDS (Coogan et al., 2005). Sexually transmitted HP-16 virus has been established as the cause of a number of oropharyngeal cancers (Marur et al., 2010; Shaw and Robinson, 2010). Dry mouth (xerostomia) is an early symptom of Sjogren's syndrome, one of the most common autoimmune disorders (Al-Hashimi, 2001); xerostomia is also a side effect for a large number of prescribed medications (Nabi et al., 2006; Uher et al., 2009; Weinberger et al., 2010).

Further, there is mounting evidence that oral health complications not only reflect general health conditions, but also exacerbate them. Infections that begin in the mouth can travel throughout the body. For example, periodontal bacteria have been found in samples removed from brain abscesses (Silva, 2004), pulmonary tissue (Suzuki and Delisle, 1984), and cardiovascular tissue (Haraszthy et al., 2000). Periodontal disease has been associated with adverse pregnancy outcomes (Albert et al., 2011; Offenbacher et al., 2006; Radnai et al., 2006; Scannapieco et al., 2003b; Tarannum and Faizuddin, 2007), respiratory disease (Scannapieco and Ho, 2001), cardiovascular disease (Blaizot et al., 2009; Offenbacher et al., 2009b; Scannapieco et al., 2003a; Slavkin and Baum, 2000), and diabetes (Chávarry et al., 2009; Löe, 1993; Taylor, 2001; Teeuw et al., 2010).

Poor oral health may be associated with several other types of morbidity (both individual and societal) including chronic pain, loss of days from school (Gift et al., 1992, 1993), and inappropriate use of emergency departments (Cohen et al., 2011; Davis et al., 2010). Oral health affects speech, nutrition, growth and function, social development, and quality of life (HHS, 2000b). In rare cases, untreated oral disease in children has led to death (Otto, 2007). The impact of poor oral health extends to a child's family and community through lost work hours and the cost of hospital admissions, for example. Figure 2-1 illustrates the range of consequences of early childhood caries in a morbidity and mortality pyramid.

OVERVIEW OF ORAL HEALTH STATUS AND ACCESS TO ORAL HEALTH CARE IN THE UNITED STATES

Although there is a wide range of diseases and conditions that manifest themselves in or near the oral cavity itself, this report will focus primarily on access to services for the prevention, diagnosis, and treatment of two diseases and their sequelae: dental caries and periodontal diseases. Dental caries, or tooth decay, is caused by a bacterial infection (most commonly *Streptococcus mutans*) that is often passed from person to person (e.g., from mother to child). *Oral Health in America* called dental caries the most common chronic disease of childhood (HHS, 2000b), and it is among the most common diseases in the world (WHO, 2010d). Despite decades of knowledge of how to prevent dental caries, they remain a significant problem for all age groups. Periodontal disease is generally broken into two categories: gingivitis and periodontitis. Gingivitis is an inflammation of the tissue surrounding the teeth that results from a buildup of dental plaque between the tissue and the teeth. It is generally due to poor oral hygiene. Untreated gingivitis can result in periodontitis, the breakdown of the ligament that connects the teeth to the jaw bone, and the destruction of the bone that supports the teeth in the jaw. At least 8.5 percent of adults (ages 20–64) and 17.2 percent of older adults (age 65 and older) in the United States have periodontal disease (NIDCR, 2011a,b).

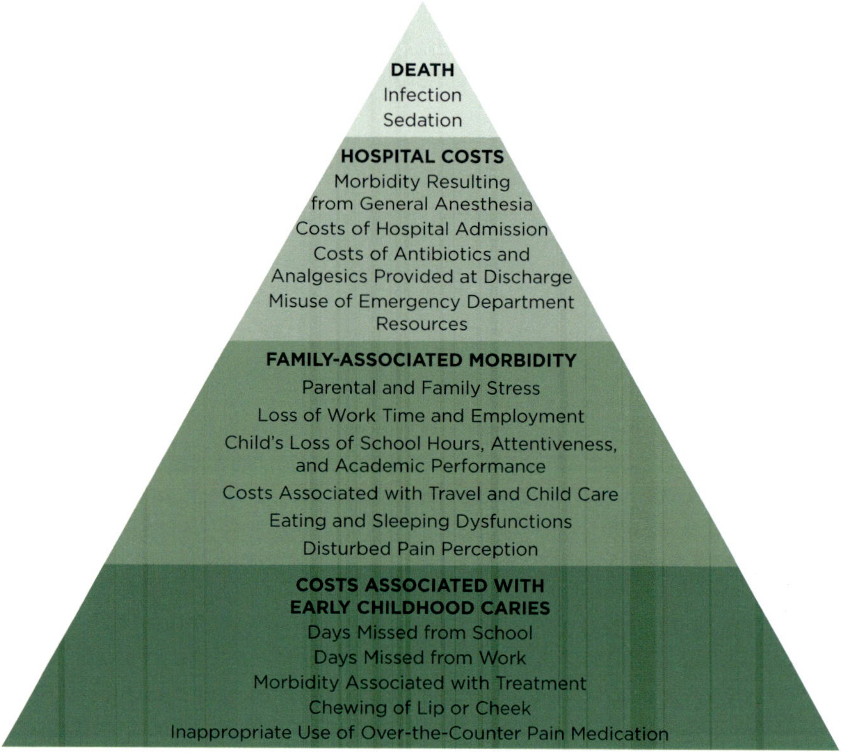
DEATH
Infection
Sedation
HOSPITAL COSTS
Morbidity Resulting from General Anesthesia
Costs of Hospital Admission
Costs of Antibiotics and Analgesics Provided at Discharge
Misuse of Emergency Department Resources
FAMILY-ASSOCIATED MORBIDITY
Parental and Family Stress
Loss of Work Time and Employment
Child's Loss of School Hours, Attentiveness, and Academic Performance
Costs Associated with Travel and Child Care
Eating and Sleeping Dysfunctions
Disturbed Pain Perception
COSTS ASSOCIATED WITH EARLY CHILDHOOD CARIES
Days Missed from School
Days Missed from Work
Morbidity Associated with Treatment
Chewing of Lip or Cheek
Inappropriate Use of Over-the-Counter Pain Medication

FIGURE 2-1
Proposed early childhood caries morbidity and mortality pyramid.

SOURCE: Casamassimo et al., 2009.

A Note on Data Sources

The following sections document the oral health status and access to care for various populations. Data was drawn from published studies that rely on a number of data sources, including the National Health and Nutrition Examination Survey (NHANES), the National Health Interview Survey, the Medical Expenditure Panel Survey (MEPS), and smaller-scale surveys. While the magnitude of disparities in oral health and access to care may differ among the various sources, similar conclusions can be drawn from them about disparities in oral health status and access to care. Other researchers have noted similar trends in the past (Macek et al., 2002). Therefore, the committee felt comfortable using a variety of data sources, both national and smaller scale. The committee did not have the ability to analyze raw data and thus relied on published sources. As a result, the committee did not always use the most recent survey data, because it has not been analyzed in the published literature. In particular, many published studies on oral health status rely on NHANES data from 1988–1994 and 1999–2004, and consequently the committee also relied heavily on those data. While NHANES has included an oral health assessment in subsequent years, the data collected is less detailed and not easily comparable to earlier data. Until 2004, NHANES collected tooth-level data, meaning that a dentist evaluated the teeth of each survey respondent to determine the number of decayed, missing, or filled teeth and surfaces (CDC, 2010b). Beginning in 2005, the oral health survey moved to person-level surveillance for caries, meaning that each survey respondent was evaluated only for the presence or absence of any decayed, missing, and filled teeth (CDC, 2010b; Dye et al., 2011a). The Patient Protection and Affordable Care Act required the Centers for Disease Control and Prevention (CDC) to return to person-level surveillance for NHANES, although funding has not been appropriated.[1]

Overall Oral Health Status

In April 2007, the National Center for Health Statistics of the CDC released a comprehensive assessment of the oral health status of the U.S. population (Dye et al., 2007). Using data provided by two iterations of NHANES (NHANES III, 1988–1994, and NHANES, 1999–2004), which is the most comprehensive survey on oral health status in the United States, the assessment concluded that "Americans of all ages continue to experience improvements in their oral health" (Dye et al., 2007). Specifically, the report noted that among older adults, edentulism (complete tooth loss) and periodontitis (gum disease) had declined. Among adults, CDC observed improvements in the prevalence of dental caries, tooth retention, and periodontal health. For adolescents and youth, dental caries decreased, while dental sealants (used to prevent tooth decay) became more prevalent. Encouragingly, the increase in dental sealants was consistent among all racial and ethnic groups, although non-Hispanic black and Mexican American children and adolescents continue to have a lower prevalence of sealants than white children and adolescents, and low-income children receive fewer dental sealants than those who live above 200 percent of the federal poverty level (FPL).

While the data from the NHANES surveys showed improvements in certain indicators of oral health status across two intervals of time, Americans' overall health status in the 1999–2004 period remained discouraging.

[1] *Patient Protection and Affordable Care Act,* Public Law 148, 111th Cong., 2nd sess. (March 23, 2010), §4102.

For example, over 25 percent of adults 20 to 64 years of age and nearly 20 percent of respondents over age 65 were experiencing untreated dental caries at the time of their examination. Even young children experienced high rates of caries: nearly 28 percent of children ages 2–5 years had caries experience, and 20 percent have untreated caries. Moreover, caries prevalence among preschool children increased between 1988–1994 and 1999–2004 (Dye et al., 2010). In addition, disturbing disparities remain in oral health status for many underserved and vulnerable populations, which will be discussed in detail later in this chapter.

Access to Oral Health Care

Limited and uneven access to oral health care contributes to both poor oral health and disparities in oral health. More than half of the population (56 percent) did not visit a dentist in 2004 (Manski and Brown, 2007), and in 2007, 5.5 percent of the population reported being unable to get or delaying needed dental care, significantly higher than the numbers that reported being unable to get or delaying needed medical care or prescription drugs (Chevarley, 2010). Nearly all measures indicate that vulnerable and underserved populations access oral health care in particularly low numbers. For example, poor children are more likely to report unmet dental need than those with higher incomes (Bloom et al., 2010), non-Hispanic black and Hispanic children and adults are less likely to have seen a dentist in the past 6 months than non-Hispanic white populations (Bloom et al., 2010; Pleis et al., 2010), and less than 20 percent of eligible Medicaid beneficiaries received preventive dental services in 2009 (CMS, 2010). These disparities and others will be discussed in more detail later in this chapter.

Healthy People: Benchmarks for Oral Health

Since 1980, the Department of Health and Human Services (HHS) has used the *Healthy People* process to set the country's health-promotion and disease-prevention agenda (Koh, 2010). *Healthy People* is a set of health objectives for the nation, consisting of (1) overarching goals for improving the overall health of all Americans, and (2) more specific objectives in a variety of focus areas, including oral health. Every 10 years, HHS evaluates the progress that has been made on *Healthy People* goals, develops new goals, and sets new benchmarks for progress. The goals are developed by relevant HHS agencies, with input from external stakeholders and the public. *Healthy People 2020* objectives were released in December 2010 and are listed in Box 2-2.

Healthy People 2010 came to a close with the announcement of the *Healthy People 2020* benchmarks in late 2010. Progress on the *Healthy*

People 2010 goals was mixed, although final data have yet to be analyzed (Koh, 2010; Sondik et al., 2010; Tomar and Reeves, 2009). At the midcourse review in 2006, no oral health objectives had met or exceeded their targets (HHS, 2006). Encouragingly, however, progress was made in a number of categories, including decreasing caries among adolescents (although not among younger children), increasing the proportion of children with dental sealants, increasing the proportion of adults with no permanent tooth loss, and increasing the proportion of the population with access to community water fluoridation (HHS, 2006; Tomar and Reeves, 2009). In contrast, several objectives moved away from their targets. For example, the proportion of children aged 2 to 4 years with dental caries increased from 18 to 22 percent, and the proportion of untreated dental caries in this population increased from 16 to 17 percent (HHS, 2006). In addition, the number of oral and pharyngeal cancers detected at an early stage decreased.

ORAL HEALTH STATUS AND ACCESS TO ORAL HEALTH CARE FOR VULNERABLE AND UNDERSERVED POPULATIONS

While there has been some improvement in the oral health of the U.S. population overall, underserved populations continue to suffer disparities in both their disease burden and access to needed services. For example, dental caries remain a significant problem in certain specific populations such as low-income children and racial and ethnic minorities (Edelstein and Chinn, 2009). According to NHANES, twice as many poor children ages 2 to 11 have at least one untreated decayed tooth, compared to nonpoor children (Dye et al., 2007). In addition, low-income children also receive fewer dental sealants (Dye et al., 2007). Minority children are more likely to have dental decay than white children, and their decay is more severe (IHS, 2002; Vargas and Ronzio, 2006). When migrant and seasonal farmworkers in Michigan were asked which health care service would benefit them the most, the most common response was dental services, ahead of pediatric care, transportation, and interpretation, among other services (Anthony et al., 2008). This section will explore the disparities in status and access to care for a variety of vulnerable and underserved populations.

Children and Adolescents

Children

While not all children are underserved, many children are vulnerable to developing oral diseases, particularly dental caries. The U.S. Government Accountability Office (GAO) recently reported that according to NHANES, dental disease in children has not decreased, noting that about

BOX 2-2
***Healthy People 2020*: Oral Health Objectives**

Oral health of children and adolescents

1. Reduce the proportion of children and adolescents who have dental caries experience in their primary or permanent teeth.
2. Reduce the proportion of children and adolescents with untreated dental decay.

Oral health of adults

3. Reduce the proportion of adults with untreated dental decay.
4. Reduce the proportion of adults who have ever had a permanent tooth extracted because of dental caries or periodontal disease.
5. Reduce the proportion of adults aged 45–74 with moderate or severe periodontitis.
6. Increase the proportion of oral and pharyngeal cancers detected at the earliest stage.

Access to preventive services

7. Increase the proportion of children, adolescents, and adults who used the oral health care system in the past year.
8 Increase the proportion of low-income children and adolescents who received any preventive dental service during the past year.
9. Increase the proportion of school-based health centers with an oral health component.
10. Increase the proportion of local health departments and Federally Qualified Health Centers that have an oral health component.

one in three children aged 2–18 enrolled in Medicaid had untreated tooth decay, and one in nine had untreated decay in three or more teeth (GAO, 2008). The lack of adequate dental treatment may affect children's speech, nutrition, growth and function, social development, and quality of life (HHS, 2000b). In spite of these significant problems, according to MEPS, only about 25 percent of children under the age of 6, 59 percent of children ages 6–12, and 48 percent of adolescents ages 13–20 had a dental visit in 2004 (Manski and Brown, 2007).

A number of factors are related to the likelihood that a child has visited the dentist in the past year, including insurance status, race, ethnicity, being born outside the United States, language spoken at home, whether the child's mother has a regular source of dental care (Grembowski et al., 2008; Lewis et al., 2007). Dentally uninsured children receive fewer dental services than insured children (Kenney et al., 2005; Lewis et al., 2007;

11. Increase the proportion of patients that receive oral health services at Federally Qualified Health Centers each year.

Oral health interventions

12. Increase the proportion of children and adolescents who have received dental sealants on their molar teeth.
13. Increase the proportion of the U.S. population served by community water systems with optimally fluoridated water.
14. Increase the proportion of adults who receive preventive interventions in dental offices.

Monitoring and surveillance systems

15. Increase the number of states and the District of Columbia that have a system for recording and referring infants and children with cleft lips and cleft palates to craniofacial anomaly rehabilitative teams.
16. Increase the number of states and the District of Columbia that have an oral and craniofacial health surveillance system.

Public health infrastructure

17. Increase the number of health agencies that have a public dental health program directed by a dental professional with public health training.

SOURCE: HHS, 2010.

Manski and Brown, 2007). The data on dental visits for publicly insured children, however, are mixed. Some data indicate that publicly insured children are less likely to receive dental services and receive fewer dental services on average than privately insured children (Manski and Brown, 2007); however, studies that control for race and income (among other factors) indicate that publicly and privately insured children are equally likely to have a preventive dental visit (Kenney et al., 2005; Lewis et al., 2007). African American and Latino children are less likely to have had a preventive dental visit (Lewis et al., 2007) or any dental contact in the past year than white children (Bloom et al., 2010). This may contribute to the low levels of dental visits among publicly insured children in uncontrolled estimates, since African American and Latino children are more likely to be enrolled in Medicaid (Kaiser Family Foundation, 2009). Children born outside the United States and children whose primary language at home is not English are both less likely than reference groups to have a preventive dental visit in the past 12 months (Lewis et al., 2007). In addition, low-income children whose parents regularly visit the dentist are more likely to visit the dentist, according to surveys done in Washington state and Detroit (Grembowski et al., 2008; Sohn et al., 2007).

Adolescents

As noted above, adolescents, generally those aged 10–19 (IOM, 2009), have a high prevalence of oral disease. Risk factors for dental caries are similar to those for other age groups, but adolescents' risk for oral and perioral injury is exacerbated by behaviors such as the use of alcohol and illicit drugs, driving without a seatbelt, cycling without a helmet, engaging in contact sports without a mouth guard, and using firearms (IOM, 2009). Other concerns among adolescent populations, which are not unique to this age group, include damage caused by the use of all forms of tobacco, erosion of teeth and damage to soft tissues caused by eating disorders, oral manifestations of sexually transmitted infections (e.g., soft tissue lesions) as a result of oral sex, and increased risk of periodontal disease during pregnancy. In an online Harris Interactive poll of nearly 1,200 adolescents, respondents frequently mentioned having access to affordable, convenient, and high-quality dental care as what they would most like to change to make health services more helpful (IOM, 2009).

Homeless Populations

Homeless people have poorer oral health than the general population. However, no national data are available on the oral health status of homeless populations, and the few available studies may skew the results due to sample size, the population surveyed (e.g., people who present at a clinic), and inability to reach the chronically homeless, among other factors. In a national survey, homeless veterans reported higher rates of oral pain, more decayed teeth, and fewer filled teeth than the general population (Gibson et al., 2003). Many homeless veterans reported having oral pain either currently or within the past year (Conte et al., 2006). Similarly, in a small survey of homeless adolescents in Seattle, over 50 percent reported having sensitive teeth, 39 percent reported a toothache, and 27 percent reported sore or bleeding gums (Chi and Milgrom, 2008). In addition, homeless people in these surveys were more likely than the general population to perceive their oral health as poor (Chi and Milgrom, 2008; Gibson et al., 2003). Homeless people also struggle to access oral health care. A national survey of homeless people found that dental care was the most commonly reported unmet health need (Baggett et al., 2010). In fact, homeless people surveyed at a free dental screening had not seen a dentist in, on average, 5.7 years (Conte et al., 2006).

Homeless populations face a multitude of barriers to both maintaining good oral health and accessing oral health care. They are more likely to engage in behaviors detrimental to oral health such as smoking and using other types of tobacco products (Conte et al., 2006; Gibson et al., 2003), heavy alcohol use (Gibson et al., 2003), and substance abuse (Chi and Milgrom, 2008). They also may lack toothbrushes, toothpaste, clean water, or a place to brush their teeth (Chi and Milgrom, 2008). Homeless people often lack dental coverage, and homeless children struggle to maintain Medicaid coverage because they do not have a permanent address. Over one-third of homeless people at a free dental screening answered that they did not know where to seek dental care if needed (Conte et al., 2006).

Low-Income Populations

Socioeconomic status, as measured by poverty status,[2] is a strong determinant of oral health (Vargas et al., 1998). In every age group, persons in the lower-income group are more likely to have had dental caries experience and more than twice as likely to have untreated dental caries in comparison to their higher-income counterparts (Dye et al., 2007). Poor children ages 2–8 have more than twice the rate of dental caries experience as nonpoor children (Dye et al., 2010). Despite the fact that most children living below the FPL are eligible to receive dental care through Medicaid, many children in this income group have untreated decay (Dye et al., 2007). Among adults, tooth extraction is a common treatment for advanced dental decay when financial resources are limited. Consistently, total tooth loss, or edentulism, among persons 65 years of age and over is more frequent among those living below the FPL than among those living at twice the FPL (Dye et al., 2007).

Poor children and adults receive significantly fewer dental services than the population as a whole (Dye et al., 2007; Lewis et al., 2007; Stanton and Rutherford, 2003). The likelihood of visiting a dentist decreases with decreasing income (Haley et al., 2008; Manski et al., 2004), and people who live below the FPL are less than half as likely to have visited a dentist in the past year as those who make over 400 percent of the FPL (Manski and Brown, 2007). Children whose families make below 200 percent of the FPL are less than half as likely to have a preventive dental visit than children living in higher-income families (Stanton and Rutherford, 2003).

[2] For the purposes of this report, poor refers to individuals and families with income below the FPL; near-poor refers income between 100 and 199 percent of FPL; and nonpoor refers to income above 200 percent of the FPL.

Low-income children also receive fewer dental sealants (Dye et al., 2007), although improvements have been made in this area. Between 1988–1994 and 1999–2004, the largest increase in sealant use was among poor children (an increase of 3 percent to 21 percent) (Dye and Thornton-Evans, 2010). Low-income populations are also more likely to receive episodic or emergency oral health care, rather than receiving preventive care and having a usual source of care (Cohen et al., 2011; Kenney et al., 2005; Lewis et al., 2007, 2010).

It is important to note that most children living below the FPL are eligible to receive dental care through Medicaid, and therefore have financing available for oral health care. Indeed, according to the Medical Expenditure Panel Survey, 83 percent of poor children had dental coverage, which is more than any other income group, although they are less likely to have private dental coverage (Manski and Brown, 2007). In contrast, over 60 percent of poor adults lacked dental coverage (Manski and Brown, 2010). Poor populations face a number of barriers to accessing oral health care, many of which will be discussed in greater detail later in this report. They include inability to pay due to lack of dental coverage (Haley et al., 2008; Lewis et al., 2007) or the size of the expense (Haley et al., 2008); difficulty finding a dentist who will accept Medicaid (Lewis et al., 2010); long waits to get appointments (Lewis et al., 2010); lack of transportation (Lewis et al., 2010); higher levels of medical care use (Kuthy et al., 1996); and parents who do not receive regular oral health care (Sohn et al., 2007). Access for low-income populations is also complicated by other factors including age, race, ethnicity, and proximity to oral health providers.

Older Adults

The prevalence of caries and periodontal disease increases steadily with age (Dye et al., 2007). Encouragingly, however, the prevalence of both diseases in older adults has decreased over time (Dye et al., 2007). In addition, the percentage of older adults who are totally edentulous has decreased over time (Lamster, 2004).

Oral health status is related to functional and other health deficiencies. Poor oral health and oral health-related quality of life in older adults are significantly associated with disability and reduction in mobility (Makhija et al., 2011; Yu et al., 2011). In addition, older adults are more likely than other segments of the population to have other diseases that may exacerbate their oral health, and vice versa, such as cardiovascular disease, diabetes, and pneumonia (CDC, 2011; El-Solh et al., 2004; NHLBI, 2010).

The Institute of Medicine (IOM) has long recognized issues related to the oral health of older adults. For example, in a 1992 study on various needs of older adults, an entire chapter was devoted to oral health, noting that oral health had improved for older adults, but that adults who retain their teeth continue to be at risk for oral diseases (IOM, 1992). At that time, the IOM recommended to assess the oral health status, risk factors for oral diseases, and use and delivery of oral health services for older adults as well as to consider methods for performing oral cancer screenings in primary care settings.

Older adults frequently do not access oral health care. According to MEPS, only 42 percent of adults age 55 and older reported visiting a dentist in 1996, ranging from 46 percent of 55- to 65-year-olds to 32 percent of adults over age 75 (Manski et al., 2004). Older adults are more likely to have serious medical issues and functional limitations, which can deter them from seeking dental care (Chen et al., 2011; Kiyak and Reichmuth, 2005). Older adults who spend more on medication and medical visits are less likely to use dental services (Kuthy et al., 1996). Additionally, the more functional limitations an older person reports, the less likely he or she is to seek dental care (Dolan et al., 1998). Admittance to long-term care (LTC) facilities creates a significant barrier to receipt of dental care. While federal law requires LTC facilities that receive Medicare or Medicaid funding to provide access to dental care, only 80 percent of facilities report doing so (Jones, 2002). Even when dental care is available, evidence indicates that many residents do not regularly receive dental care and many oral health problems go undetected (Dolan et al., 2005). For example, according to a 1999 survey, only 13 percent of nursing home residents over age 65 received dental services in the billing year of their discharge (Jones, 2002).

Multiple factors contribute to low access to oral health services for older adults. LTC facilities may underestimate the importance of oral health. For example, in a survey of Ohio nursing home executives, 49 percent rated their residents' oral health as fair or poor but 64 percent were still satisfied with the oral health care provided at their facilities (Pyle et al., 2005). In addition, LTC facilities have difficulty finding dentists to care for their patients. One study showed that the perceived willingness of dentists to treat LTC residents either in the facility or in private offices was the greatest barrier to providing dental care in Michigan alternative LTC facilities (Smith et al., 2010). In the absence of dentists, nursing home staff must identify residents' oral health needs, but nurses and nursing assistants are not adequately trained to identify many oral health issues (Coleman and Watson, 2006; Jablonski, 2010; Jablonski et al., 2009).

Another significant reason that older adults have difficulty accessing oral health care is the relative lack of training of the health care workforce in the special needs of older adults (Ettinger, 2010). In a 2008 report on the care of older adults (IOM, 2008), the IOM noted that in 1987 the National Institute on Aging predicted a need for 1,500 geriatric dental academicians and 7,500 dental practitioners with training in geriatric dentistry by the year 2000 (NIA, 1987). By the mid-1990s, however, only about 100 dentists in total had completed advanced training in geriatrics (HRSA, 1995), and little has changed since then. Of the dental students graduating in 2001, almost 20 percent did not feel prepared to care for older adults and 25 percent felt the geriatric dental curriculum was inadequate (Mohammad et al., 2003). The American Dental Association (ADA) currently does not recognize geriatric dentistry as a separate specialty, board certification by the American Board of General Dentistry does not explicitly require questions on geriatric dental care, and none of the 509 residencies recognized by the American Dental Education Association are specifically devoted to the care of geriatric patients (IOM, 2008).

People with Special Health Care Needs

It appears that both children and adults with special health care needs (SHCN)[3] have poorer oral health than the general population (Anders and Davis, 2010; Owens et al., 2006). Most, though not all, studies indicate that the overall prevalence of dental caries in people with SHCN is either the same as the general population or slightly lower (Anders and Davis, 2010; López Pérez et al., 2002; Tiller et al., 2001). But available data indicate that people with SHCN suffer disproportionately from periodontal disease and edentulism, have more untreated dental caries, poorer oral hygiene, and receive less care than the general population (Anders and Davis, 2010; Armour et al., 2008; Havercamp et al., 2004; Owens et al., 2006). However, little high-quality data exists on the oral health of people with SHCN. People with SHCN are a difficult population to assess, in part because of their diversity, and also because they are geographically dispersed. Moreover, it is also difficult to analyze national data on this population because their numbers are not large enough to produce reliable statistics. The few available studies of people with SHCN are conducted with populations that are not representative of the SHCN community as a whole (Feldman et al., 1997; Owens et al., 2006; Reid et al., 2003).

Access to care for people with SHCN appears to vary with age. While children with SHCN receive preventive dental care at similar or higher rates than children without SHCN (Kenney et al., 2008; Newacheck and Kim, 2005; Van Cleave and Davis, 2008), adults with SHCN are less likely to have seen a dentist in the past year than people without SHCN (Armour

[3] Consensus appears to have developed around a definition for children with special health care needs: "those who have, or are at increased risk for, a chronic physical, developmental, behavioral, or emotional condition and who also require health and related services of a type or amount beyond that required by children generally" (MCHB, 2011). For the purposes of this report, the definition will also be used for adults.

et al., 2008). Despite the similar rates of dental care visits, dental care is the most commonly reported unmet health care need among children with SHCN (Lewis et al., 2005; Newacheck et al., 2000), and children with SHCN are more likely to report experiencing a toothache in the last 6 months than children without SHCN, with more severely affected children more likely to report a toothache (Lewis and Stout, 2010).

Disparities in oral health for people with SHCN are due to a variety of reasons. First, they often take medications that reduce saliva flow, which promotes dental caries and periodontal disease (HHS, 2000b). Additionally, people with SHCN often have impaired dexterity and thus rely on others for oral hygiene (Shaw et al., 1989). They also face systematic barriers to oral health care such as transportation barriers (especially for those with physical disabilities), cost, and health care professionals who are not trained to work with SHCN patients or dental offices that are not physically suited for them (Ettinger, 2010; Glassman and Subar, 2008; Glassman et al., 2005; Stiefel, 2002; Yuen et al., 2010). In addition, the current oral health care system has limited capacity to care for children with SHCN (Ciesla et al., 2011; Kerins et al., 2011). It is likely that children and adults with SHCN experience different barriers to care; however, not enough information exists to divide the populations.

Pregnant Women and Mothers

Oral health problems are common among pregnant women and follow similar disparities with respect to race, ethnicity, income, insurance, and age. However, pregnant women have several unique oral health needs. Pregnant women are susceptible to periodontitis, loose teeth, and pyogenic granulomas, also known as pregnancy oral tumors (Silk et al., 2008; Steinberg et al., 2008). Periodontal disease has been identified in observational studies as a potential factor contributing to adverse pregnancy outcomes, such as preterm birth and low birth weight (Albert et al., 2011; Radnai et al., 2006; Vergnes and Sixou, 2007).

The oral health of pregnant women is important not only for their own health, but because there is a strong relationship between the oral health status and oral health care habits of a mother and her children's oral health status and habits. The bacteria that cause dental caries are transmissible from caregivers, especially mothers, to children (Douglass et al., 2008). Moreover, children of mothers with untreated dental caries and tooth loss are between two and more than three times as likely to have untreated dental caries compared to children whose mothers had no untreated dental caries or no tooth loss (Dye et al., 2011b; Weintraub et al., 2010). Children enrolled in Medicaid are more likely to receive oral health care when their mothers have a regular source of oral health care (Grembowski et al., 2008). The provision of oral health services for pregnant women and mothers may include education about how their own oral health relates to their children's oral health as well as how to prevent dental caries in their young children.

Recently, states and health care organizations have promoted the importance and safety of oral health care for pregnant women. The American Academy of Pediatrics and the American College of Obstetricians and Gynecologists agree that it is very important for pregnant women to continue usual oral health care (AAP and ACOG, 2007). Both the New York State Department of Health and the California Dental Association have released evidence-based guidelines for treating pregnant women (California Dental Association, 2010; New York State Department of Health, 2006). Both sets of guidelines recommend that prenatal care providers educate women about the importance of oral health and refer them for oral health care, and that oral health care professionals provide routine and necessary oral health care to pregnant women (California Dental Association, 2010; New York State Department of Health, 2006). Recently, several randomized clinical trials of pregnant women with periodontal disease have been performed to examine the effect of receiving treatment during pregnancy or postpartum (Macones et al., 2010; Michalowicz et al., 2006; Offenbacher et al., 2009a). Results of these trials suggest that periodontal treatment is safe for pregnant women and their fetuses and effective in reducing the level of periodontal disease (Michalowicz et al., 2006). However, periodontal treatment during pregnancy does not necessarily reduce the incidence of poor birth outcomes (Macones et al., 2010; Michalowicz et al., 2006; Offenbacher et al., 2009a).

Although oral health care is considered both safe and effective for pregnant women and their fetuses (Michalowicz et al., 2008), many women do not receive dental care during pregnancy (Boggess et al., 2010; Gaffield et al., 2001; Hunter and Yount, 2011; Marchi et al., 2010). Even when women report having an oral health problem during the pregnancy, only about half of them visit a dentist (California Dental Association, 2010; Gaffield et al., 2001; Marchi et al., 2010). Among women with oral health problems, the likelihood of visiting a dentist during the pregnancy is associated with dental coverage status and timing of the first prenatal care visit (Gaffield et al., 2001). Although over 40 percent of all pregnant women have medical insurance through Medicaid (Kaiser Family Foundation, 2007), many of them are not covered for oral health care because only about half of state Medicaid programs pay for the oral health care of pregnant women. In addition, some women report being erroneously informed to not visit the dentist during pregnancy (Boggess et al., 2010).

Racial and Ethnic Minorities

As will be described in more detail below, racial and ethnic minorities experience significant disparities in oral health status and access to oral health care compared to the U.S. population as a whole. These disparities can be attributed to a number of complex societal factors, including lower incomes, a lower prevalence of dental coverage, and a dearth of dentists located in communities where racial and ethnic minorities live, among many other factors.

African Americans

African Americans have poorer oral health than the overall U.S. population throughout the life cycle. African American children and adolescents are have slightly more dental caries and more untreated dental caries than white children and adolescents (Dye et al., 2007). African American adults (ages 20–64) have approximately the same prevalence of dental caries as white adults; however, dental caries in African Americans is much more likely to be untreated (Dye et al., 2007). In addition, African American adults are significantly more likely to have periodontal disease than white adults (Dye et al., 2007). African American older adults have, on average, fewer teeth than whites (Dye et al., 2007). African Americans also perceive their oral health as worse than whites; parents of non-Hispanic black children are twice as likely as parents of white children to rate their child's oral health as fair or poor (Dietrich et al., 2008); and African American adults are less than half as likely as white adults to rate their oral health as excellent or very good (Dye et al., 2007). Encouragingly, the oral health of African Americans appears to be improving for many, though not all, of these measures. For example, 17 percent of African American adults had periodontal disease in the 1999–2004 NHANES survey, down from 26 percent in the 1988–1994 survey (Dye et al., 2007).

African Americans also experience disparities in access to oral health care. In 2003, 72 percent of African American children received preventive oral health care, compared to 84 percent of white children (Dietrich et al., 2008). In 2009, 53 percent of African American adults reported seeing a dentist or other dental professional in the past year, compared to 61 percent of the overall population (Pleis et al., 2010).

American Indians and Alaskan Natives

American Indians and Alaskan Natives (AI/AN) also have poorer oral health than the overall U.S. population throughout the life cycle. In 1999, the Indian Health Service (IHS) surveyed its patients to determine the burden of dental caries on the AI/AN population and compare AI/AN oral health to the overall populations' oral health (IHS, 2002). The survey found that AI/AN children and adolescents, ages 2 to 19, are more likely to suffer from dental caries and are more likely to have untreated dental caries as compared to the overall population. The rate of dental caries for AI/AN children ages 2 to 5, for example, is five times the U.S. average, and more than two-thirds of AI/AN children suffer from dental caries (IHS, 2002). AI/AN adults ages 35 to 44 also have more teeth with untreated dental caries, but fewer missing teeth, and about the same number of filled teeth as the overall population. AI/AN adults over age 55 have fewer teeth, higher rates of dental caries, and more periodontal disease, but fewer root caries than the overall population. AI/AN elders are more likely to be edentulous; two surveys found that at least 40 percent of AI/AN adults between the ages of 65 and 74 were edentulous, compared to 29 percent of the overall population (Jones et al., 2000).

AI/AN populations face complex barriers to attaining good oral health, including a lack of sources of fluoridated water, instability in IHS dental programs, and geographic barriers to care. Historically, IHS has supported water fluoridation on Indian reservations for the prevention of dental caries, but the number of reservation systems submitting fluoridation monitoring reports to IHS dropped from 700 in the early 1990s to fewer than 500 in 1995 (Martin, 2000).

Asian Americans

Although Asian Americans make up a growing proportion of the U.S. population, they have received little attention in the oral health literature. Asian Americans comprise many ethnic subgroups with varying age, education, income, and nativity statuses, and varying abilities to access oral health care (Qiu and Ni, 2003). Underutilization of oral health care among Asian Americans is associated with poverty, lack of dental coverage, and residing in the United States for less than 5 years (Qiu and Ni, 2003).

Latinos

Latinos have poorer oral health and receive fewer dental services as compared to white populations. These disparities exist independently of income level, education, dental coverage status, and attitude toward preventive care (Dietrich et al., 2008). While Latinos are a diverse population, comprising numerous subgroups, more is known about the oral health of Mexican Americans than other subgroups because NHANES oversamples Mexican Americans. Thus, the focus here will be on the oral health status of Mexican Americans, but it should be noted that the experience of Mexican Americans may not be representative of all Latino subpopulations. Both dental caries experience and untreated dental caries are significantly more prevalent in Mexican American children (ages 2–11) than in both non-Hispanic white and black children (Dye et al., 2007). Mexican American adults have fewer dental caries experiences than white non-Hispanic adults; however, they have higher rates of untreated dental caries (Dye et al., 2007). Disparities in the oral health of Mexican Americans persist throughout the life cycle, in adolescents through older adults (Dye et al., 2007).

Latinos also experience disparities in access to oral health care. They are less likely to report any dental visit in the past year, either for preventive, restorative, or emergency care (Manski and Magder, 1998). Latino children are less likely than white children to have ever seen a dentist or to have seen a dentist in the last year (Dietrich et al., 2008). In 2003, only 67 percent of Latino children received preventive dental care, compared to 84 percent of white children (Dietrich et al., 2008). In 2009, 48 percent of Hispanic and Latino adults reported seeing a dentist or other dental professional in the past year, compared to 61 percent of the adults overall (Pleis et al., 2010).

Acculturation is associated with disparities in Latino oral health,[4] indicating that reducing oral health disparities for Latinos requires linguistically and culturally appropriate oral health care and promotion. Latinos who primarily speak Spanish at home are less likely to report a dental visit in the past 12 months than those who speak English (Jaramillo et al., 2009) and are also less likely to have a dental home (Graham et al., 2005). The association between acculturation and oral health disparities persists throughout diverse groups of Latino Americans. Less acculturated Mexican American, Cuban American, and Puerto Rican Americans are all significantly less likely to report receiving recent oral health care than those who are more acculturated (Stewart et al., 2002). Acculturation is likely to be related to access to care rather than overall oral health, because acculturation is associated with missing teeth and untreated decayed surfaces but not with overall experience with dental caries (Cruz et al., 2004).

Rural and Urban Populations

High-quality data on oral health status and access to care by geographic location are sparse. Some data indicate that rural residents have poorer oral health than urban residents (Vargas et al., 2002, 2003b,c), while others indicate that urban residents have more oral health needs (Maserejian et al.,

[4] Surveys generally use language as a proxy for acculturation, treating individuals who regularly speak English as more acculturated than those who primarily speak Spanish.

2008). Similarly, some analyses indicate that rural residents access less oral health care or report more problems accessing oral health care than urban residents (NCHS, 2011; Vargas et al., 2003a); however, that association disappears after controlling for supply of dentists (Allison and Manski, 2007). More complex, multivariate analyses are needed to assess whether oral health status and access to care are related to place of residence, or instead to income, education level, supply of dentists, or other predisposing factors.

Rural residents may not access oral health care for a number of reasons. Fewer dentists work in rural areas than urban areas (Doescher et al., 2009; Eberhardt et al., 2001). In addition, a smaller proportion of rural residents have dental coverage, which is a good predictor of receipt of dental care (DeVoe et al., 2003; Lewis et al., 2007). Finally, the water in rural communities is less likely to be fluoridated than city water, which means rural residents are more susceptible to dental caries.

In 2005, the IOM examined the quality of general health care in rural communities (IOM, 2005). The committee specifically noted the role of IHS and the Health Resources and Services Administration (HRSA) in providing scholarships and loan repayment for practice in rural areas as well as the efforts of individual programs by dental schools and others in providing exposure to care in rural settings. The committee concluded that "fundamental change in health professions education programs will be needed to produce an adequate supply of properly educated health care professionals for rural and frontier communities." They recommended that schools (specifically including dental schools) make greater efforts to recruit students from rural areas, to locate a meaningful portion of the formal educational experience in rural settings, to recruit faculty with experience in caring for rural populations, and to develop education programs that are relevant to rural practice.

FACTORS THAT CONTRIBUTE TO POOR ORAL HEALTH AND LACK OF ACCESS TO ORAL HEALTH CARE

Underserved and vulnerable populations experience significant barriers to accessing oral health care and improving oral health. Barriers that are unique or particularly significant to a specific population have been discussed, but others cut across demographic lines and affect the oral health of many different populations. Those are discussed here. This list is not intended to be exhaustive, but is intended to highlight areas the committee believes are of importance and where significant progress can be made.

Social Determinants of Oral Health

Social determinants also affect oral health and contribute to inequalities in oral health (Patrick et al., 2006). The World Health Organization describes social determinants of health as a combination of structural determinants ("the unequal distribution of power, income, goods, and services") and daily living conditions ("the conditions in which people are born, grow, live, work, and age") (Commission on Social Determinants of Health, 2008). Social gradients in dental decay, periodontal disease, oral cancer, and tooth loss have all been reported (Kwan and Petersen, 2010). Income inequality has also been shown to be related to oral health (Bernabé and Marcenes, 2011). Recognizing the relationship between social determinants of health and oral health outcomes is important for developing interventions.

Social determinants of health create significant barriers to reducing and ultimately eliminating disparities in oral health. Progress will require changes in the social and physical environment, such as public education, working and living conditions, health system, and the natural environment (Patrick et al., 2006; Williams, 2005). Interventions will need to focus on the individual, families, and communities (Fisher-Owens et al., 2007). Unfortunately, not enough is known about bridging the science, practice, and policy of social determinants of health so that scientific knowledge can be translated into practical policies that will reduce disparities in oral health (Dankwa-Mullan et al., 2010a,b).

Oral Health Literacy

This section provides a brief overview of oral health literacy. The Committee on an Oral Health Initiative was specifically charged to address oral health literacy, and thus a more complete discussion of oral health literacy can be found in its report *Advancing Oral Health in America* (see Appendix D). The Committee on Oral Health Access to Services recognizes that oral health literacy is an essential component of access to care, and the brevity of the discussion here is not meant to deemphasize its importance.

Nearly all aspects of oral health care require literacy (e.g., realizing the importance of self-care, understanding that dental caries is an infectious disease, scheduling a dental appointment, completing insurance forms). However, little is known specifically about oral health literacy. The National Institute of Dental and Craniofacial Research Workgroup on Oral Health Literacy proposed a research agenda for oral health literacy in 2005 (NIDCR, 2005), but little progress has been made since then.

Available data indicate that the public's oral health literacy (and general health literacy) is poor (Jones et al., 2007; Kutner et al., 2006). Poor oral health literacy is strongly associated with self-reported lower oral health status, lower dental knowledge, and fewer dental visits. The public has little knowledge about the best ways to prevent oral diseases. Fluoride and dental sealants have long been acknowledged as the most effective ways to prevent dental caries, yet the public consistently answers that toothbrushing and flossing are more effective (Ahovuo-Saloranta et al., 2008; Gift et al., 1994; Marinho et al., 2003a). Although each year 30,000 Americans are diagnosed with oral cancers and nearly 8,000 people die from them, the public's knowledge about the risk factors and symptoms of oral cancers is low (ACS, 2009; Cruz et al., 2002; Horowitz et al., 1998, 2002; Patton et al., 2004).

The public's lack of knowledge about oral health may, in part, be due to low oral health literacy among health care professionals themselves, including both dental and nondental health care professionals. This includes both general health literacy and communication skills (Neuhauser, 2010; Rozier et al., 2011; Schwartzberg et al., 2007; Williams et al., 2002), as well as specific knowledge related to oral health and oral health care (Caspary et al., 2008; Forrest et al., 2000; Quijano et al., 2010; Yellowitz et al., 2000).

Prevention of Oral Diseases and Maintenance of Oral Health

Many oral diseases can be prevented through a combination of steps taken at home, in the dental office or other health care settings, or on a community-wide basis. Increasing access to preventive services is an important component of improving access to oral health care for vulnerable and underserved populations. IOM's concurrent Committee on an Oral Health Initiative was directly charged to address the role of preventive services in oral health; therefore, a fuller discussion of this topic can be found in its report *Advancing Oral Health in America* (see Appendix D). So as not to duplicate that committee's work, this committee chose to provide a brief, broad overview of the prevention of oral diseases.

Fluoride

The oral health benefits of fluoride have been well known for more than 75 years (CDC, 2010a). Fluoride reduces the risk of dental caries in both children and adults (Griffin et al., 2007; IOM, 1997; Marinho, 2009; Marinho et al., 2002, 2003a; NRC, 1989; Twetman, 2009; WHO, 2010c). Fluoride works through a variety of mechanisms, including incorporating into enamel before teeth erupt, inhibiting demineralization and enhancing remineralization of teeth,[5] and inhibiting bacterial activity in dental plaque (CDC, 2001; HHS, 2000b).

[5] Dental caries work through a process of demineralization: bacteria in the mouth breaks down dietary carbohydrates to form acids, which demineralize the dental enamel and form cavities. Before a tooth becomes fully demineralized and cavitated, it can remineralize if the proper combination of calcium and phosphate (generally from saliva) is present (Featherstone, 2009).

Some modes of fluoride delivery to whole communities involve the addition of very low levels of fluoride to public water systems, salt, or milk. Community water fluoridation is credited with significantly reducing the incidence of dental caries in the United States and is recognized as one of the 10 great public health achievements of the 20th century (CDC, 1999a). Evidence continues to reaffirm that community water fluoridation is effective, safe, inexpensive, and is associated with significant cost savings (CDC, 1999b, 2001; Griffin et al., 2001a,b; HHS, 2000b; Horowitz, 1996; Kumar et al., 2010; O'Connell et al., 2005; Parnell et al., 2009; Yeung, 2008). The Task Force on Community Preventive Services recommends community water fluoridation (Task Force on Community Preventive Services, 2002), and dental professional associations support water fluoridation (ADA, 2010; ADHA, 2011; APHA, 2008). Over 70 percent of the U.S. population had access to optimally fluoridated water in 2008; *Healthy People 2020* set a goal of 79.6 percent by 2020 (HHS, 2010).

Other forms of fluoride are applied personally, by a caretaker, or by an oral health care professional; these include toothpastes, mouth rinses, gels, and varnishes. Fluoride supplements, such as drops and chewable tablets, also may be prescribed or dispensed by oral health care professionals. Fluoride varnish is easily and quickly applied by both dental and nondental health professionals, including medical assistants (commonly during well-child visits) (Grossman, 2010). It has been shown to be effective in the prevention of dental caries in both deciduous and permanent teeth (Autio-Gold and Courts, 2001; Beltran-Aguilar et al., 2000; Marinho et al., 2002). The interval for frequency of application of fluoride varnish varies depending on the risk of the patient (ADA, 2006).

Dental Sealants

Dental sealants ("sealants") prevent dental caries from developing in the pits and fissures of teeth,[6] where dental caries is most prevalent (Ahovuo-Saloranta et al., 2008). A Cochrane review of sealant studies found that resin-based sealants were effective at preventing dental caries, ranging from an 87 percent reduction in dental caries after 12 months to 60 percent at 48–54 months (Ahovuo-Saloranta et al., 2008). Sealants can also be placed over noncavitated carious lesions to slow the progression of the lesions (Griffin et al., 2008).

Despite their effectiveness, few children have sealants. The most recent NHANES (1999–2004) data indicate that 32 percent of 8-year-olds and 21 percent of 14-year-olds have sealants on their permanent molars (Dye et al.,

[6] A dental sealant is a thin, protective coating of plastic resin or glass ionomer that is applied to the biting surfaces of teeth to prevent food particles and bacteria from collecting in the normal pits and fissures and developing into caries.

2007). This is a significant increase from 1988–1994, when 23 percent of 8-year-olds and 15 percent of 14-year-olds had sealants, but it falls short of the *Healthy People 2010* goal of 50 percent for both groups (Dye et al., 2007; HHS, 2000a). In addition, low-income children, who are most likely to have dental caries, are the least likely to receive sealants (Dye et al., 2007).

Sealants can be applied in a dental office or in community-based programs, such as school-based sealant programs. Many sealant programs target high-risk populations, which have proven to be effective for the prevention of dental caries as well as demonstrate cost savings (Kitchens, 2005; Pew Center on the States, 2010; Weintraub, 1989, 2001; Weintraub et al., 1993, 2001). The Task Force on Community Preventive Services recommends school-based sealant programs, although evidence is insufficient to comment on the effectiveness of similar state- or community-wide programs (Truman et al., 2002). School-based sealant programs are discussed further in Chapter 4.

Oral Health and Personal Health Behaviors

While community and dental-office based interventions are important for preventing oral diseases, personal behaviors also play an important role. A healthy diet is important for maintaining oral health. Dietary carbohydrates, sugar-rich foods and drinks, and carbonated beverages all are implicated in the formation of dental caries (Burt et al., 1988; Ehlen et al., 2008; Grindefjord et al., 1996; Heller et al., 2001; HHS, 2000b; Kitchens and Owens, 2007; Moynihan and Petersen, 2004; Sundin et al., 1992; WHO, 2010a). Fruits and vegetable consumption, however, can protect against oral cancer (HHS, 2000b; Pavia et al., 2006; WHO, 2010a). In addition, an insufficient level of folic acid is a risk factor in the development of birth defects such as cleft lip and palate (HHS, 2000b).

Both tobacco use and excessive alcohol consumption are risk factors for oral cancers, and when used together they act synergistically as carcinogens (HHS, 2000b; WHO, 2010a). Together, tobacco use and excessive alcohol consumption account for 90 percent of all oral cancers (Truman et al., 2002). In addition, tobacco use is associated with the development and progression of periodontal disease, oral candidiasis in HIV-positive individuals, oral cancer recurrence, and congenital birth defects such as cleft lip and palate (Burns, 1996; Conley et al., 1996; Gelskey, 1999; HHS, 2000b; Palacio et al., 1997; WHO, 2010b; Wyszynski et al., 1997).

Personal hygiene includes toothbrushing, flossing, and the use of mouth rinses. Regular toothbrushing with fluoridated toothpaste reduces caries risk for both dental caries and gingival inflammation (Deery et al., 2004; Marinho, 2009; Marinho et al., 2003a,b; Robinson et al., 2005; Walsh et al., 2010). However, the relationship between self-care, supragingival plaque, and periodontal disease development and disease prognosis is weak (Lindhe et al., 1989).

Disease Management

While the committee prioritizes prevention in its vision, it recognizes that many individuals have existing diseases that must be treated. Traditionally, dental treatment has focused on surgical interventions and standardized patient education. But recently some oral health educators and practitioners have adopted personalized chronic disease and risk assessment models for oral health diseases, particularly dental caries (Edelstein, 2010; Featherstone et al., 2003; Fontana and Zero, 2007; Lindskog et al., 2010; Yorty et al., 2011). Although caries has often been considered an infectious disease, it has many features of a chronic disease that make it a promising candidate for management through risk assessment, including a complex etiology, long duration, unresponsiveness to acute management, and progressive destruction (Edelstein, 2010). A full discussion is beyond the scope of this report, but this section will provide a brief introduction to caries chronic disease and risk management models.

Caries risk-management models recognize that patients have different risks for developing caries and thus should be treated differently. Risk-assessment tools instruct the provider to assess the patient's caries history, bacteria levels, diet, saliva flow, and access to fluoridated water, among many other factors, and base the treatment on the patient's risk factors (Featherstone et al., 2007; Jenson et al., 2007; Ramos-Gomez et al., 2007). For example, a patient with a low bacteria count, a history of few caries, and who regularly drinks fluoridated water and brushes with fluoridated toothpaste should receive different interventions than a patient with a high bacteria count, many previous caries, and less access to fluoride. The first patient may not need as many dental visits or as many professional fluoride applications, while the second patient may need more tailored health education and more frequent dental visits and services (Featherstone et al., 2007; Jenson et al., 2007; Ramos-Gomez et al., 2007). In the risk-assessment model, patients may be advised to deviate from the standard semi-annual dental recall visit; patients with higher risk may need to see an oral health provider more frequently, while patients with low risk may only need to visit the dentist yearly (Patel et al., 2010). Early evidence indicates that risk-management models are successful at reducing cariogenic bacteria and future caries compared to conventional care (Featherstone and Gansky, 2005).

Quality Assessment

Despite the current interest in the quality of general health care, little is known about the quality of oral health care. While significant efforts are being made in medicine to develop quality measures, understanding about measurement and assessment of the quality of oral health care lags far behind (Stanton and Rutherford, 2003). A review of current National Quality Forum-endorsed measures of quality finds no measures related to oral health (National Quality Forum, 2010). Further, the annual AHRQ National Healthcare Quality Report and the National Healthcare Disparities Report currently include only information about access to dental services and not about the state of quality in oral health care (AHRQ, 2010). This is not to say that oral health quality measures do not exist, but that they lag far behind quality measures in other health care fields. None of the existing quality measures in oral health care assess long-term patient outcomes; they are limited to measures of technical excellence, patient satisfaction (as opposed to patient experience), service use, and structure and process measures (Bader, 2009a). However, the ADA has recently convened a group of stakeholders, including the Centers for Medicare and Medicaid Services, in a Dental Quality Alliance, which is charged with developing pediatric oral health quality measures (Rich, 2010).

Two significant barriers prevent the further development of quality measures in oral health: a dearth of evidence-based standards and guidelines, and the lack of universally accepted and used diagnosis codes in dentistry. The development of new measures depends on evidence-based standards and guidelines from which to create metrics. Quality measurement in dentistry is hampered by the absence of a strong evidence base for most dental treatments and, therefore, a lack of evidence-based guidelines (Bader, 2009b; Crall et al., 1999). In fact, many Cochrane reviews in dentistry did not have enough evidence to answer the research question posed (Ashley et al., 2009; Bader, 2009a,b; Bonner et al., 2006; Esposito et al., 2007; Fedorowicz et al., 2009; Hiiri et al., 2010; Rickard et al., 2004; Yeung et al., 2005). Dental research is challenged in part because with the typical small practice design, it can be difficult to collect outcomes data due to the need to gather data from multiple practices as well as integrate the variety of forms that are used to collect the same data (Bader, 2009a). The practice design also makes it difficult to disseminate evidence when it exists; most dentists work alone, so information sharing is limited, and few have chairside access to journals or computers (Bader, 2009b).

The absence of a universally accepted set of diagnosis codes among dentists also is a barrier to developing quality measures (Bader, 2009a; Crall et al., 1999; Garcia et al., 2010). Several code sets are available for oral health, but they have not been put into general use (Kalenderian et al.,

2011; Leake, 2002). The ADA has developed a comprehensive system of diagnostic codes, the Systematized Nomenclature of Dentistry (SNODENT), but it is yet to be released. Several closed-panel delivery systems have also developed oral health code sets for use inside their systems, but they are not available to the general public (Bader, 2009a). Ideally, the diagnostic codes used by dentists would be compatible with codes used by other health care professionals, so that consistent oral health information could be collected from all types of providers. In addition, oral health quality measures need to be developed in the context of available data sources. Finally, in addition to the barriers discussed here, many other factors beyond the scope of this report will contribute to the complexity of developing better quality measures for oral health. They include the privacy and confidentiality requirements of the Health Insurance Portability and Accountability Act (and electronic health record standards, among others).

FINDINGS AND CONCLUSIONS

The committee noted the following key findings and conclusions:

- Oral health is inextricably linked to overall health.
- The overall oral health status of the U.S. population has improved; however, significant disparities exist for vulnerable populations, including people with low incomes, racial and ethnic minorities, children, rural populations, pregnant women, older adults, people with special health care needs, and homeless people.
- Many populations with poor oral health are underserved by the current oral health system.
- Many complex and interrelated factors contribute to poor oral health and lack of access to oral health care, including social determinants of health, poor health literacy, a lack of emphasis on preventive oral health interventions, and a lack of quality measures by which to evaluate and improve oral health care.

REFERENCES

AAP (American Academy of Pediatrics) and ACOG (American College of Obstetrics and Gynecology). 2007. *Guidelines for perinatal care*. 6th ed. Elk Grove, IL: American Academy of Pediatrics and American College of Obstetricians and Gynecologists.

ACS (American Cancer Society). 2009. *Cancer facts and figures 2009*. Atlanta, GA: American Cancer Society.

ADA (American Dental Association). 2006. Professionally applied topical fluoride: Evidence-based clinical recommendations. *Journal of the American Dental Association* 137(8):1151-1159.

ADA. 2010. *Fluoride & fluoridation*. http://www.ada.org/2467.aspx (accessed September 16, 2010).

ADHA (American Dental Hygienists Association). 2011. *Public health*. http://www.adha.org/publichealth/index.html (accessed March 17, 2011).

Ahovuo-Saloranta, A., A. Hiiri, A. Nordblad, H. Worthington, and M. Mäkelä. 2008. Pit and fissure sealants for preventing dental decay in the permanent teeth of children and adolescents. *Cochrane Database of Systematic Reviews* (4):CD001830.

AHRQ (Agency for Healthcare Research and Quality). 2010. *National healthcare quality & disparities reports: NHQRDRnet*. http://nhqrnet.ahrq.gov/nhqrdr/jsp/nhqrdr.jsp (accessed November 29, 2010).

Albert, D. A., M. D. Begg, H. F. Andrews, S. Z. Williams, A. Ward, M. Lee Conicella, V. Rauh, J. L. Thomson, and P. N. Papapanou. 2011. An examination of periodontal treatment, dental care, and pregnancy outcomes in an insured population in the United States. *American Journal of Public Health* 101(1):151-156.

Al-Hashimi, I. 2001. The management of Sjögren's syndrome in dental practice. *Journal of the American Dental Association* 132(10):1409-1417.

Allison, R. A., and R. J. Manski. 2007. The supply of dentists and access to care in rural Kansas. *Journal of Rural Health* 23(3):198-206.

Anders, P. L., and E. L. Davis. 2010. Oral health of patients with intellectual disabilities: A systematic review. *Special Care in Dentistry* 30(3):110-117.

Anthony, M., J. M. Williams, and A. M. Avery. 2008. Health needs of migrant and seasonal farmworkers. *Journal of Community Health Nursing* 25(3):153-160.

APHA (American Public Health Association). 2008. *Community water fluoridation in the United States*. http://www.apha.org/advocacy/policy/policysearch/default.htm?id=1373 (accessed September 28, 2010).

Armour, B. S., M. Swanson, H. B. Waldman, and S. P. Perlman. 2008. A profile of state-level differences in the oral health of people with and without disabilities, in the U.S., in 2004. *Public Health Reports* 123(1):67-75.

Ashley, P. F., C. E. C. S. Williams, D. R. Moles, and J. Parry. 2009. Sedation versus general anaesthesia for provision of dental treatment in under 18 year olds. *Cochrane Database of Systematic Reviews* (1):CD006334.

Autio-Gold, J. T., and F. Courts. 2001. Assessing the effect of fluoride varnish on early enamel carious lesions in the primary dentition. *Journal of the American Dental Association* 132(9):1247-1253.

Bader, J. D. 2009a. Challenges in quality assessment of dental care. *Journal of the American Dental Association* 140(12):1456-1464.

Bader, J. D. 2009b. Stumbling into the age of evidence. *Dental Clinics of North America* 53(1):15-22.

Baggett, T. P., J. J. O'Connell, D. E. Singer, and N. A. Rigotti. 2010. The unmet health care needs of homeless adults: A national study. *American Journal of Public Health* 100(7):1326-1333.

Beltran-Aguilar, E. D., J. W. Goldstein, and S. A. Lockwood. 2000. Fluoride varnishes: A review of their clinical use, cariostatic mechanism, efficacy and safety. *Journal of the American Dental Association* 131(5):589-596.

Bernabé, E., and W. Marcenes. 2011. Income inequality and tooth loss in the United States. *Journal of Dental Research*. Published electronically April 20, 2011. doi: 10.1177/0022034511400081.

Blaizot, A., J. N. Vergnes, S. Nuwwareh, J. Amar, and M. Sixou. 2009. Periodontal diseases and cardiovascular events: Meta-analysis of observational studies. *International Dental Journal* 59(4):197-209.

Bloom, B., R. A. Cohen, and G. Freeman. 2010. *Summary health statistics for U.S. children: National Health Interview Survey, 2009*. Hyattsville, MD: Department of Health and Human Services.

Boggess, K. A., D. M. Urlaub, K. E. Massey, M.-K. Moos, M. B. Matheson, and C. Lorenz. 2010. Oral hygiene practices and dental service utilization among pregnant women. *Journal of the American Dental Association* 141(5):553-561.

Bonner, B., J. Clarkson, L. Dobbyn, and S. Khanna. 2006. Slow-release fluoride devices for the control of dental decay. *Cochrane Database of Systematic Reviews* (4):CD005101.

Burns, D. N., D. Hillman, J. D. Neaton, R. Sherer, T. Mitchell, L. Capps, W. G. Vallier, M. D. Thurnherr, and F. M. Gordin. 1996. Cigarette smoking, bacterial pneumonia, and other clinical outcomes in HIV-1 infection. *Journal of Acquired Immune Deficiency Syndromes and Human Retrovirology* 13(4):374-383.

Burt, B. A., S. A. Eklund, K. J. Morgan, F. E. Larkin, K. E. Guire, L. O. Brown, and J. A. Weintraub. 1988. The effects of sugars intake and frequency of ingestion on dental caries increment in a three-year longitudinal study. *Journal of Dental Research* 67(11):1422-1429.

California Dental Association. 2010. *Oral health during pregnancy and early childhood: Evidence-based guidelines for health professionals*. Sacramento, CA: California Dental Association.

Casamassimo, P. S., S. Thikkurissy, B. L. Edelstein, and E. Maiorini. 2009. Beyond the DMFT: The human and economic cost of early childhood caries. *Journal of the American Dental Association* 140(6):650-657.

Caspary, G., D. M. Krol, S. Boulter, M. A. Keels, and G. Romano-Clarke. 2008. Perceptions of oral health training and attitudes toward performing oral health screenings among graduating pediatric residents. *Pediatrics* 122(2):e465-e471.

CDC (Centers for Disease Control and Prevention). 1999a. Ten great public health achievements—United States, 1900-1999. *Morbidity and Mortality Weekly Report* 48(12):241-243.

CDC. 1999b. Water fluoridation and costs of medicaid treatment for dental decay—Louisiana, 1995-1996. *Morbidity and Mortality Weekly Report* 48(34):753-757.

CDC. 2001. Recommendations for using fluoride to prevent and control dental caries in the United States. *MMWR Recommendations and Reports* 50(RR14):1-42.

CDC. 2010a. *CDC honors 65 years of community water fluoridation*. http://www.cdc.gov/fluoridation/65_years.htm (accessed September 16, 2010).

CDC. 2010b. *National Health and Nutrition Examination Survey: 1999-2010 survey content*. U.S. Department of Health and Human Services.

CDC. 2011. *National diabetes fact sheet, 2011*. http://www.cdc.gov/diabetes/pubs/factsheet11.htm (accessed May 2, 2011).

Chávarry, N., M. V. Vettore, C. Sansone, and A. Sheiham. 2009. The relationship between diabetes mellitus and destructive periodontal disease: A meta-analysis. *Oral Health & Preventive Dentistry* 7(2):107-127.

Chen, H., J. Moeller, and R. J. Manski. 2011. The influence of comorbidity and other health measures on dental and medical care use among Medicare beneficiaries 2002. *Journal of Public Health Dentistry*. Published electronically May 11, 2011. doi: 10.1111/j.1752-7325.2011.00251.x.

Chevarley, F. M. 2010. *Percentage of persons unable to get or delayed in getting needed medical care, dental care, or prescription medicines: United States, 2007*. Statistical brief #282. Rockville, MD: Agency for Healthcare Research and Quality.

Chi, D., and P. Milgrom. 2008. The oral health of homeless adolescents and young adults and determinants of oral health: Preliminary findings. *Special Care in Dentistry* 28(6):237-242.

Ciesla, D., C. A. Kerins, N. S. Seale, and P. S. Casamassimo. 2011. Characteristics of dental clinics in U.S. children's hospitals. *Pediatric Dentistry* 33(2):100-106.

CMS (Centers for Medicare and Medicaid Services). 2010. *Annual EPSDT participation report form CMS-416, fiscal year 2009*. https://www.cms.gov/MedicaidEarlyPeriodicScrn/Downloads/2009National.pdf (accessed March 15, 2011).

Cohen, L. A., A. J. Bonito, C. Eicheldinger, R. J. Manski, M. D. Macek, R. R. Edwards, and N. Khanna. 2011. Comparison of patient visits to emergency departments, physician offices, and dental offices for dental problems and injuries. *Journal of Public Health Dentistry* 71(1):13-22.

Coleman, P., and N. M. Watson. 2006. Oral care provided by certified nursing assistants in nursing homes. *Journal of the American Geriatrics Society* 54(1):138-143.

Commission on Social Determinants of Health. 2008. *Closing the gap in a generation: Health equity through action on the social determinants of health*. Geneva, Switzerland: WHO.

Conley, L. J., T. J. Bush, S. P. Buchbinder, K. A. Penley, F. N. Judson, and S. D. Holmberg. 1996. The association between cigarette smoking and selected HIV-related medical conditions. *AIDS* 10(10):1121-1126.

Conte, M., H. L. Broder, G. Jenkins, R. Reed, and M. N. Janal. 2006. Oral health, related behaviors and oral health impacts among homeless adults. *Journal of Public Health Dentistry* 66(4):276-278.

Coogan, M. M., J. Greenspan, and S. J. Challacombe. 2005. Oral lesions in infection with human immunodeficiency virus. *Bulletin of the World Health Organization* 83(9):700-706.

Crall, J. J., C. I. Szlyk, and D. A. Schneider. 1999. Pediatric oral health performance measurement: Current capabilities and future directions. *Journal of Public Health Dentistry* 59(3):136-141.

Cruz, G. D., R. Z. Le Geros, J. S. Ostroff, J. L. Hay, H. Kenigsberg, and D. M. Franklin. 2002. Oral cancer knowledge, risk factors and characteristics of subjects in a large oral cancer screening program. *Journal of the American Dental Association* 133(8):1064-1071.

Cruz, G. D., R. Shore, R. Z. Le Geros, and M. Tavares. 2004. Effect of acculturation on objective measures of oral health in Haitian immigrants in New York City. *Journal of Dental Research* 83(2):180-184.

Dankwa-Mullan, I., K. B. Rhee, D. M. Stoff, J. R. Pohlhaus, F. S. Sy, N. Stinson, Jr., and J. Ruffin. 2010a. Moving toward paradigm-shifting research in health disparities through translational, transformational, and transdisciplinary approaches. *American Journal of Public Health* 100(S1):S19-S24.

Dankwa-Mullan, I., K. B. Rhee, K. Williams, I. Sanchez, F. S. Sy, N. Stinson Jr., and J. Ruffin. 2010b. The science of eliminating health disparities: Summary and analysis of the NIH summit recommendations. *American Journal of Public Health* 100(S1):S12.

Davis, E. E., A. S. Deinard, and E. W. H. Maïga. 2010. Doctor, my tooth hurts: The costs of incomplete dental care in the emergency room. *Journal of Public Health Dentistry* 70(3):205-210.

Deery, C., M. Heanue, S. Deacon, P. Robinson, A. Walmsley, H. Worthington, W. Shaw, and A. Glenny. 2004. The effectiveness of manual versus powered toothbrushes for dental health: A systematic review. *Journal of Dentistry* 32(3):197-211.

DeVoe, J. E., G. E. Fryer, R. Phillips, and L. Green. 2003. Receipt of preventive care among adults: Insurance status and usual source of care. *American Journal of Public Health* 93(5):786-791.

Dietrich, T., C. Culler, R. I. Garcia, and M. M. Henshaw. 2008. Racial and ethnic disparities in children's oral health: The National Survey of Children's Health. *Journal of the American Dental Association* 139(11):1507-1517.

Doescher, M. P., G. A. Keppel, S. M. Skillman, and R. A. Rosenblatt. 2009. *The crisis in rural dentistry*. Seattle, WA: WWAMI Rural Health Research Center.

Dolan, T. A., C. W. Peek, A. E. Stuck, and J. C. Beck. 1998. Functional health and dental service use among older adults. *Journal of Gerontology. Series A Biological Sciences and Medical Sciences* 53A(6):M413-M418.

Dolan, T. A., K. Atchison, and T. N. Huynh. 2005. Access to dental care among older adults in the United States. *Journal of Dental Education* 69(9):961-974.

Douglass, J. M., Y. Li, and N. Tinanoff. 2008. Association of mutans streptococci between caregivers and their children. *Pediatric Dentistry* 30(5):375-387.

Dye, B., and G. Thornton-Evans. 2010. Trends in oral health by poverty status as measured by Healthy People 2010 objectives. *Public Health Reports* 125(6):817-830.

Dye, B. A., S. Tan, V. Smith, B. G. Lewis, L. K. Barker, G. Thornton-Evans, P. I. Eke, E. D. Beltran-Aguilar, A. M. Horowitz, and L. Chien-Hsun. 2007. *Trends in oral health status: United States, 1988-1994 and 1999-2004*. Hyattsville, MD: National Center for Health Statistics.

Dye, B. A., O. Arevalo, and C. M. Vargas. 2010. Trends in paediatric dental caries by poverty status in the United States, 1988–1994 and 1999–2004. *International Journal of Paediatric Dentistry* 20(2):132-143.

Dye, B. A., L. K. Barker, X. Li, B. G. Lewis, and E. D. Beltrán-Aguilar. 2011a. Overview and quality assurance for the oral health component of the national health and nutrition examination survey (NHANES), 2005-08. *Journal of Public Health Dentistry* 71(1):54-61.

Dye, B. A., C. M. Vargas, J. J. Lee, L. Magder, and N. Tinanoff. 2011b. Assessing the relationship between children's oral health status and that of their mothers. *Journal of the American Dental Association* 142(2):173-183.

Eberhardt, M. S., D. D. Ingram, and D. M. Makuc. 2001. *Urban and rural health chartbook: Health, United States, 2001*. Hyattsville, MD: National Center for Health Statistics.

Edelstein, B. L. 2010 (unpublished). *Lessons from medicine: Opportunities and constraints for oral disease management*. Commissioned by the IOM Committee on Oral Health Access to Services.

Edelstein, B. L., and C. H. Chinn. 2009. Update on disparities in oral health and access to dental care for America's children. *Academic Pediatrics* 9(6):415-419.

Ehlen, L. A., T. A. Marshall, F. Qian, J. S. Wefel, and J. J. Warren. 2008. Acidic beverages increase the risk of in vitro tooth erosion. *Nutrition Research* 28(5):299-303.

El-Solh, A. A., C. Pietrantoni, A. Bhat, M. Okada, J. Zambon, A. Aquilina, and E. Berbary. 2004. Colonization of dental plaques: A reservoir of respiratory pathogens for hospital-acquired pneumonia in institutionalized elders. *Chest* 126(5):1575-1582.

Esposito, M., G. M. Grusovin, H. Maghaireh, P. Coulthard, and H. V. Worthington. 2007. Interventions for replacing missing teeth: Management of soft tissues for dental implants. *Cochrane Database of Systematic Reviews* (3):CD006697.

Ettinger, R. L. 2010. Meeting oral health needs to promote the well-being of the geriatric population: Educational research issues. *Journal of Dental Education* 74(1):29-35.

Featherstone, J. D. B. 2009. Remineralization, the natural caries repair process—The need for new approaches. *Advances in Dental Research* 21(1):4-7.

Featherstone, J. D. B., and S. A. Gansky. 2005. A randomized clinical trial of caries management by risk assessment. *Caries Research* 39(4):295 (abstract #225).

Featherstone, J. D. B., S. M. Adair, M. H. Anderson, R. J. Berkowitz, W. F. Bird, J. J. Crall, P. K. D. Besten, K. J. Donly, P. Glassman, and P. Milgrom. 2003. Caries management by risk assessment: Consensus statement, April 2002. *Journal of the California Dental Association* 31(3):257-269.

Featherstone, J. D. B., S. Domejean-Orliaguet, L. Jenson, M. Wolff, and D. A. Young. 2007. Caries risk assessment in practice for age 6 through adult. *Journal of the California Dental Association* 35(10):703-713.

Fedorowicz, Z., M. Nasser, and N. Wilson. 2009. Adhesively bonded versus non-bonded amalgam restorations for dental caries. *Cochrane Database of Systematic Reviews* (4):CD007517.

Feldman, C., M. Giniger, M. Sanders, R. Saporito, H. Zohn, and S. Perlman. 1997. Special Olympics, special smiles: Assessing the feasibility of epidemiologic data collection. *Journal of the American Dental Association* 128(12):1687-1696.

Fisher-Owens, S. A., S. A. Gansky, L. J. Platt, J. A. Weintraub, M. J. Soobader, M. D. Bramlett, and P. W. Newacheck. 2007. Influences on children's oral health: A conceptual model. *Pediatrics* 120(3):e510-e520.

Fontana, M., and D. Zero. 2007. Bridging the gap in caries management between research and practice through education: The Indiana University experience. *Journal of Dental Education* 71(5):579-591.

Forrest, J. L., A. M. Horowitz, and Y. Shmuely. 2000. Caries preventive knowledge and practices among dental hygienists. *Journal of Dental Hygiene* 74(3):183-195.

Gaffield, M. L., B. J. Colley, D. M. Malvitz, and R. Romaguera. 2001. Oral health during pregnancy: An analysis of information collected by the pregnancy risk assessment monitoring system. *Journal of the American Dental Association* 132(7):1009-1016.

GAO (Government Accountability Office). 2008. *Extent of dental disease in children has not decreased, and millions are estimated to have untreated tooth decay.* Washington, DC: U.S. Government Accountability Office.

Garcia, R. I., R. E. Inge, L. Niessen, and D. P. DePaola. 2010. Envisioning success: The future of the oral health care delivery system in the United States. *Journal of Public Health Dentistry* 70(Supp. 1):S58-S65.

Gelskey, S. C. 1999. Cigarette smoking and periodontitis: Methodology to assess the strength of evidence in support of a causal association. *Community Dentistry and Oral Epidemiology* 27(1):16-24.

Gibson, G., R. Rosenheck, J. Tullner, R. Grimes, C. Seibyl, A. Rivera-Torres, H. Goodman, and M. Nunn. 2003. A national survey of the oral health status of homeless veterans. *Journal of Public Health Dentistry* 63(1):30-37.

Gift, H. C., S. T. Reisine, and D. C. Larach. 1992. The social impact of dental problems and visits. *American Journal of Public Health* 82(12):1663-1668.

Gift, H. C., S. T. Reisine, and D. C. Larach. 1993. Erratum: The social impact of dental problems and visits. *American Journal of Public Health* 83(6):816.

Gift, H. C., S. B. Corbin, and R. E. Nowjack-Raymer. 1994. Public knowledge of prevention of dental disease. *Public Health Reports* 109(3):397-404.

Glassman, P., and P. Subar. 2008. Improving and maintaining oral health for people with special needs. *Dental Clinics of North America* 52(2):447-461.

Glassman, P., T. Henderson, M. Helgeson, C. Meyerowitz, R. Ingraham, R. Isman, D. Noel, R. Tellier, and K. Toto. 2005. Oral health for people with special needs: Consensus statement on implications and recommendations for the dental profession. *Journal of the California Dental Association* 33(8):619-623.

Graham, M. A., S. L. Tomar, and H. L. Logan. 2005. Perceived social status, language and indentified dental home among Hispanics in Florida. *Journal of the American Dental Association* 136(11):1572-1582.

Grembowski, D., C. Spiekerman, and P. Milgrom. 2008. Linking mother and child access to dental care. *Pediatrics* 122(4):e805-e814.

Griffin, S. O., B. F. Gooch, S. A. Lockwood, and S. L. Tomar. 2001a. Quantifying the diffused benefit from water fluoridation in the United States. *Community Dentistry and Oral Epidemiology* 29(2):120-129.

Griffin, S. O., K. Jones, and S. L. Tomar. 2001b. An economic evaluation of community water fluoridation. *Journal of Public Health Dentistry* 61(2):78-86.

Griffin, S. O., E. Regnier, P. M. Griffin, and V. Huntley. 2007. Effectiveness of fluoride in preventing caries in adults. *Journal of Dental Research* 86(5):410-415.

Griffin, S. O., E. Oong, W. Kohn, B. Vidakovic, B. F. Gooch, J. Bader, J. Clarkson, M. R. Fontana, D. M. Meyer, R. G. Rozier, J. A. Weintraub, and D. T. Zero. 2008. The effectiveness of sealants in managing caries lesions. *Journal of Dental Research* 87(2):169-174.

Grindefjord, M., G. Dahllöf, B. Nilsson, and T. Modeer. 1996. Stepwise prediction of dental caries in children up to 3.5 years of age. *Caries Research* 30(4):256-266.

Grossman, D. C. 2010. *Oral health promotion in well child care: The group health experience.* Paper presented at Meeting of the Committee on Oral Health Access to Services, July 27, San Francisco, CA.

Haley, J., G. Kenney, and J. Pelletier. 2008. *Access to affordable dental care: Gaps for low-income adults.* Menlo Park, CA: Kaiser Commission on Medicaid and the Uninsured.

Haraszthy, V. I., J. J. Zambon, M. Trevisan, M. Zeid, and R. J. Genco. 2000. Identification of periodontal pathogens in atheromatous plaques. *Journal of Periodontology* 71(10):1554-1560.

Havercamp, S. M., D. Scandlin, and M. Roth. 2004. Health disparities among adults with developmental disabilities, adults with other disabilities, and adults not reporting disability in North Carolina. *Public Health Reports* 119(4):418-426.

Heller, K. E., B. A. Burt, and S. A. Eklund. 2001. Sugared soda consumption and dental caries in the United States. *Journal of Dental Research* 80(10):1949-1953.

HHS (Department of Health and Human Services). 2000a. *Healthy People 2010: Understanding and improving health.* 2nd ed. Washington, DC: U.S. Government Printing Office.

HHS. 2000b. *Oral health in America: A report of the surgeon general.* Rockville, MD: National Institute of Dental and Craniofacial Research.

HHS. 2006. *Midcourse review: Healthy People 2010.* Washington, DC: U.S. Department of Health and Human Services.

HHS. 2010. *Healthy People 2020: Oral health objectives.* http://www.healthypeople.gov/2020/topicsobjectives2020/objectiveslist.aspx?topicid=32 (accessed December 27, 2010).

Hiiri, A., A. Ahovuo-Saloranta, A. Nordblad, and M. Mäkelä. 2010. Pit and fissure sealants versus fluoride varnishes for preventing dental decay in children and adolescents. *Cochrane Database of Systematic Reviews* (3):CD003067.

Horowitz, A. M., H. S. Moon, H. S. Goodman, and J. A. Yellowitz. 1998. Maryland adults' knowledge of oral cancer and having oral cancer examinations. *Journal of Public Health Dentistry* 58(4):281-287.

Horowitz, A. M., M. T. Canto, and W. L. Child. 2002. Maryland adults' perspectives on oral cancer prevention and early detection. *Journal of the American Dental Association* 133(8):1058-1063.

Horowitz, H. S. 1996. The effectiveness of community water fluoridation in the United States. *Journal of Public Health Dentistry* 56(5):253-258.

HRSA (Health Resources and Services Administration). 1995. *A national agenda for geriatric education: White papers.* Washington, DC: U.S. Department of Health and Human Services.

Hunter, L. P., and S. M. Yount. 2011. Oral health and oral health care practices among low-income pregnant women. *Journal of Midwifery and Women's Health* 52(2):103-109.

IHS (Indian Health Service). 2002. *An oral health survey of American Indian and Alaska Native dental patients: Findings, regional differences, and national comparisons.* Rockville, MD: Indian Health Service, Division of Dental Services.

IOM (Institute of Medicine). 1992. *The second fifty years: Promoting health and preventing disability.* Washington, DC: National Academy Press.

IOM. 1997. *Dietary reference intakes.* Washington, DC: National Academy Press.

IOM. 2005. *Quality through collaboration: The future of rural health care*. Washington, DC: The National Academies Press.

IOM. 2008. *Retooling for an aging America: Building the health care workforce*. Washington, DC: The National Academies Press.

IOM. 2009. *Adolescent health services: Missing opportunities*. Washington, DC: The National Academies Press.

IOM. 2011. *Advancing oral health in America*. Washington, DC: The National Academies Press.

Jablonski, R. 2010. *Nursing education and research (geriatrics)*. Presentation at meeting of the Committee on an Oral Health Initiative, Washington, DC. June 28, 2010.

Jablonski, R. A., C. L. Munro, M. J. Grap, C. M. Schubert, M. Ligon, and P. Spigelmyer. 2009. Mouth care in nursing homes: Knowledge, beliefs, and practices of nursing assistants. *Geriatric Nursing* 30(2):99-107.

Jaramillo, F., P. I. Eke, G. O. Thornton-Evans, and S. O. Griffin. 2009. Acculturation and dental visits among Hispanic adults. *Public Health Research, Practice, and Policy* 6(2):A50.

Jenson, L., A. W. Budenz, J. D. B. Featherstone, F. J. Ramos-Gomez, V. W. Spolsky, and D. A. Young. 2007. Clinical protocols for caries management by risk assessment. *Journal of the California Dental Association* 35(10):714-723.

Jones, A. 2002. *The national nursing home survey: 1999 summary.* Hyattsville, MD: United States Department of Health and Human Services, National Center for Health Statistics.

Jones, D. B., W. J. Niendorff, and E. B. Broderick. 2000. A review of the oral health of American Indian and Alaska Native elders. *Journal of Public Health Dentistry* 60(Supp. 1):256-260.

Jones, M., J. Y. Lee, and R. G. Rozier. 2007. Oral health literacy among adult patients seeking dental care. *Journal of the American Dental Association* 138(9):1199-1208.

Kaiser Family Foundation. 2007. *Number of births financed by Medicaid, 2003*. http://www.statehealthfacts.org/comparemaptable.jsp?ind=222&cat=4 (accessed February 1, 2011).

Kaiser Family Foundation. 2009. *Distribution of the nonelderly with Medicaid by race/ethnicity, states (2008-2009), U.S.* http://www.statehealthfacts.org/comparebar.jsp?ind=158&cat=3 (accessed May 3, 2011).

Kalenderian, E., R. L. Ramoni, J. M. White, M. E. Schoonheim-Klein, P. C. Stark, N. S. Kimmes, G. G. Zeller, G. P. Willis, and M. F. Walji. 2011. The development of a dental diagnostic terminology. *Journal of Dental Education* 75(1):68-76.

Kenney, G. M., J. R. McFeeters, and J. Y. Yee. 2005. Preventive dental care and unmet dental needs among low-income children. *American Journal of Public Health* 95(8):1360-1366.

Kenney, M. K., M. D. Kogan, and J. J. Crall. 2008. Parental perceptions of dental/oral health among children with and without special health care needs. *Ambulatory Pediatrics* 8(5):312-320.

Kerins, C., P. S. Casamassimo, D. Ciesla, Y. Lee, and N. S. Seale. 2011. A preliminary analysis of the US dental health care system's capacity to treat children with special health care needs. *Pediatric Dentistry* 33(2):107-112.

Kitchens, D. H. 2005. The economics of pit and fissure sealants in preventive dentistry: A review. *Journal of Contemporary Dental Practice* 6(3):95-103.

Kitchens, M., and B. M. Owens. 2007. Effect of carbonated beverages, coffee, sports and high energy drinks, and bottled water on the in vitro erosion characteristics of dental enamel. *Journal of Clinical Pediatric Dentistry* 31(3):153-159.

Kiyak, H. A., and M. Reichmuth. 2005. Barriers to and enablers of older adults' use of dental services. *Journal of Dental Education* 69(9):975-986.

Koh, H. 2010. A 2020 vision for healthy people. *New England Journal of Medicine* 362(18):1653-1656.

Kumar, J. V., O. Adekugbe, and T. A. Melnik. 2010. Geographic variation in Medicaid claims for dental procedures in New York State: Role of fluoridation under contemporary conditions. *Public Health Reports* 125(5):647-654.

Kuthy, R. A., M. S. Strayer, and R. J. Caswell. 1996. Determinants of dental user groups among an elderly, low-income population. *Health Services Research* 30(6):809-825.

Kutner, M., E. Greenberg, Y. Jin, and C. Paulsen. 2006. *The health literacy of America's adults: Results from the 2003 National Assessment of Adult Literacy.* Washington, DC: National Center for Health Statistics, U.S. Department of Education.

Kwan, S., and P. E. Petersen. 2010. Oral health: Equity and social determinants. In *Equity, social determinants and public health programmes*, edited by E. Blas and A. S. Kurup. Geneva, Switzerland: World Health Organization Press.

Lamster, I. B. 2004. Oral health care services for older adults: A looming crisis. *American Journal of Public Health* 94(5):699-702.

Leake, J. 2002. Diagnostic codes in dentistry-definition, utility and developments to date. *Journal-Canadian Dental Association* 68(7):403-407.

Lewis, C., and J. Stout. 2010. Toothache in U.S. children. *Archives of Pediatrics and Adolescent Medicine* 164(11):1059-1063.

Lewis, C., A. S. Robertson, and S. Phelps. 2005. Unmet dental care needs among children with special health care needs: Implications for the medical home. *Pediatrics* 116(3):e426-e431.

Lewis, C., W. Mouradian, R. Slayton, and A. Williams. 2007. Dental insurance and its impact on preventative dental care visits for U.S. children. *Journal of the American Dental Association* 138(3):369-380.

Lewis, C. W., K. A. Linsenmayer, and A. Williams. 2010. Wanting better: A qualitative study of low-income parents about their children's oral health. *Pediatric Dentistry* 32(7):518-524.

Lindhe, J., H. Okamoto, T. Yoneyama, A. Haffajee, and S. S. Socransky. 1989. Longitudinal changes in periodontal disease in untreated subjects. *Journal of Clinical Periodontology* 16(10):662-670.

Lindskog, S., J. Blomlöf, I. Persson, A. Niklason, A. Hedin, L. Ericsson, M. Ericsson, B. Järncrantz, U. Palo, and G. Tellefsen. 2010. Validation of an algorithm for chronic periodontitis risk assessment and prognostication: Risk predictors, explanatory values, measures of quality, and clinical use. *Journal of Periodontology* 81(4):584-593.

Löe, H. 1993. Periodontal disease. The sixth complication of diabetes mellitus. *Diabetes Care* 16(1):329-334.

López Pérez, R., S. A. Borges Yáñez, G. Jiménez García, and G. Maupomé. 2002. Oral hygiene, gingivitis, and periodontitis in persons with Down syndrome. *Special Care in Dentistry* 22(6):214-220.

Macek, M. D., R. J. Manski, C. M. Vargas, and J. F. Moeller. 2002. Comparing oral health care utilization estimates in the United States across three nationally representative surveys. *Health Services Research* 37(2):499-521.

Macones, G. A., S. Parry, D. B. Nelson, J. F. Strauss, J. Ludmir, A. W. Cohen, D. M. Stamilio, D. Appleby, B. Clothier, M. D. Sammel, and M. Jeffcoat. 2010. Treatment of localized periodontal disease in pregnancy does not reduce the occurrence of preterm birth: Results from the Periodontal Infections and Prematurity Study (PIPS). *American Journal of Obstetrics and Gynecology* 202(2):147.e141-147.e148.

Makhija, S. K., G. H. Gilbert, O. J. Clay, J. C. Matthews, P. Sawyer, and R. M. Allman. 2011. Oral health–related quality of life and life-space mobility in community-dwelling older adults. *Journal of the American Geriatrics Society* 59(3):512-518.

Manski, R. J., and E. Brown. 2007. *Dental use, expenses, private dental coverage, and changes, 1996 and 2004.* Rockville, MD: Agency for Healthcare Research and Quality.

Manski, R. J., and E. J. Brown. 2010. *Dental coverage of adults ages 21-64, United States, 1997 and 2007.* Rockville, MD: Agency for Healthcare Research and Quality.

Manski, R. J., and L. S. Magder. 1998. Demographic and socioeconomic predictors of dental care utilization. *Journal of the American Dental Association* 129(2):195-200.

Manski, R. J., H. S. Goodman, B. C. Reid, and M. D. Macek. 2004. Dental insurance visits and expenditures among older adults. *American Journal of Public Health* 94(5):759-764.

Marchi, K., S. Fisher-Owens, J. Weintraub, Z. Yu, and P. Braveman. 2010. Most pregnant women in California do not receive dental care: Findings from a population-based study. *Public Health Reports* 125(6):831-842.

Marinho, V. C. 2009. Cochrane reviews of randomized trials of fluoride therapies for preventing dental caries. *European Archives of Paediatric Dentistry* 10(3):183-191.

Marinho, V. C., J. P. Higgins, S. Logan, and A. Sheiham. 2002. Fluoride varnishes for preventing dental caries in children and adolescents. *Cochrane Database of Systematic Reviews* (3):CD002279.

Marinho, V. C., J. P. Higgins, S. Logan, and A. Sheiham. 2003a. Topical fluoride (toothpastes, mouthrinses, gels or varnishes) for preventing dental caries in children and adolescents. *Cochrane Database of Systematic Reviews* (4):CD002782.

Marinho, V. C. C., J. P. T. Higgins, S. Logan, and A. Sheiham. 2003b. Fluoride toothpastes for preventing dental caries in children and adolescents. *Cochrane Database of Systematic Reviews* (1):CD002278.

Martin, R. F. 2000. The IHS dental program: A historical perspective. *Journal of Public Health Dentistry* 60(Supp. 1):238-242.

Marur, S., G. D'Souza, W. H. Westra, and A. A. Forastiere. 2010. HPV-associated head and neck cancer: A virus-related cancer epidemic. *The Lancet Oncology* 11(8):781-789.

Maserejian, N. N., M. A. Tavares, C. Hayes, J. A. Soncini, and F. L. Trachtenberg. 2008. Rural and urban disparities in caries prevalence in children with unmet dental needs: The New England children's amalgam trial. *Journal of Public Health Dentistry* 68(1):7-13.

MCHB (Maternal and Child Health Bureau). 2011. *Maternal and child health research program strategic research issues: FY 2004-2009.* http://mchb.hrsa.gov/programs/research/issues.htm (accessed March 16, 2011).

Michalowicz, B. S., J. S. Hodges, A. J. Diangelis, V. R. Lupo, M. J. Novak, J. E. Ferguson, W. Buchanan, J. Bofill, P. N. Papapanou, D. A. Mitchell, S. Matseoane, and P. A. Tschida. 2006. Treatment of periodontal disease and the risk of preterm birth. *New England Journal of Medicine* 355:1885-1894.

Michalowicz, B. S., A. J. DiAngelis, M. J. Novak, W. Buchanan, P. N. Papapanou, D. A. Mitchell, A. E. Curran, V. R. Lupo, J. E. Ferguson, J. Bofill, S. Matseoane, A. S. Deinard, Jr., and T. B. Rogers. 2008. Examining the safety of dental treatment in pregnant women. *Journal of the American Dental Association* 139(6):685-695.

Mohammad, A. R., P. M. Preshaw, and R. L. Ettinger. 2003. Current status of predoctoral geriatric education in U.S. dental schools. *Journal of Dental Education* 67(5):509-514.

Moynihan, P., and P. Petersen. 2004. Diet, nutrition and the prevention of dental diseases. *Public Health Nutrition* 7(1a):201-226.

Nabi, G., J. Cody, G. Ellis, P. Herbison, and J. Hay-Smith. 2006. Anticholinergic drugs versus placebo for overactive bladder syndrome in adults. *Cochrane Database of Systematic Reviews*(4):CD003781.

National Quality Forum. 2010. *NQF-endorsed standards.* http://www.qualityforum.org/Measures_List.aspx (accessed November 29, 2010).

NCHS (National Center for Health Statistics). 2011. *Health, United States, 2010: With special feature on death and dying.* Hyattsville, MD: U.S. Department of Health and Human Services.

Neuhauser, L. 2010. *Communicating with patients: A survey of dental team members—preliminary results.* Paper presented at meeting of the Committee on an Oral Health Initiative, June 28, Washington, DC.

New York State Department of Health. 2006. *Oral health care during pregnancy and early childhood: Practice guidelines*. Albany, NY: New York State Department of Health.

Newacheck, P. W., and S. E. Kim. 2005. A national profile of health care utilization and expenditures for children with special health care needs. *Archives of Pediatrics and Adolescent Medicine* 159(1):10-17.

Newacheck, P. W., M. McManus, H. B. Fox, Y.-Y. Hung, and N. Halfon. 2000. Access to health care for children with special health care needs. *Pediatrics* 105(4):760-766.

NHLBI (National Heart, Lung, and Blood Institute). 2010. *NHLBI FY 2010 fact book*. Washington, DC: U.S. Department of Health and Human Services.

NIA (National Institute on Aging). 1987. *Personnel for health needs of the elderly through the year 2020*. Bethesda, MD: U.S. Department of Health and Human Services.

NIDCR (National Institute of Dental and Craniofacial Research). 2005. The invisible barrier: Literacy and its relationship with oral health. *Journal of Public Health Dentistry* 65(3):174-192.

NIDCR. 2011a. *Periodontal disease in adults (age 20 to 64)*. http://www.nidcr.nih.gov/DataStatistics/FindDataByTopic/GumDisease/PeriodontaldiseaseAdults20to64 (accessed February 14, 2011).

NIDCR. 2011b. *Periodontal disease in seniors (age 65 and over)*. http://www.nidcr.nih.gov/DataStatistics/FindDataByTopic/GumDisease/PeriodontaldiseaseSeniors65over (accessed February 14, 2011).

NRC (National Research Council). 1989. *Diet and health: Implications for reducing chronic disease risk*. Washington, DC: National Academy Press.

O'Connell, J. M., D. Brunson, T. Anselmo, and P. W. Sullivan. 2005. Costs and savings associated with community water fluoridation programs in Colorado. *Preventing Chronic Disease* 2(Special issue):1-13.

Offenbacher, S., D. Lin, R. Strauss, R. McKaig, J. Irving, S. P. Barros, K. Moss, D. A. Barrow, A. Hefti, and J. D. Beck. 2006. Effects of periodontal therapy during pregnancy on periodontal status, biologic parameters, and pregnancy outcomes: A pilot study. *Journal of Periodontology* 77(12):2011-2024.

Offenbacher, S., J. D. Beck, H. L. Jared, S. M. Maurriello, L. C. Mendoza, D. J. Couper, D. D. Stewart, A. P. Murtha, D. L. Cochran, D. J. Dudley, M. S. Reddy, N. C. Geurs, and J. C. Hauth. 2009a. Effects of periodontal therapy on rate of preterm delivery: A randomized controlled trial. *Obstetrics and Gynecology* 114(3):551-559.

Offenbacher, S., J. D. Beck, K. Moss, L. Mendoza, D. W. Paquette, D. A. Barrow, D. J. Couper, D. D. Stewart, K. L. Falkner, S. P. Graham, S. Grossi, J. C. Gunsolley, T. Madden, G. Maupome, M. Trevisan, T. E. V. Dyke, and R. J. Genco. 2009b. Results from the Periodontitis and Vascular Events (PAVE) study: A pilot multicentered, randomized, controlled trial to study effects of periodontal therapy in a secondary prevention model of cardiovascular disease. *Journal of Periodontology* 80(2):190-201.

Otto, M. 2007. For want of a dentist. *Washington Post*, February 28, B01.

Owens, P. L., B. D. Kerker, E. Zigler, and S. M. Horwitz. 2006. Vision and oral health needs of individuals with intellectual disability. *Mental Retardation and Developmental Disabilities Research Reviews* 12(1):28-40.

Palacio, H., J. F. Hilton, A. J. Canchola, and D. Greenspan. 1997. Effect of cigarette smoking on HIV-related oral lesions. *Journal of Acquired Immune Deficiency Syndromes and Human Retrovirology* 14(4):338-342.

Parnell, C., H. Whelton, and D. O'Mullane. 2009. Water fluoridation. *European Archives of Paediatric Dentistry* 10(3):141-148.

Patel, S., R. C. Bay, and M. Glick. 2010. A systematic review of dental recall intervals and incidence of dental caries. *Journal of the American Dental Association* 141(5):527-539.

Patrick, D., R. Lee, M. Nucci, D. Grembowski, C. Jolles, and P. Milgrom. 2006. Reducing oral health disparities: A focus on social and cultural determinants. *BMC Oral Health* 6(Supp. 1):S4.

Patton, L. L., R. Agans, J. R. Elter, and J. H. Southerland. 2004. Oral cancer knowledge and examination experiences among North Carolina adults. *Journal of Public Health Dentistry* 64(3):173-180.

Pavia, M., C. Pileggi, C. G. A. Nobile, and I. F. Angelillo. 2006. Association between fruit and vegetable consumption and oral cancer: A meta-analysis of observational studies. *American Journal of Clinical Nutrition* 83(5):1126-1134.

Pew Center on the States. 2010. *The cost of delay: State dental policies fail one in five children.* Washington, DC: Pew Center on the States.

Pleis, J. R., B. W. Ward, and J. W. Lucas. 2010. *Summary health statistics for U.S. adults: National Health Interview Survey, 2009.* Hyattsville, MD: Department of Health and Human Services.

Pyle, M. A., T. R. Jasinevicius, D. R. Sawyer, and J. Madsen. 2005. Nursing home executive directors' perception of oral care in long-term care facilities. *Special Care in Dentistry* 25(2):111-117.

Qiu, Y., and H. Ni. 2003. *Utilization of dental care services by Asians and Native Hawaiian or other Pacific Islanders: United States, 1997-2000.* Hyattsville, MD: National Center for Health Statistics.

Quijano, A., A. J. Shah, A. I. Schwarcz, E. Lalla, and R. J. Ostfeld. 2010. Knowledge and orientations of internal medicine trainees toward periodontal disease. *Journal of Periodontology* 81(3):359-363.

Radnai, M., I. Gorzó, E. Urbán, J. Eller, T. Novák, and A. Pál. 2006. Possible association between mother's periodontal status and preterm delivery. *Journal of Clinical Periodontology* 33(11):791-796.

Ramos-Gomez, F. J., J. Crall, S. A. Gansky, R. L. Slayton, and J. D. Featherstone. 2007. Caries risk assessment appropriate for the age 1 visit (infants and toddlers). *Journal of the California Dental Association* 35(10):687-702.

Reid, B. C., R. Chenette, and M. D. Macek. 2003. Prevalence and predictors of untreated caries and oral pain among special Olympic athletes. *Special Care in Dentistry* 23(4):139-142.

Rich, K. 2010. *Dental quality alliance.* Paper presented at National Oral Health Conference, St. Louis, MO.

Rickard, G. D., R. J. Richardson, T. M. Johnson, D. C. McColl, and L. Hooper. 2004. Ozone therapy for the treatment of dental caries. *Cochrane Database of Systematic Reviews* (3):CD004153.

Robinson, P., S. A. Deacon, C. Deery, M. Heanue, A. D. Walmsley, H. V. Worthington, A. M. Glenny, and B. C. Shaw. 2005. Manual versus powered toothbrushing for oral health. *Cochrane Database of Systematic Reviews* (1):CD002281.

Rozier, R. G., A. M. Horowitz, and G. Podschun. 2011. Dentist-patient communication techniques used in the United States. *Journal of the American Dental Association* 142(5): 518-530.

Scannapieco, F. A., and A. W. Ho. 2001. Potential associations between chronic respiratory disease and periodontal disease: Analysis of National Health and Nutrition Examination Survey III. *Journal of Periodontology* 72(1):50-56.

Scannapieco, F. A., R. B. Bush, and S. Paju. 2003a. Associations between periodontal disease and risk for atherosclerosis, cardiovascular disease, and stroke. A systematic review. *Annals of Periodontology* 8(1):38-53.

Scannapieco, F. A., R. B. Bush, and S. Paju. 2003b. Periodontal disease as a risk factor for adverse pregnancy outcomes. A systematic review. *Annals of Periodontology* 8(1):70-78.

Schwartzberg, J. G., A. Cowett, J. VanGeest, and M. S. Wolf. 2007. Communication techniques for patients with low health literacy: A survey of physicians, nurses, and pharmacists. *American Journal of Health Behavior* 31(Supp. 1):S96-S104.

Shaw, L., M. Shaw, and T. Foster. 1989. Correlation of manual dexterity and comprehension with oral hygiene and periodontal status in mentally handicapped adults. *Community Dentistry and Oral Epidemiology* 17(4):187-189.

Shaw, R., and M. Robinson. 2010. The increasing clinical relevance of human papillomavirus type 16 (HPV-16) infection in oropharyngeal cancer. *British Journal of Oral and Maxillofacial Surgery*. Published electronically August 19, 2010. doi:10.1016/j.bjoms.2010.06.023.

Silk, H., A. B. Douglass, J. M. Douglass, and L. Silk. 2008. Oral health during pregnancy. *American Family Physician* 77(8):1139-1144.

Silva, R. M. D. 2004. Characterization of *Streptococcus constellatus* strains recovered from a brain abscess and periodontal pockets in an immunocompromised patient. *Journal of Periodontology* 75(12):1720-1723.

Slavkin, H. C., and B. J. Baum. 2000. Relationship of dental and oral pathology to systemic illness. *Journal of the American Medical Association* 284(10):1215-1217.

Smith, B. J., E. M. Ghezzi, M. C. Manz, and C. P. Markova. 2010. Oral healthcare access and adequacy in alternative long-term care facilities. *Special Care in Dentistry* 30(3):85-94.

Sohn, W., A. Ismail, A. Amaya, and J. Lepkowski. 2007. Determinants of dental care visits among low-income African-American children. *Journal of the American Dental Association* 138(3):309-318.

Sondik, E. J., D. T. Huang, R. J. Klein, and D. Satcher. 2010. Progress toward the Healthy People 2010 goals and objectives. *Annual Review of Public Health* 31(1):271-281.

Stanton, M. W., and M. K. Rutherford. 2003. *Dental care: Improving access and quality.* Rockville, Maryland: Agency for Healthcare Research and Quality.

Steinberg, B. J., L. Minsk, J. I. Gluch, and S. K. Giorgio. 2008. Women's oral health issues. In *Women's health in clinical practice*. Totowa, NJ: Humana Press. Pp. 273-293.

Stewart, D. C. L., A. N. Ortega, D. Dausey, and R. Rosenheck. 2002. Oral health and use of dental services among Hispanics. *Journal of Public Health Dentistry* 62(2):84-91.

Stiefel, D. J. 2002. Oral health and dental care access challenges. *Special Care in Dentistry* 22(3):26S-39S.

Sundin, B., L. Granath, and D. Birkhed. 1992. Variation of posterior approximal caries incidence with consumption of sweets with regard to other caries related factors in 15–18 year olds. *Community Dentistry and Oral Epidemiology* 20(2):76-80.

Suzuki, J. B., and A. L. Delisle. 1984. Pulmonary actinomycosis of periodontal origin. *Journal of Periodontology* 55(10):581-584.

Tarannum, F., and M. Faizuddin. 2007. Effect of periodontal therapy on pregnancy outcome in women affected by periodontitis. *Journal of Periodontology* 78(11):2095-2103.

Task Force on Community Preventive Services. 2002. Recommendations on selected interventions to prevent dental caries, oral and pharyngeal cancers, and sports-related craniofacial injuries. *American Journal of Preventive Medicine* 23(Supp. 1):16-20.

Taylor, G. W. 2001. Bidirectional interrelationships between diabetes and periodontal diseases: An epidemiologic perspective. *Annals of Periodontology* 6(1):99-112.

Teeuw, W. J., V. E. A. Gerdes, and B. G. Loos. 2010. Effect of periodontal treatment on glycemic control of diabetic patients: A systematic review and meta-analysis. *Diabetes Care* 33(2):421-427.

Tiller, S., K. I. Wilson, and J. E. Gallagher. 2001. Oral health status and dental service use of adults with learning disabilities living in residential institutions and in the community. *Community Dental Health* 18(3):167-171.

Tomar, S. L., and A. F. Reeves. 2009. Changes in the oral health of U.S. children and adolescents and dental public health infrastructure since the release of the Healthy People 2010 objectives. *Academic Pediatrics* 9(6):388-395.

Truman, B. I., B. F. Gooch, I. Sulemana, H. C. Gift, A. M. Horowitz, C. A. Evans Jr., S. O. Griffin, and V. G. Carande-Kulis. 2002. Reviews of evidence on interventions to prevent dental caries, oral and pharyngeal cancers, and sports-related craniofacial injuries. *American Journal of Preventive Medicine* 23(1 Supp.):21-54.

Twetman, S. 2009. Caries prevention with fluoride toothpaste in children: An update. *European Archives of Paediatric Dentistry Dentistry* 10(3):162-167.

Uher, R., A. Farmer, N. Henigsberg, M. Rietschel, O. Mors, W. Maier, D. Kozel, J. Hauser, D. Souery, A. Placentino, J. Strohmaier, N. Perroud, A. Zobel, A. Rajewska-Rager, M. Z. Dernovsek, E. R. Larsen, P. Kalember, C. Giovannini, M. Barreto, P. McGuffin, and K. J. Aitchison. 2009. Adverse reactions to antidepressants. *The British Journal of Psychiatry* 195(3):202-210.

Van Cleave, J., and M. M. Davis. 2008. Preventive care utilization among children with and without special health care needs: Associations with unmet need. *Ambulatory Pediatrics* 8(5):305-311.

Vargas, C. M., and C. R. Ronzio. 2006. Disparities in early childhood caries. *BMC Oral Health* 6(Supp. 1):S3-S7.

Vargas, C., J. Crall, and D. Schneider. 1998. Sociodemographic distribution of pediatric dental caries: NHANES III, 1988-1994. *Journal of the American Dental Association* 129(9):1229.

Vargas, C. M., B. A. Dye, and K. L. Hayes. 2002. Oral health status of rural adults in the United States. *Journal of the American Dental Association* 133(12):1672-1681.

Vargas, C. M., B. A. Dye, and K. L. Hayes. 2003a. Oral health care utilization by U.S. rural residents, National Health Interview Survey 1999. *Journal of Public Health Dentistry* 63(3):150-157.

Vargas, C. M., C. R. Ronzio, and K. L. Hayes. 2003b. Oral health status of children and adolescents by rural residence, United States. *Journal of Rural Health* 19(3):260-268.

Vargas, C. M., J. A. Yellowitz, and K. L. Hayes. 2003c. Oral health status of older rural adults in the United States. *Journal of the American Dental Association* 134(4):479-486.

Vergnes, J. N., and M. Sixou. 2007. Preterm low birth weight and maternal periodontal status: A meta-analysis. *American Journal of Obstetrics and Gynecology* 196(2):135.e131-135.e137.

Walsh, T., H. V. Worthington, A. M. Glenny, P. Appelbe, V. C. Marinho, and X. Shi. 2010. Fluoride toothpastes of different concentrations for preventing dental caries in children and adolescents. *Cochrane Database of Systematic Reviews* (1):CD007868.

Weinberger, A. H., E. L. Reutenauer, P. I. Jatlow, S. S. O'Malley, M. N. Potenza, and T. P. George. 2010. A double-blind, placebo-controlled, randomized clinical trial of oral selegiline hydrochloride for smoking cessation in nicotine-dependent cigarette smokers. *Drug and Alcohol Dependence* 107(2-3):188-195.

Weintraub, J. A. 1989. The effectiveness of pit and fissure sealants. *Journal of Public Health Dentistry* 49(5):317-330.

Weintraub, J. A. 2001. Pit and fissure sealants in high-caries-risk individuals. *Journal of Dental Education* 65(10):1084-1090.

Weintraub, J. A., S. C. Stearns, B. A. Burt, E. Beltran, and S. A. Eklund. 1993. A retrospective analysis of the cost-effectiveness of dental sealants in a children's health center. *Social Science and Medicine* 36(11):1483-1493.

Weintraub, J. A., S. C. Stearns, R. G. Rozier, and C. C. Huang. 2001. Treatment outcomes and costs of dental sealants among children enrolled in Medicaid. *American Journal of Public Health* 91(11):1877-1881.

Weintraub, J. A., P. Prakash, S. G. Shain, M. Laccabue, and S. A. Gansky. 2010. Mothers' caries increases odds of children's caries. *Journal of Dental Research* 89(9):954-958.

WHO (World Health Organization). 2010a. *Oral health: Risks to oral health and intervention*. http://www.who.int/oral_health/action/risks/en/index.html (accessed September 15, 2010).

WHO. 2010b. *Oral health: Tobacco*. http://www.who.int/oral_health/action/risks/en/index2.html (accessed September 15, 2010).

WHO. 2010c. *Oral health: Fluorides*. http://www.who.int/oral_health/action/risks/en/index1.html (accessed September 15, 2010).

WHO. 2010d. Oral health: What is the burden of oral disease? http://www.who.int/oral_health/disease_burden/global/en/index.html (accessed December 27, 2010).

Williams, D. R. 2005. Patterns and causes of disparities in health. In *Policy challenges in modern health care*, edited by D. Mechanic, L. Rogut, D. C. Colby, and J. R. Knickman. New Brunswick, NJ: Rutgers University Press.

Williams, M. V., T. Davis, R. M. Parker, and B. D. Weiss. 2002. The role of health literacy in patient-physician communication. *Family Medicine* 34(5):383-389.

Wyszynski, D. F., D. L. Duffy, and T. H. Beaty. 1997. Maternal cigarette smoking and oral clefts: A meta-analysis. *Cleft Palate-Craniofacial Journal* 34(3):206-210.

Yellowitz, J. A., A. M. Horowitz, T. F. Drury, and H. S. Goodman. 2000. Survey of U.S. dentists' knowledge of opinions about oral pharyngeal cancer. *Journal of the American Dental Association* 131(5):653-661.

Yeung, A., J. L. Hitchings, T. V. Macfarlane, A. Threlfall, M. Tickle, and A. Glenny. 2005. Fluoridated milk for preventing dental caries. *Cochrane Database of Systematic Reviews* (3):CD003876.

Yeung, C. A. 2008. A systematic review of the efficacy and safety of fluoridation. *Evidence-Based Dentistry* 9(2):39-43.

Yorty, J. S., A. T. Walls, and S. Wearden. 2011. Caries risk assessment/treatment programs in U.S. dental schools: An eleven-year follow-up. *Journal of Dental Education* 75(1):62-67.

Yu, Y.-H., Y.-L. Lai, W. S. Cheung, and H.-K. Kuo. 2011. Oral health status and self-reported functional dependence in community-dwelling older adults. *Journal of the American Geriatrics Society* 59(3):519-523.

Yuen, H. K., B. J. Wolf, D. Bandyopadhyay, K. M. Magruder, A. W. Selassie, and C. F. Salinas. 2010. Factors that limit access to dental care for adults with spinal cord injury. *Special Care in Dentistry* 30(4):151-156.

3

The Oral Health Care Workforce

The oral health care workforce is a critical component of access to care for vulnerable and underserved populations in that access is dependent, in part, on the availability of a sufficient supply of competent oral health care professionals. The extent to which the different professionals interact with each other can vary greatly. In addition, the services that may be delivered by each professional often vary by state. These issues are not dissimilar to those which have been faced in other health care professions.

This chapter gives an overview of the oral health workforce including basic demographics, how professionals are educated, what kind of care they provide, and how they interact. The chapter continues with a discussion of the regulation of the health care workforce in general, and the dental workforce specifically. Finally the chapter concludes with descriptions of a variety of innovations in workforce education, training, and use to improve access and care for underserved and vulnerable populations. The capacity and efficiency of the oral health care system (including consideration of the adequacy of the workforce) is discussed in Chapter 4.

THE DENTAL WORKFORCE

As with other health care professions, it can be difficult to definitively quantify the dental workforce for a variety of reasons including changes in employment status, differing measures (e.g., licensed vs. active professionals), the holding of more than one position per professional, and the presence of multiple and overlapping job titles. Aside from sheer numbers, consideration is needed for geographic distribution and racial, ethnic, and gender diversity. This section provides a general overview of the basic demographics of the dental workforce.

General Description

Most professionally active dentists are general dentists (ADA, 2009d) (see Box 3-1 for types of dentists). Recognized specialties include orthodontics and dentofacial orthopedics, oral and maxillofacial surgery, pediatrics, periodontics, prosthodontics, endodontics, oral and maxillofacial pathology, oral and maxillofacial radiology, and dental public health. Almost all professionally active dentists (92 percent) work in the private practice set-

BOX 3-1
Types of Dentists

A *professionally active dentist* is primarily or secondarily occupied in a private practice, dental school faculty/staff, armed forces, or other federal service (e.g., Veterans Administration, U.S. Public Health Service); or is a state or local government employee, hospital staff dentist, graduate student/intern/resident, or other health/dental organization staff member.

An *active private practitioner* is someone whose primary and/or secondary occupation is private practice.

A *new dentist* is anyone who has graduated from dental school within the last 10 years.

An *independent dentist* is a dentist running a sole proprietorship or one who is involved in a partnership.

A *solo dentist* is an independent dentist working alone in the practice he or she owns.

A *nonowner dentist* does not share in ownership of the practice.

An *employed dentist* works on a salary, commission, percentage, or associate basis.

An independent contractor contracts with owner(s) for use of space and equipment.

A *nonsolo dentist* works with at least one other dentist and can be an independent or nonowner dentist.

NOTE: Each of these types can be either general or specialty practitioners.
SOURCES: ADA, 2009b,d.

ting (ADA, 2009d). (See Chapter 4 for more on the private practice setting of care.) Occupations of other professionally active dentists include[1]

- Dental school faculty/staff member (1.7 percent)
- Armed forces (0.9 percent)
- Graduate student/intern/resident (1.3 percent)
- Hospital staff dentist (0.4 percent)
- State or local government employee (0.8 percent)
- Other federal service (0.8 percent)
- Other health/dental organization staff (1.0 percent)

In 2009, 48 percent of dental school graduates planned to enter private practice immediately while 30 percent planned to pursue advanced education, 10 percent planned to enter some form of government service, and less than one-half of 1 percent planned to enter the fields of teaching, research, or administration[2] (Okwuje et al., 2010).

Dental hygienists are found in most settings where oral health services are provided, but they are mainly employed in private dental practices. They also work in educational institutions and in public health settings such as school-based clinics, prisons, long-term care, and other institutional care facilities (ADHA, 2009b; Mertz and Glassman, 2011). In private dental practice, the work of dental hygienists is generally billed under the dentist's contractual agreement with an insurance company using the supervising dentist's provider number. However, as of June 2010, 15 states allowed their state Medicaid departments to directly reimburse dental hygienists for their services (ADHA, 2010c).

Dental assistants primarily work in a clinical capacity, but other roles include front-office positions, practice management, and education (McDonough, 2007). Most dental assistants work in private practices and as assistants to general dentists, but many dental assistants work in specialty practices. Currently, there are multiple job titles for dental assistants across the country in different states (ADAA/DANB Alliance, 2005; DANB, 2007). These titles are generally grouped into four categories: entry level (e.g., trainees), dental assistants, certified or registered dental assistants, and expanded functions dental assistants (EFDAs) (DANB, 2007). Each of these categories includes multiple titles, depending on the state. For example, while the title of EFDA is commonly used to describe all dental assistants who can perform extended duties, there are many other titles used (e.g., expanded duties dental assistant, advanced dental assistant, registered restorative assistant in extended functions), and many states permit dental

[1] Does not total 100 percent due to rounding.
[2] The remaining graduates reported "other/undecided" for their future plans.

assistants to perform specific extended functions (e.g., coronal polishing, administration or monitoring of sedation, pit and fissure sealants) (DANB, 2007). In fact, some states permit certified dental assistants to act at the level of an EFDA, even though titles such as *certified dental assistant* or *registered dental assistant* are used (DANB, 2007). As stated by the Dental Assistant National Board, "Without a single, nationally accepted set of guidelines that govern the practice of dental assisting in the country, it is difficult to execute a concise overview" of the profession (DANB, 2007). (EFDAs are discussed further later in this chapter.)

Dental laboratory technicians (also known as dental technicians) create bridges, dentures, and other dental prosthetics. Dental technicians work in a variety of settings including dentists' offices, their own private businesses, or small privately owned offices (BLS, 2010e). While dental technicians create devices based on the prescription of a dentist, denturists are trained and licensed in some states to work independently in taking impressions and making, fitting, and repairing dentures. Denturists were first recognized as a profession in Oregon, where licensure began in 1980 (Oregon State Denturist Association, 2011). Seven states currently regulate denturists (National Denturist Association, 2011). Denturists are not typically considered part of the traditional dental team.

Current Numbers and Future Demand

As mentioned previously, determining the exact number of professionals can be difficult because of differences in terminology, differing measures, and employment characteristics. According to the Bureau of Labor Statistics (BLS), dentists held approximately 141,900 jobs in 2008, with about 85 percent of those practitioners being general dentists (see Table 3-1). In that same year, an American Dental Association (ADA) survey found that there were 181,725 professionally active dentists, of which 79 percent were general dentists and 21 percent were new dentists (graduated within the previous 10 years) (ADA, 2009d). Similarly, it can be difficult to estimate the dental hygiene workforce. As shown in Table 3-1, dental hygienists held just over 174,000 jobs in 2008, but this is likely an overestimate, since many dental hygienists hold more than one job. A 2007 survey commissioned by the American Dental Hygienists' Association (ADHA) found that there were about 152,000 licensed dental hygienists in the United States and that 130,000 were actively practicing (ADHA, 2009b). About half of all dental hygienists work part time (ADHA, 2009b; BLS, 2010c).

Table 3-1 also shows the BLS estimates of numbers of jobs held by and increases in growth of all dental professions. The BLS predicts a 36 percent growth in the employment of both dental hygienists and dental assistants

TABLE 3-1
Employment of Dental Professions and Occupations, 2008 and Projected 2018

Profession/ Occupation	Number of Jobs, 2008	Number of Jobs, 2018	Projected Increase in Growth (%), 2008-2018
Dentists	141,900	164,000	16
General dentists	120,200	138,600	15
Dental hygienists	174,100	237,000	36
Dental assistants	295,300	400,900	36
Dental laboratory technicians	46,000	52,400	14

SOURCES: BLS, 2010b,c,d,e.

between 2008 and 2018, ranking them among the fastest growing of all occupations.

Income

The BLS reports a mean annual wage of almost $143,000 for salaried general dentists (BLS, 2010d). This is similar to the ADA estimate of the average net income (from the primary private practice) for employed dentists of $132,000 (ADA, 2009c); however, as noted above, employed dentists account for only a small portion of all dentists. Dentists' income can vary depending on setting and type of employment (see Table 3-2). Incomes also vary slightly depending on whether the practice is incorporated or unincorporated, the age of practitioner, the number of years since graduation, and the number of hours worked per year. In comparison, a survey of executive directors of health centers reported an average salary for the highest-paid dentist on staff of $125,000; the average budgeted salary for a dentist with 10 or more years of experience was $145,000 (Bolin, 2010).

In 2008, dental hygienists had a median annual wage of about $66,500 and dental assistants had a median annual wage of about $32,000 (BLS, 2010b, 2010c). Nearly 30 percent of dental hygienists do not receive any benefits (ADHA, 2009b). In 2008, dental technicians had a median annual wage of about $34,000 (BLS, 2010e).

Age

The ADA estimates that 35 percent of all professionally active dentists are age 55 and older, with an average age of 49.6 years (ADA, 2009d). Among independent dentists in private practice, 43 percent are age 55 or

TABLE 3-2
Private Practice Dentists' Net Income by Type of Employment, 2007

Practitioner	Net Income from Primary Private Practice ($)	Total Net Income from Dentistry ($)
All independent dentists	234,000	237,000
Independent general practitioners	206,000	208,000
Independent nonsolo general practitioners	232,000	237,000
Independent specialists	353,000	360,000
Independent nonsolo specialists	392,000	405,000
Solo general practitioners	195,000	196,000
Solo specialists	334,000	338,000
Employed dentists (weighted)	132,000	n/a[a]
Employed general practitioners	122,000	n/a
Employed specialists	181,000	n/a
New employed dentists	114,000	n/a
Independent contractors (weighted)	114,000	n/a

[a]N/A = not available.
SOURCE: ADA, 2009c.

older, with an average age of 52.3 years (ADA, 2009b). This may add to the burden of need for dentists as these practitioners near retirement. The mean age of dental hygienists is about 44 years of age (ADHA, 2009b), which, like dentists, may lead to concerns about the numbers nearing retirement.

Gender

About 79 percent of all professionally active dentists are male (ADA, 2009d). However, the gender gap is slowly closing; 63 percent of new professionally active dentists are male, and only 56 percent of first-year dental students in the 2008–2009 academic year were male (ADA, 2009d, 2010a). Overall, dental hygienists and dental assistants are virtually all female (ADHA, 2009b; McDonough, 2007). This is not likely to change drastically in the near future; among all students enrolled in accredited programs in 2008–2009, 97 percent of dental hygiene students and 95 percent of dental-assisting students were female (ADA, 2009a).

Racial and Ethnic Diversity

The racial and ethnic profile of the dental workforce is not representative of the overall population (see Table 3-3). While diversity among the dental professions students has increased in the previous decade (see Table 3-4), the numbers still are not significantly changed.

Evidence shows that a diverse health professions workforce (including race and ethnicity, gender, and geographic distribution) leads to improved access for underserved populations, greater patient satisfaction, and better

TABLE 3-3
Dental Professions by Percentage of Race and Hispanic Ethnicity, 2000

	General Population	Dentists	Dental Hygienists	Dental Assistants
White[a]	75.1	82.8	90.9	75.8
Black or African American[a]	12.3	3.3	2.3	5.6
Asian[a]	3.6	8.8	2.0	3.6
Hispanic or Latino Origin	12.5	3.6	3.7	12.6

[a]Category excludes Hispanic origin.
SOURCES: U.S. Census Bureau, 2000, 2002.

TABLE 3-4
Percentage of Dental Professions School and Program Enrollment by Race and Hispanic Ethnicity, 2000-2001 and 2008-2009

	Enrolled Dental Students		Enrolled Dental Hygiene Students		Enrolled Dental Assistant Students[a]	
	2000-2001	2008-2009	2000-2001	2008-2009	2000-2001	2008-2009
White	63.4	59.9	82.3	78.6	68.4	60.2
Black	4.8	5.8	4.2	4.4	12.5	15.1
Asian	24.8	23.4	4.6	7.0	2.9	4.8
Hispanic	5.3	6.2	5.7	7.3	9.7	11.1

[a]Includes only dental assistant students enrolled in CODA-approved programs. Racial and ethnic diversity of entire dental assistant workforce may be different.
SOURCES: ADA, 2002, 2009a, 2010a.

communication (HRSA, 2006; IOM, 2004). The Agency for Healthcare Research and Quality 2010 *National Healthcare Disparities Report* (AHRQ, 2010) stated:

> Workforce diversity increases the opportunities for race- and language-concordant health care visits. It also can improve cultural competency at the system, organization, and provider levels in several ways. These include appropriate program design and policies, organizational commitment to culturally competent care, and cross-cultural education of colleagues [Nickens, 1992]. As such, diversity is an important element of a patient-centered health care encounter.

Health care professionals from underrepresented minority (URM) populations, in part due to patient preference, often account for a disproportionate amount of the services provided to URM and low-income populations (Brown et al., 2000; HRSA, 2006; IOM, 2003; Mitchell and Lassiter, 2006). For example, a 1996 survey by the ADA revealed that nearly 77 percent of white dentists' patients were white, while 62 percent of African American dentists' patients were African American and only 27 percent were white (ADA, 1998; Brown et al., 2000). More recently, among dental students graduating in 2008, 80 percent of African American students and 75 percent of Hispanic students expected at least one-quarter of their patients would be from underserved racial and ethnic populations; nearly 37 percent of the African American students and 27 percent of the Hispanic students expected at least half their practice would come from these populations (Okwuje et al., 2009). In comparison, only 43.5 percent of white students expected at least one quarter of their patients to come from underserved racial and ethnic populations, and only 6.5 percent expected at least half of their practice to comprise these populations (Okwuje et al., 2009). It is important to note that the recruitment of low-income students (regardless of race or ethnicity) may also be important for the care of vulnerable and underserved patients (Andersen et al., 2010). A 2011 study of dental students found that students who were female, from URM populations, or had low socioeconomic status expressed greater attitudes of altruism than other students (Carreon et al., 2011).

Several factors complicate recruitment of URM students including lack of exposure to and knowledge of the dental profession, minimal opportunities for mentorship from dental professionals, and competition from other health professions for underrepresented minority students who are academically qualified (Haden et al., 2003). Other barriers may include lack of financial resources or knowledge of available financial aid.

Several Title VII grants are specifically targeted to increase the diversity of the health care workforce. Dental schools with significant enrollment of URM students are eligible for Centers of Excellence grants to improve recruitment and training of URM students.[3] Health Careers Opportunity Program grants are available to dental and dental hygiene schools to establish or extend programs to identify, recruit, and support students from disadvantaged backgrounds.[4] Scholarships for Disadvantaged Students grants provide funding to dental and dental hygiene schools for financial aid to disadvantaged students.[5] Experiences with bridge and pipeline programs to recruit students from URM, low-income, and rural populations are discussed later in this chapter.

Distribution of the Dental Workforce

The distribution of the dental workforce, both in geographic dispersion as well as specialization, is a long-recognized challenge (Brown, 2001; Hart-Hester and Thomas, 2003; Mertz and Grumbach, 2001; Saman et al., 2010). In 1957, Dr. Wesley Young stated, "A recurrent problem in dental manpower is the tendency of dentists to concentrate in urban areas, leaving sparsely settled sections of the state understaffed" (Young, 1958). In 2001, Brown noted that while the workforce may be adequate at the national level, there are imbalances at the regional level (Brown, 2001). Part of the reason for maldistribution has to do with the ability of a dentist to support private practices in rural areas because of population size or income (Allison and Manski, 2007; Wall and Brown, 2007; Wendling, 2010). These same issues may affect the development of independent dental hygiene practices (Brown et al., 2005). One way to estimate geographic distribution is to look at the ratio of dentists per population. In 2007, there was an average of about 59 professionally active dentists per 100,000 population, ranging from about 40 dentists per 100,000 population in Mississippi and Arkansas to about 102 dentists per 100,000 population in the District of Columbia (ADA, 2009d; U.S. Census Bureau, 2010). The lowest ratios occur across the southernmost states in the United States (Kaiser Family Foundation, 2011).

Within these numbers, there are variations in the types of dentists available in each region and across the country. For example, there are 0.7 professionally active periodontists per 100,000 adult population (age 18 and above), or more than 144,000 adults per professionally active periodontist. In contrast, there are about nine pediatric dentists per 100,000 population of children aged 17 and under, translating to more than 11,000 patients per pediatric dentist (about 3,200 children under age 5 for each pediatric dentist). But this varies even more when looking at individual states. For ex-

---

[3] 42 U.S.C. §293.
[4] 42 U.S.C. §293c.
[5] 42 U.S.C. §293a.

ample, Massachusetts has one pediatric dentist for every 6,000 children age 17 and under (one for every 1,600 children under age 5), but West Virginia has only about one pediatric dentist for every 23,000 children age 17 and under (one for every 6,200 children under age 5). Similarly, Massachusetts has one periodontist for every 18,500 adults, while West Virginia has one periodontist for every 84,000 adults.

Concurrently, the dental hygiene workforce may also be experiencing challenges owing to the maldistribution of dentists and the downturn in the economy. For example, a 2009 survey of dental hygienists showed that 68 percent of respondents reported finding sufficient employment was somewhat or very difficult in their geographic area, and of these, 80 percent felt that there were too many hygienists living in the area (ADHA, 2009a). Based on the number of providers per population, another way to measure the distribution of the dental workforce is to examine the designation of Health Professional Shortage Areas (HPSAs). By regulation, the secretary of the Department of Health and Human Services (HHS) has the responsibility of defining HPSAs.

> *Health Professional(s) Shortage Area* means any of the following that the Secretary determines has a shortage of health professional(s): (1) An urban or rural area (which need not conform to the geographic boundaries of a political subdivision and which is a rational area for the delivery of health services); (2) a population group; or (3) a public or nonprofit private medical facility.[6]

Box 3-2 delineates the specific requirements for designation of a dental HPSA.

As of March 13, 2011, there were 4,639 dental HPSAs with 33.3 million unserved individuals; it is estimated that 9,933 new dentists would be needed to achieve the target ratio for these populations to be adequately served, defined as 1 dentist per 3,000 individuals (HRSA, 2011b). The number of dental HPSAs and need for dentists is on the rise; in 2009, there were 4,230 dental HPSAs and a need for 9,642 new dentists to meet unserved needs (HRSA, 2010c). Two-thirds of current dental HPSAs are in nonmetropolitan areas (HRSA, 2011b). Among all dental HPSAs, 17 percent are designated by geographic area, 34 percent are designated by population group, and 49 percent are designated by facility (HRSA, 2011b). Figure 3-1 shows the array of dental HPSAs across the country for both geographic areas (including areas in which the entire county is a dental HPSA) and population groups.

As discussed in Chapter 1, making estimates of underservice and unmet

---

[6] *Code of Federal Regulations*, Public Health Service, Department of Health and Human Services, title 42, chapter 1, part 5 (2010).

BOX 3-2
Requirements for Dental HPSA Designation

Geographic areas must meet these requirements:

- Be rational areas for the delivery of dental services.
- Meet one of the following conditions:
    - o Have a population to full-time equivalent (FTE) dentist ratio of at least 5,000:1, or
    - o Have a population to FTE dentist ratio of less than 5,000:1 but greater than 4,000:1 and unusually high needs for dental services or insufficient capacity.
- Dental professionals in contiguous areas must be overutilized, excessively distant, or inaccessible to the population.

Population groups must meet these requirements:

- Reside in a rational service area for the delivery of dental care services,
- Have access barriers that prevent the population group from use of the area's dental providers,
- Have a ratio of the number of persons in the population group to the number of dentists practicing in the area and serving the population group of at least 4,000:1, and
- Members of certain federally recognized American Indian tribes are automatically designated. Other American Indian or Alaska Native groups may be designated if the meet the basic criteria described above.

Facilities must meet these requirements:

- Be either federal and/or state correctional institutions or public and/or nonprofit medical facilities, and meet specific criteria.
- Federal or state correctional facilities must:
    - o have at least 250 inmates, and
    - o have a ratio of the number of internees per year to the number of FTE dentists serving the institution of at least 1,500:1.
- Public and/or nonprofit private dental facilities must:
    - o provide general dental care services to an area or population group designated as having a dental HPSA, and
    - o have insufficient capacity to meet the dental care needs of that area or population group.

SOURCE: HRSA, 2011a.

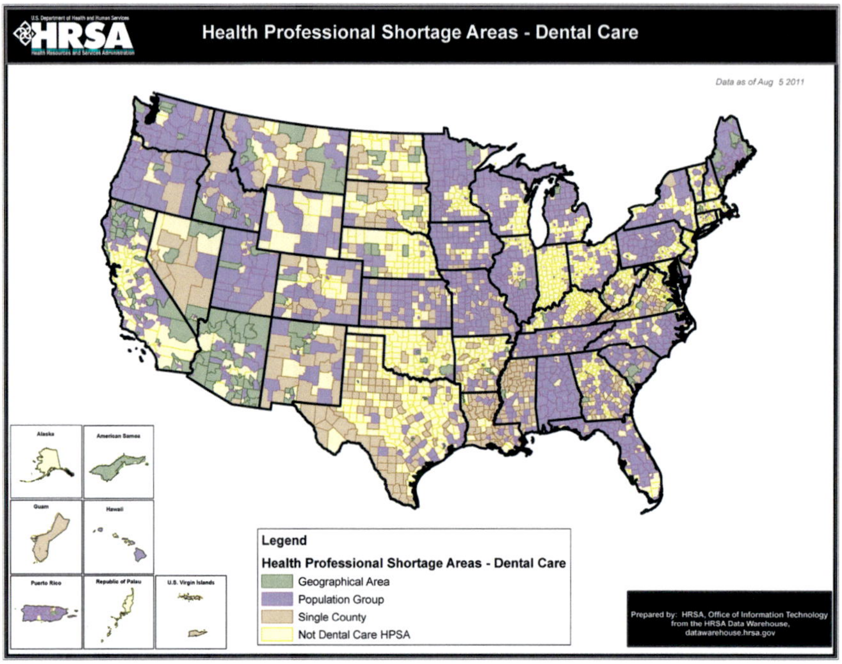

FIGURE 3-1
Dental Health Professional Shortage Areas designated by geographic area and population group.

SOURCE: HRSA, 2011c.

need are complicated. The committee recognizes that ratios of provider per population and designation of HPSAs alone do not fully depict access issues and do not on their own determine the availability of or utilization of care. For example, an increase in the number of providers per population does not necessarily translate into improved access to care. In addition, shortcomings in the current criteria and methodologies used to make HPSA designations have been identified (GAO, 2006; Orlans et al., 2002). However, until improved methodologies and criteria are developed, these measures serve as some of the only resources to help inform discussions about the availability of services, and serve as the basis for many policy decisions.

EDUCATION AND TRAINING OF THE DENTAL WORKFORCE

Over time, the education of dental professionals has largely evolved from apprenticeships to formalized programs in a variety of locations including dental schools, 4-year colleges and universities, community colleges, and technical schools (Haden et al., 2003). The U.S. Department of Education recognizes the Commission on Dental Accreditation (CODA) as the accrediting agency for predoctoral dental education programs; programs for dental hygienists, dental assistants, and dental laboratory technicians; and advanced dental educational programs (e.g., residencies) (U.S. Department of Education, 2010). Federal support for dental education allowed dental schools to expand dramatically between 1960 and 1980, but this support has lagged in recent years (HRSA, 2005). Title VII training grants for dentistry currently take two forms: grants to increase the workforce that is prepared to care for vulnerable populations and grants to diversify the workforce, though the public policy goals of the Title VII grants have varied over time (HRSA, 2005; Reynolds, 2008).

Dentists

Most U.S. dental schools offer a 4-year curriculum, after which graduates are awarded a degree as either a Doctor of Dental Medicine (D.M.D.), or a Doctor of Dental Surgery (D.D.S.) (ADA, 2010a). The number of dental schools in the United States is increasing, and more dentists are being produced. As of 2011, there were 61 predoctoral dental education programs in the United States and Puerto Rico, up from 57 schools in 2009 (ADA, 2010a; ADEA, 2011b). About 4,800 new dentists graduated in 2008, up from 4,095 in 1999 (ADA, 2010a). The number of dental schools is currently on the rise. (See Chapter 4 for further discussion.)

Cost of Education

The cost of dental education is a barrier to entry, especially for low-income and URM students (IOM, 2004; Pyle et al., 2006; Sullivan Commission, 2004; Walker et al., 2008). In 2008–2009, the average annual tuition for dental schools was $27,961 for state residents and $41,561 for nonresidents (ADA, 2010a); the difference is significant considering many states do not have a single dental school. As this problem exists for several professions, the Western Interstate Commission for Higher Education created the Professional Student Exchange Program in which students from certain states may receive assistance to attend health professional schools (including dental schools) in other states (WICHE, 2011).

In 2009, average dental education debt was $164,000, ranging from $141,000 for graduates of public schools to $195,000 for graduates of private schools (Okwuje et al., 2010). Overall, 77 percent of graduates had at least $100,000 in debt, and 62 percent had at least $150,000 in debt (Okwuje et al., 2010). The average educational debt for all medical school graduates in 2010 was comparable; debt for medical students was approximately $158,000, with 78 percent of graduates having at least $100,000 in debt and 42 percent having at least $150,000 in debt (AMA, 2011b). However, these groups may not be exactly comparable, as medical students typically spend several years after graduation in internship, residency, and fellowship programs that may add to their subsequent accumulated debt.

Debt varies greatly among dental graduates and may affect future career choices. Twenty percent of graduates report having little to no debt (almost 10 percent had no debt); at the other end of the spectrum, another 20 percent report graduating with more than $250,000 in debt (Okwuje et al., 2010). Even within these numbers, there are variations; for example, 38 percent of graduates from private schools had more than $250,000 in debt, compared to 6.5 percent of graduates from public schools (Okwuje et al., 2010). Among graduates with no debt, 40 percent planned to enter private practice compared to 56 percent of those with $250,000 or more of debt; additionally, 33 percent of those with no debt planned to pursue advanced education compared to only 24 percent of those with $250,000 or more of debt (Okwuje et al., 2010). However, among all graduates, only 33 percent said that their educational debt had "much" or "very much" influence on their plans upon graduation (Okwuje et al., 2010).

One strategy that has been used to ameliorate the burden of student debt is the provision of financial incentives to care for vulnerable and underserved populations. The National Health Service Corps, developed in the 1970s, offers both scholarships and loan repayment to clinicians, including dentists and dental hygienists, who agree to serve for 2 to 4 years in an HPSA (HRSA, 2010b). In FY 2009, 464 dentists and 66 dental hygienists served in the National Health Service Corps (Anderson, 2010).

Community-Based Education

Traditionally, dental schools own and operate their own patient care clinics, where students receive most of their clinical training. These clinics operate as teaching laboratories in that their primary goal is to educate students; the care that patients receive is a secondary outcome and the patients served in those clinics may not be representative of a broad populations. (See Chapter 4 for more on dental school clinics as a site of care.) For both educational and financial reasons, many dental schools are now moving from the traditional clinical education model to community-based education where students rotate through off-site locations to provide care to vulnerable and underserved populations (Bailit et al., 2007; Ballweg et al., 2011; Berg et al., 2010; Formicola et al., 2008; Hood, 2009; Walker et al., 2008).

Community-based education is associated with greater confidence in performing procedures and caring for underserved and vulnerable populations (Bailit, 1999; McQuistan et al., 2010). These experiences have also been associated with smoother transition into professional practice; improved clinical skills; greater appreciation for social, ethical, and cultural issues; and increased willingness to care for vulnerable and underserved populations (Atchison et al., 2009; Baumeister et al., 2007; Berg et al., 2010; DeCastro et al., 2005; Holtzman and Seirawan, 2009; Johnson et al., 2007; McAndrew, 2010; Strauss et al., 2010). Community-based dental education has also been shown to have financial benefits for both the dental schools and the community settings (Bailit, 2010). However, a survey of dental students graduating in 2009 showed a varied response as to whether these experiences would affect their choice in practice location as well as their interest in treating URM patients (Okwuje et al., 2010).

Community surveys of graduating dental students show that the cumulative time students spend in extramural clinics has been steadily increasing; between 2003 and 2008, the percentage of students providing 4 or more weeks of care on extramural clinical rotations (cumulatively over the 4 years of dental school) increased from 47 percent to 62 percent (Okwuje et al., 2009). However, the survey of 2009 graduating dental students asked about the time spent in these sites on an annual basis (rather than cumulative time over the 4 years of school). The majority of students reported spending little time in extramural clinical rotations, with most of it occurring in the last year of school (see Table 3-5).

Support for community-based education is growing. In 2001, the ADA said "Dental schools should develop programs in which students, residents, and faculty provide care for members of the underserved populations in community clinics and practices" (ADA, 2001). In January 2010, the Advisory Committee on Training in Primary Care Medicine and Dentistry

TABLE 3-5
Percentage of Time Spent in Extramural Clinics for Each Year in Dental School Reported by 2009 Dental School Graduates

Year	Less Than 1 Week	1 to 2 Weeks	3 to 4 Weeks	1 Month or More
First year	87.7	9.2	1.9	1.3
Second year	78.4	15.7	4.0	1.9
Third year	32.0	33.5	19.4	15.1
Fourth year	8.4	30.7	21.5	39.5

SOURCE: Okwuje et al., 2010.

(established by law and supported by HRSA's Bureau of Health Professions) recommended that Congress and the Centers for Medicare and Medicaid Services (CMS) "should revise funding policies for Graduate Medical Education and other educational programs to foster and support the use of community-based (nonhospital) sites for primary care training for physicians, dentists, and physician assistants" (Advisory Committee on Training in Primary Care Medicine and Dentistry, 2010). In addition, they recommended the provision of training grants to support and recruit community-based clinician educators for health care trainees, including dentists.

In August 2010, CODA adopted a new resolution that includes a requirement for schools to make service learning and/or community-based learning opportunities available and encourage students to participate in these opportunities (ADA, 2010c; ADEA, 2011a). The stated intent of this requirement is

> Service learning experiences and/or community-based learning experiences are essential to the development of a culturally competent oral health care workforce. The interaction and treatment of diverse populations in a community-based clinical environment adds a special dimension to clinical learning experience and engenders a life-long appreciation for the value of community service. (ADA, 2010c)

Over 90 percent of dental schools now offer community-based rotations for dental students (Haden et al., 2010). However, the breadth and depth of these experiences remains unknown. Additionally, many considerations are needed when establishing community-based dental programs such as the best time in the academic schedule to participate, transportation and housing issues, cultural competence of the students to work with diverse populations, legal liability, and developing partnerships with community sites (Mascarenhas and Henshaw, 2010). An additional challenge, as discussed in general previously, is the recruitment of experienced and available faculty in these settings, or the development of academic skills for those willing to become community educators (Hood, 2009; Mascarenhas and Henshaw, 2010; McAndrew, 2010).

Experiences with Specific Populations

Associated with community-based dental education, dental students' exposure to specific vulnerable and underserved populations and students' perception of the quality of the education they receive regarding those populations affects their confidence in caring for those populations (Baumeister et al., 2007; McQuistan et al., 2010; Vainio et al., 2011; Weil and Inglehart, 2010). For example, hands-on experiences with caring for children with special health care needs (Casamassimo et al., 2004), homeless populations

(Habibian et al., 2010), and patients with autism (Weil and Inglehart, 2010) has been associated with improvement in perceptions of those populations, increased confidence in caring for them, and greater likelihood to care for special populations in the future. However, among dental students graduating in 2008, 23 percent felt less than prepared to care for older adults and almost 31 percent felt less than prepared to care for patients with disabilities (Okwuje et al., 2009).

CODA's accreditation standards state "graduates must be competent in assessing the treatment needs of patients with special needs" but does not require specific education or clinical experiences with caring for these populations (ADA, 2010c). The standards clarify the intent of the above requirement as

> appropriate patient pool should be available to provide experiences that may include patients who's [sic] medical, physical, psychological, or social situations make it necessary to consider a wide range of assessment and care options. The assessment should emphasize the importance of non-dental considerations. These individuals include, but are not limited to, people with developmental disabilities, cognitive impairment, complex medical problems, significant physical limitations, and the vulnerable elderly. Clinical instruction and experience with the patients with special needs should include instruction in proper communication techniques and assessing the treatment needs compatible with the special need. (ADA, 2010c)

Training in the care of specific populations may affect dentists' practice patterns. For example, one study of general dentists in Michigan and pediatric dentists across the country showed that only 41 percent of the general dentists reported performing infant oral health examinations compared to more than 80 percent of pediatric dentists, and that the general dentists were less engaged in prevention activities than the pediatric dentists (Ananaba et al., 2010). Other studies show examples of both pediatric dentists and general dentists not routinely encouraging or performing dental examinations or treatments before the age of one (Brickhouse et al., 2008; Malcheff et al., 2009; Salama and Kebriaei, 2010), which could indicate a need for improvements in dental education regarding the care of infants. One study from 2001 showed that the education of dental students in caring for infants varied widely among dental schools (McWhorter et al., 2001).

Residency Programs

Upon completion of dental school, students may have had few opportunities to integrate their skills and knowledge with practical hands-on experience and may not feel adequately prepared for independent practice, especially to care for underserved and vulnerable populations. Dental residencies provide further training in general dentistry or specialization in one of the nine recognized dental specialty areas. In 2008–2009, there were 5,864 total dentists enrolled in 723 advanced dental education programs in the United States (3,009 in first-year enrollments), including dental residencies and fellowship programs (ADA, 2010b). About half of these programs were sponsored by dental schools (ADA, 2010b). Among enrollees, 61 percent were male, and the racial and ethnic diversity mirrored their proportion in dental schools (see Table 3-4) (ADA, 2010b). Currently, two states require a residency as a requirement for licensure: New York and Delaware.[7]

In the 1995 IOM report *Dental Education at the Crossroads* (*Crossroads*) report, noting the lack of time in the curricula of undergraduate programs to develop critical skills, the committee concluded that "all graduates of U.S. dental schools should have the opportunity to round out and refine their predoctoral work through a supervised and accredited postgraduate experience," leading to a formal recommendation for the development of postdoctoral educational programs to be made available for every graduate (IOM, 1995). A survey of deans of dental schools performed for that report found that three-quarters of the deans agreed that building or sustaining a strong postdoctoral general dentistry program was a priority, and slightly more than 60 percent agreed that a year of postgraduate training should be required within 10 years.

Additional training has been attributed to the better preparation of dentists to care for underserved and vulnerable populations (IOM, 1995). Postgraduate dental education in particular is seen as an opportunity to address these needs (Garrison, 1991; Glassman and Meyerowitz, 1999; Lefever et al., 2003; Morris et al., 1982). Dentists who have completed general dentistry residency programs report feeling more comfortable caring for underserved patients and patients with complex health care needs, and care for those patients more often, even after completing residency (Atchison et al., 2002; Dixon et al., 2002; Gatlin et al., 1993; Lam et al., 2009; Tejani et al., 2002).

The advantages and disadvantages of dental residency have been debated for decades. Advantages of dental residency include enhanced status of the profession and the opportunity to address both dissatisfaction with the breadth of undergraduate education and lack of student confidence in preparedness for practice (Hillenbrand, 1981; Lefever et al., 2003). In particular, many have noted that given the advances in science and technology,

---

[7] Del. Code. Ann. tit. 24, s. 1122 (2011); N.Y. Comp. Codes R. & Regs. tit.8, s. 61.18 (2010).

the nation's changing demographics, and the rising challenges in caring for vulnerable and underserved populations, the 4-year undergraduate education is inadequate to fully prepare students not only with sufficient knowledge, but with the skills to integrate this knowledge into practice (Atchison et al., 2002; Glassman and Meyerowitz, 1999; Hillenbrand, 1981; Kennedy and Tedesco, 1999; Lefever et al., 2003; Thierer and Meyerowitz, 2005; Yeager, 2001). Disadvantages of dental residency include the increased cost of education and the opportunity costs related to the delay of professional practice (Atchison et al., 2002; Hillenbrand, 1981; IOM, 1995; Lefever et al., 2003).

A survey of several cohorts of dentists showed that the respondents were evenly split regarding support of a mandatory fifth year of training (Lefever et al., 2003). Those who supported the extra year were more likely to have completed a residency themselves or to work in a setting such as a hospital or nursing home. Those who did not support the year argued that alternatively, curricular reform of dental school education would be preferable; they also cited autonomy—that is was the right of each dentist to decide if he or she needed additional training (Lefever et al., 2003). Both groups agreed that the extra year needed to be a practical, real-world experience rather than an extension of the undergraduate education program.

Barriers to expanding residency opportunities include the fact that funding sources, especially for the creation of new programs, may be tenuous, availability of training sites and faculty may be lacking, and adequate supportive staff is needed (Hillenbrand, 1981; IOM, 1995; Lam et al., 2009; Ng et al., 2008; Thierer and Meyerowitz, 2005). The 1995 *Crossroads* report found that "creating appropriately structured, stipend-paying residency positions demands a substantial investment of administrative and faculty time—and favorable local conditions" (IOM, 1995). Also, in 1981, Hilllenbrand expressed concern for the basis of such programs in the hospital setting, noting that "too much emphasis may be placed on the hospital aspects of the program at the risk of producing less than a comprehensively trained general practitioner" (Hillenbrand, 1981).

In comparison, other doctoral-level health care professions (e.g., allopathic medicine, osteopathic medicine, podiatric medicine) have requirements for residency training. The *Crossroads* report noted

> [I]n contrast to medicine, substantial numbers of dental students do not pursue residency training after graduation. Yet, the emphasis in most dental schools on preparing students to be competent, entry-level general practitioners upon graduation puts a considerable burden on both schools and students. (IOM, 1995)

Students of allopathic and osteopathic medicine both complete 4 years of general graduate education. After this, these physicians complete between 3 and 8 years of internship and residency training (AMA, 2011a; AOA, 2011; BLS, 2009c). Further, some physicians receive additional fellowship training in a subspecialty (e.g., child and adolescent psychiatry as a subspecialty of psychiatry) (AMA, 2011a). Like dental students, students of podiatric medicine complete 4 years of graduate education geared toward their disciplines. However, after this, podiatrists then complete 2 or more years of postgraduate education in residency programs (APMA, 2011). Most states require at least 2 years of postgraduate training as a prerequisite for licensure in podiatric medicine (BLS, 2009d).

The role of dental residency programs in providing direct care for vulnerable and underserved populations is discussed further in Chapter 4.

HHS Financial Support of Dental Residency Programs

Title VII has been successful at expanding residencies in general and pediatric dentistry, which were, until recently, the only dental disciplines for which the grants were available (Ng et al., 2008). Title VII–funded dental residencies have been successful at recruiting and training URM students, and graduates of Title VII–funded medical residencies are more likely to provide care to underserved communities and populations, and are more prepared to provide culturally competent care (Edelstein et al., 2003; Green et al., 2008; HHS, 2003; Ng et al., 2008). A review of the impact of Title VII-funded dental residency programs found that

> Title VII grantees have been instrumental in promoting community-based training to increase access to oral health services to underserved and vulnerable populations in the medically and dentally underserved communities where they reside. (Ng et al., 2008)

Title VII–funded programs have also been credited with developing curricula regarding the oral health needs of many vulnerable and underserved populations and developing interprofessional training approaches (Ng et al., 2008).

The Patient Protection and Affordable Care Act (ACA) significantly expanded the number of grants available for dental training, including funds for residencies in general, pediatric, and public health dentistry, as well as technical assistance to pediatric dentistry training programs. In addition to Title VII funds, several individual HHS divisions provide support for residency training (CDC, 2011; HRSA, 2010a).

Graduate Medical Education (GME) payments are also available to help train dental residents.[8] Direct Graduate Medical Education (DGME)

---

[8] *Code of Federal Regulations*, Centers for Medicare and Medicaid Services, Department of Health and Human Services, title 42, sec. 413.75 (2009).

payments cover a portion of the cost of resident stipends and expenses, and indirect medical education (IME) payments cover the additional costs associated with training (Iglehart, 2010). When dental residencies are located in a hospital setting, the hospital receives both DGME and IME payments from CMS. Dental school–based residencies are much more limited in their ability to receive GME funds. In 2003, CMS issued a regulation clarifying its policy on GME payments for residents trained outside the hospital: CMS would no longer provide any GME payments for residents whose training had historically been paid for by dental schools.[9] As a result of this rule, 26 dental schools lost funding for most or all of their residency programs (Bresch, 2010).

Dental Hygienists

In the 2008–2009 academic year, there were 301 CODA-accredited dental hygiene education programs (ADA, 2009a). Most of these programs award associate degrees (82 percent), but others award bachelor degrees, diplomas, and certificates. In 2008, there were 6,723 dental hygiene graduates (up from 5,345 in 1999) (ADA, 2009a). In the early years of the profession, dental hygiene education programs were often co-located with dental education programs in schools of dentistry (Haden et al., 2003). Today, about two-thirds of dental hygiene education programs are located in community, junior, and technical colleges (ADHA, 2006), which may decrease the amount of interaction between dentists and dental hygienists during their training, and therefore not prepare them to work as a team. Annual tuition can vary widely. For example, community colleges have an average annual tuition of $3,145 while the average annual tuition for programs co-located with dentals schools is $12,659 (ADA, 2009a). While the educational admissions requirements for dental hygiene education programs vary widely, more than 80 percent of first-year students have completed at least 2 years of college (ADA, 2009a). Faculty in dental hygiene education programs are mostly dental hygienists (76 percent) and dentists (21 percent) (ADA, 2009a). Recently, the ACA extended Title VII grant funding to dental hygiene programs in general, pediatric, and public health dentistry.

As with dental students, dental hygiene students need to be prepared to care for special populations and work in the community setting, but little is known about the extent of the education and training of dental hygienists for a variety of such populations (e.g., infants, diverse populations, older adults). A recent survey of dental hygiene programs revealed that nearly all programs (98 percent) present information on special needs

[9] *Code of Federal Regulations*, Centers for Medicare and Medicaid Services, Department of Health and Human Services, title 42, sec. 413.81 (2009).

BOX 3-3
Competencies for Entry into the Professions of Dental Hygiene and Dental Assisting: Community Involvement (CM)

CM.1 Assess the oral health needs and services of the community to determine action plans and availability of resources to meet the health care needs.

CM.2 (Hygienists) Provide screening, referral, and educational services that allow patients to access the resources of the health care system.

CM.2 (Assistants) Provide educational services that allow patients to access the resources of the health care system.

CM.3 Provide community oral health services in a variety of settings.

CM.4 Facilitate patient access to oral health services by influencing individuals or organizations for the provision of oral health care.

CM.5 Evaluate reimbursement mechanisms and their impact on the patient's access to oral health care.

CM.6 Evaluate the outcomes of community-based programs, and plan for future activities.

CM.7 Advocate for effective oral health care for underserved populations.

SOURCE: ADEA, 2010.

populations through lectures, but only 42 percent require related clinical experiences (Dehaitem et al., 2008). Most cited challenges with space in curricula, but nearly 30 percent expressed support for increasing these clinical experiences, and accreditation standards now require competence in assessing the needs of these populations. Dental hygiene programs are also embracing community-based education. In 2010, the American Dental Education Association House of Delegates redefined competencies for entry into the allied dental professions. Box 3-3 lists the competencies that focus on community involvement.

As will be discussed later in this chapter, some dental hygienists perform expanded duties in various sites of care and under different levels of supervision. As these duties expand, further consideration will be needed for the adequacy of dental hygiene education to practice in these settings, or if advanced training will be needed.

Dental Assistants

Dental assistants are trained on the job or in formal education programs. Education programs in dental assisting may be located in postsecondary institutions (that may or may not be accredited by CODA), high schools, vocational programs, and technical schools (ADAA/DANB Alliance, 2005). Dental assistants may also be trained on the job by their employers. Considering the numerous educational pathways and the fact that most states do not license dental assistants, it is difficult to generalize a description of the workforce as a whole or to assess the impact of the various training alternatives (ADAA/DANB Alliance, 2005; Neumann, 2004). Little is known about the wide variety of programs that are not accredited by CODA.

In 2008–2009, there were 273 CODA-accredited dental assisting programs, almost all of which (87 percent) were in public institutions (ADA, 2009a). Average cost for tuition and fees of these programs for in-district students was $6,791 (ADA, 2009a). In 2008, there were about 6,100 graduates from CODA-accredited programs (ADA, 2009a). Virtually all CODA-accredited programs (88 percent) require a high school diploma for admission, and 9 percent require even more (ADA, 2009a). Most CODA-accredited programs are 1 year in length leading to a certificate or diploma. However, a few have a 2-year curriculum resulting in an associate degree. About 14 percent of faculty[10] in CODA-accredited programs are dentists, 70 percent are dental assistants, and 28 percent are dental hygienists (ADA, 2009a).

Dental Laboratory Technicians

There are no formal education or training requirements for dental technicians, and most learn required skills through on-the-job training; however, some formal programs exist in universities, community and junior colleges, vocational schools, and in the military (BLS, 2010e). In the 2008–2009 academic year, there were 20 CODA-accredited programs (ADA, 2009a). Most accredited programs last 2 years, and 13 confer an associate's degree. In the last 5 years, applications to these programs decreased by nearly 13 percent (ADA, 2009a). Average total tuition and fees range from $7,838 for in-district students to $18,214 for out-of-state students (ADA, 2009a). In 2008, there were 234 total graduates from accredited programs (ADA, 2009a).

THE NONDENTAL WORKFORCE

As oral health has become recognized as integral to overall health, nondental health care professionals have become increasingly involved in the prevention, diagnosis, and treatment of oral diseases. Training primary

[10] Some faculty members reported more than one discipline, so these numbers do not total 100 percent.

care clinicians in oral health leads to their increased ability to recognize oral disease and may help to increase their referrals to dentists (Dela Cruz et al., 2004; Pierce et al., 2002). In addition, practice changes resulting from this training can lead to increased access to preventive services and decreased dental disease (Chu et al., 2007; Kressin et al., 2009; Rozier et al., 2010). This section considers the education, training, and potential role of several nondental health care professions in the oral health care of the nation. The specific role of nondental health care professionals in the delivery of preventive services is discussed later in this chapter.

Physicians

The need for physicians to learn about oral health has been recognized for nearly a century. In 1926, Gies stated

> [A] policy of health service . . . which ignores oral hygiene, or neglects dental maladies . . . cannot be expected to commend itself to enlightened public opinion. Fortunately this disregard in the medical profession is gradually being replaced by serious attention to oral conditions, especially among the physicians who are engaged in public health services, and among . . . public-health nurses and teachers acting in their behalf. . . . This desirable movement promises to attain its logical development among practitioners of medicine in general when medical schools give to their students suitable instruction in oral hygiene, and in the correlations between clinical medicine and clinical dentistry. (Gies, 1926)

By the mid-20th century, this had become even more widely recognized (Ast, 1952; Bender and Seltzer, 1963; Bigler, 1951). In 1940, Dunning stated "It is amazing, at times, to realize how little many excellent physicians know about dental pathology and the modern treatment of dental lesions" (Dunning, 1941). Today, many physicians still do not receive education or training in oral health either during medical school, during residency training, or in continuing education programs (Krol, 2010; Mouradian et al., 2003). In addition, the breadth and depth of existing education and training efforts is highly variable (Douglass et al., 2009a; Ferullo et al., 2011).

Evidence on the ability of physicians to deliver oral health care is mixed. Even though many physicians recognize the importance of oral health, they often do not feel prepared to provide oral health care. Other barriers to the incorporation of oral health care into medical care include the ability to be reimbursed for services, availability of time in the practice schedule, and difficulty in making dental referrals (Close et al., 2010; Lewis et al., 2009). The following sections describe the education and training in oral health and the delivery of oral health care by several medical specialties.

Medical Schools

Few medical schools include curriculum on oral health, despite the presence of oral health topics on medical licensing exams (Ferullo et al., 2011; Krol, 2004; Mouradian et al., 2005; USMLE, 2010a,b). Almost 70 percent of medical schools include 4 hours or less of oral health in their curricula, and more than 10 percent have no oral health education at all (Ferullo et al., 2011). Fewer than 50 percent of schools that teach oral health cover the risks of dental caries (Ferullo et al., 2011). In 2004, the Josiah Macy, Jr. Foundation funded a 3-year grant to examine oral health education (Formicola et al., 2005; Machen, 2008). One of the project's reports emphasized the role for physicians in the identification and referral of patients with oral health needs (Mouradian et al., 2008). Subsequently, the American Association of Medical Colleges published learning objectives for oral health (AAMC, 2008). Courses that incorporate these objectives result in significantly increased student knowledge of oral health topics, even after 6 months (Silk et al., 2009). Efforts of the University of Washington to improve the oral health education of medical students are discussed later in this chapter.

Pediatricians

A 2000 national survey of pediatricians found that more than 90 percent believed they had an important role in the recognition of oral diseases and the provision of counseling regarding the prevention of caries, and three-quarters expressed interest in the application of fluoride varnish in their practices (Lewis et al., 2000). However, half reported no oral health training in either medical school or residency. In spite of efforts to improve upon this, little has changed in the last decade. A recent survey of pediatricians on the care of children age 0–3 showed that more than 90 percent agreed they should examine these patients' teeth but only 54 percent reported actually doing so (Lewis et al., 2009). In addition, 41 percent of respondents cited a lack of training as a barrier to incorporating oral health care into their practices. A 2006 survey found that two-thirds of graduating pediatrics residents thought they should be performing oral health assessments on their patients, but only about one-third received any oral health training during their residencies, and of those that did, two-thirds got less than 3 hours of training (Caspary et al., 2008). Only about 14 percent had clinical observation time with a dentist.

The American Academy of Pediatrics, the professional society for pediatricians, has developed explicit educational guidelines for oral health training in pediatric residency and the Accreditation Council for Graduate Medical Education (ACGME) requires that all residents must be able to "implement age-appropriate screening, including oral health" (AAP, 2011c; ACGME, 2007b). In addition, the pediatric board exam has questions about oral health (ABP, 2009).

Family Medicine Physicians

In 2006, the residency review committee for family medicine residencies added oral health as a requirement (ACGME, 2007a; STFM, 2011b). Yet, a recent survey showed only three-quarters of the residency directors knew of this requirement, and only about two-thirds of the programs were actually including oral health content, with the most common training time being 2 hours per year (Douglass et al., 2009a). The development of an oral health curriculum for family medicine residency programs is discussed later in this chapter.

Internal Medicine Physicians

Oral health education is not a requirement for internal medicine residencies, although the geriatrics subspecialty requires education in oral health prevention, and the sleep medicine subspecialty requires residents to have experience receiving consults from oral maxillofacial surgeons (ACGME, 2008b, 2009a,b). In a survey of internal medicine trainees, 90 percent reported receiving no training on periodontal disease during medical school, and 23 percent said they never referred patients to dentists (Quijano et al., 2010).

Obstetrics-Gynecology

Little is known about advanced education and training in oral health for obstetrician-gynecologists and oral health education is not a requirement for residencies in obstetrics and gynecology (ACGME, 2008a). There is some limited evidence that while obstetrician-gynecologists recognize the importance of good oral health during pregnancy, they may not incorporate it fully into their practice patterns (Morgan et al., 2009; Strafford et al., 2008; Wilder et al., 2007). For example, a national survey of obstetrician-gynecologists showed that while 84 percent of respondents agreed that routine dental care is important during pregnancy, 69 percent do not routinely provide oral care information to their pregnant patients, 77 percent do not advise pregnant patients to get routine dental care, and only 54 percent reported performing an oral examination as part of their prenatal care (Morgan et al., 2009). In this same survey, 85 percent of respondents said "the quality of their training in oral health issues was inadequate to nonexistent" (Morgan et al., 2009).

Nurses

The nursing workforce is composed of 3.1 million nurses including over 140,000 nurse practitioners (NPs) (ANA, 2011a,b). Basic professional nursing education includes mouth care and nurses could be educated to do oral health assessments as part of routine basic care for patients across the life span. However, in general, nurses have not placed a high priority on oral health (Clemmens and Kerr, 2008), and the training of nurses in oral health and hygiene is highly variable and often inadequate (Jablonski, 2010). Criteria set by the National Task Force on Quality Nurse Practitioner Education do not delineate any specific competencies for oral health (National Task Force on Quality Nurse Practitioner Education, 2008).

NPs in particular may have an important role to play in oral health care as a recent study found "substantial parallels" in the education and practice of dentists and nurses (Spielman et al., 2005). NPs have been defined as primary care providers (IOM, 1996) and can see patients independently and perform histories and physicals, perform lab tests, and diagnose and treat both acute and chronic conditions. NPs emphasize health promotion and disease prevention and especially focus on the health of individuals in the context of their families and communities. NPs commonly practice in rural areas and HPSAs, and the growth of the profession, in part, is due to their role in caring for underserved populations (Everett et al., 2009; Grumbach et al., 2003; Harper and Johnson, 1998). As such, they may serve as a frontline screening source for oral health disease. NPs have been shown to provide high-quality care (as compared with physicians), be cost effective, have high levels of patient satisfaction with their care, and contribute to increased productivity (Hooker and Berlin, 2002; Hooker et al., 2005; Lenz et al., 2004; Mezey et al., 2005; Mundinger et al., 2000; Sox Jr., 1979; Todd et al., 2004; Wilson et al., 2005).

In addition to NPs, there are over 3 million assistive personnel (e.g., nurse aides) who work in places where dental professionals generally do not (e.g., assisted living facilities, home health agencies) (PHI, 2010). In nursing home settings, certified nursing assistants often provide oral hygiene care for residents, but they may be unprepared for this task, having inadequate knowledge, and thus may make it a low priority (Chalmers, 1996; Coleman and Watson, 2006; Jablonski et al., 2009). For example, one survey of nursing assistants in nursing homes found they generally regarded tooth loss as "a natural consequence of aging" (Jablonski et al., 2009).

In 2005, a group of faculty from the Arizona School of Health Sciences and the Arizona School of Dentistry and Oral Health developed a set of eight general oral health competencies for NPs and physician assistants (PAs) (see Box 3-4). While these competencies have not been approved by any professional body, they reflect a combination of the evidence base

BOX 3-4
General Oral Health Competencies for Physician Assistants and Nurse Practitioners

1. Have the ability to do a thorough and competent oral examination
2. Be able to discern between normal and abnormal structures
3. Be able to discern obvious pathology and conditions of the oral cavity (e.g., oral cancers, fungal infections, traumatic conditions, dental diseases, congenital conditions)
4. Be able to inform adults and parents of young children what to expect in eruption patterns of primary and permanent teeth
5. Be able to recognize symptoms and manifestations of common diseases of the oral cavity
6. Be able to recognize oral symptoms of systemic diseases (e.g., anemia, syphilis, tuberculosis, thyroid dysfunction, Sjogren's disease, xerostomia)
7. Understand what various dental specialties can do for your patients
8. Improve PA/NP-dental interface and referrals

SOURCE: Danielsen et al., 2006.

as well as the knowledge and skills that dentists think these professionals should have.

A survey of NPs regarding these proposed competencies showed that the majority do not feel prepared for basic competencies such as performing a thorough oral exam (58 percent), recognizing oral symptoms of systemic disease (78 percent), or discerning obvious oral pathology (60 percent) (Danielsen et al., 2006). In the same survey, PAs and NPs (answering together) thought they should have competence in performing the exam (77 percent), recognizing oral symptoms of systemic disease (79 percent), and discerning obvious pathology (88 percent). Further, in a different survey of NPs, only 19 percent thought their knowledge of oral cancers was current (Siriphant et al., 2001).

Pharmacists

As health care professionals in community settings, pharmacists are often involved in health promotion and disease prevention activities such as public health education, health screenings, and the provision of vaccines. In 2008, pharmacists held almost 270,000 jobs; about 65 percent worked in retail settings and 22 percent worked in hospitals (BLS, 2009a). The BLS notes a likely increase in the need for pharmacists to provide services in settings such as doctors' offices and nursing facilities as well as to increasingly offer patient care services, such as the administration of vaccines (BLS, 2009a).

In regards to oral health specifically, customers may approach pharmacists regarding the treatment of oral health conditions such as mouth ulcers, cold sores, and persistent pain (Cohen et al., 2009; Macleod et al., 2003; Sowter and Raynor, 1997; Weinberg and Maloney, 2007). Pharmacists can have an important role in the management and treatment of oral disease such as through education on selection and use of daily oral hygiene products as well as referrals to dentists. No formal assessment has been done to evaluate the extent and depth of education and instruction that pharmacy students receive regarding oral health.

Physician Assistants

As primary care providers, PAs also have great opportunities and responsibilities to be involved in oral health care (Berg and Coniglio, 2006; Danielsen et al., 2006). PAs work under the supervision of a physician, but they can often work apart from the physician's direct presence and can prescribe medications and bill for health care services. The BLS projects the PA profession to be the seventh fastest growing occupation between 2008 and 2018 (BLS, 2010a). In 2008, PAs held about 74,800 jobs (BLS, 2009b). More than half of these jobs were located in physicians' offices, and about one-quarter were in hospitals.

About half of PAs work in family medicine or general medicine (Brugna et al., 2007; Hooker and Berlin, 2002). Like NPs, PAs are an especially important source of care for rural communities, low-income and minority populations, and in HPSAs (Everett et al., 2009; Grumbach et al., 2003) and have been shown to produce cost-effective care with quality of care comparable with physicians (Ackermann and Kemle, 1998; Brugna et al., 2007; Jones and Cawley, 1994; Sox, 1979; Wilson et al., 2005).

Most PA programs follow the traditional curricula of medical schools (Hooker and Berlin, 2002), and while some PAs receive advanced training, the bulk of the advanced programs focus on surgical and emergency care (APPAP, 2008). Very little is known about the extent of oral health education in the PA curricula. As in nurse practitioner programs, standards set by the Accreditation Review Commission on Education for the Physician Assistant (ARC-PA) do not delineate any specific competencies for oral health (ARC-PA, 2010). A survey of PA program directors found "over 74 [percent] believed that dental disease prevention should be addressed in PA education, yet only 21 [percent] of programs actually did so" (Jacques et al., 2010). The number of curriculum hours dedicated to oral health ranged from 0 to 14 hours, with an average of 3.6 hours.

In the previously mentioned survey regarding proposed competencies (see Box 3-4), only 53 percent of PAs indicated they were competent at performing an oral exam, 63 percent could "discern obvious pathology and conditions of the oral cavity," and 34 percent could "recognize oral symptoms of systemic diseases" (Danielsen et al., 2006). Interestingly, 10 percent of PAs did not think it was important for them to understand what the various dental specialties could do for their patients (compared to 2 percent of NPs) (Danielsen et al., 2006).

The PA profession has started to address its lack of attention to oral health care. For example, the Duke University Physician Assistant Program has developed two online modules for oral health (Duke University, 2011). Further, as part of its 2010–2012 strategic plan, the American Academy of Physician Assistants (AAPA) cited one of its goals as being to "improve access to preventive health services by increasing the proportion of PAs in all specialties who are delivering oral health care" (AAPA, 2010). In addition, in 2010 the AAPA held a Physician Assistant Leadership Oral Health Summit that included leaders from the physician assistant profession as well as from dentistry and family medicine (Statler, 2010). A second summit will be held in July 2011.[11]

PUBLIC HEALTH WORKERS

Public health workers include many of the professions previously mentioned, including both dental and nondental health care professionals. Public health generally refers to efforts to promote health and prevent disease for populations. As with other segments of the health care workforce, the public health workforce is difficult to enumerate due to the variety of professions involved, lack of a common taxonomy for job titles and duties, and a lack of a single comprehensive licensure or certification process for public health (HRSA, 2000). Little is known about the extent of training in oral health among schools of public health. A 2001 survey of schools of public health showed that 60 percent of schools had no faculty with a degree in dentistry or dental hygiene (Tomar, 2006). In addition, only 15 percent of schools offered a master of public health degree with a concentration in dental public health.

The predecessor to the present-day American Association of Public Health Dentistry was established in 1937, and represents a variety of public health professionals involved in oral health care (AAPHD, 2004). In 1948, the Association of State and Territorial Dental Directors was established to

[11] Personal communication, C. Evans, University of Illinois, Chicago, February 9, 2011.

represent the directors and staff of state dental public health programs and is currently an affiliate of the Association of State and Territorial Health Officials (ASTDD, 2011). In 1951, the ADA recognized dental public health as a specialty of dentistry (AAPHD, 2004). In 2005, estimates of the number of public health dentists ranged from 153 (the number of diplomats of the American Board of Public Health Dentistry) to 498 (the number of dentist members of the American Association of Public Health Dentistry) to 543 (the number of members in the ADA directory reporting a specialty of dental public health) (Tomar, 2005). The role of state and local health departments is discussed further in Chapter 4.

Members of the community themselves also contribute to health improvement through the efforts of individuals who become part of the public health workforce. For example, in communities across the United States, community health workers (known as *promotoras* in the Hispanic community) link community members to systems of care, help to mobilize communities to change the conditions for health, and conduct health education. Community workers seem to be most effective when they are selected from among individuals who are respected and trusted by their communities. In addition to their knowledge of the community's needs, their formal participation in the public health enterprise may also reassure community groups that are wary of government systems or health care providers for political, economic, or other reasons. In general health care, the use of community health workers has been shown to increase utilization of health care services and improve outcomes (Babamoto et al., 2009; Brownstein et al., 2005; Lewin et al., 2010; O'Brien et al., 2010; Rosenthal et al., 2010; Viswanathan et al., 2010; Whitley et al., 2006).

INTERPROFESSIONAL EDUCATION, TRAINING, AND CARE

The importance of the interaction between dentists and other health care professionals has been recognized for nearly a century (Dunning, 1958; Rauh, 1917). More recently, in 2001, the ADA stated that "A formal dialogue among all health care professions should be established to develop a plan for greater cooperation and integration of knowledge in medical and dental predoctoral education, hospital settings, continuing education programs, and research facilities" (ADA, 2001). Still, health care professionals are typically trained separately by discipline. As a result, professionals may gain little understanding of or appreciation for the expertise of other professionals or the skills needed to effectively participate on a team, including how and when to refer patients to each other and how to best communicate with each other.

The Value of Interprofessional Care

The value of interprofessional care, especially to care for patients with complex care needs, and the importance of interprofessional education and training has been increasingly acknowledged (Baum and Axtell, 2005; Blue et al., 2010; Buelow et al., 2008; Dodds et al., 2010; Dyer, 2003; Fulmer et al., 2005; Hall and Weaver, 2001; Howe and Sherman, 2006; Lerner et al., 2009; Misra et al., 2009; O'Leary et al., 2010; Wilder et al., 2008; Williams et al., 2006). In particular, evidence is growing that interprofessional care leads to better care coordination, and, ultimately, better patient outcomes, improved satisfaction, and cost savings (Hammick et al., 2007; HHS, 2010; McKinnon and Jorgenson, 2009; Reeves et al., 2008, 2010; Snyder et al., 2010). While more professionals are gaining experience in interprofessional training, little evidence exists to determine which methods are best for imparting the knowledge and skills necessary to work as a team member, how such training affects patterns of practice, or how it affects patient outcomes (Cooper et al., 2001; Hall and Weaver, 2001; Remington et al., 2006; Thistlethwaite and Moran, 2010).

HHS supports interprofessional education and training through such vehicles as the Title VII interdisciplinary, community-based grant programs that are designed to promote interdisciplinary care and increase access to care for underserved populations and in underserved areas. In January 2010, the Advisory Committee on Training in Primary Care Medicine and Dentistry recommended that "training grants should provide funds to develop, implement, and evaluate training programs that promote interprofessional practice in the Patient-Centered Medical-Dental Home model of care" (HHS, 2010). They also stated that "funding should support clinical sites that prepare trainees for inter-professional practice by educating medical, dental, physician assistant, and other trainees together on health care teams."

Interprofessional Care in Oral Health

Within oral health, two levels of team care may exist—first among dental professionals and second among various health care professionals. The federal government has a history of training dental professionals to work together more effectively. For example, in the 1960s, the predecessor to the modern-day HHS was actively involved in promoting workforce innovations such as dental auxiliary utilization, otherwise known as four-handed dentistry, and dental school-based training in expanded auxiliary management programs (Gladstone and Garcia, 2007; Johnson, 1969). These educational initiatives were designed to spur the adoption of team care in dentistry with each member of the dental team working up to the capacity of his or her training, in order to provide more care at less cost. More research will be needed for understanding the dynamics of the dental team as new types of dental professionals emerge. For example, a recent study of registered dental hygienists in alternative practice (RDHAP) in independent practice in California showed that nearly 48 percent found it "difficult" or "somewhat difficult" to find a dentist willing to accept their referrals (Mertz and Glassman, 2011).

Little research exists on the education and training of dental professionals and nondental professionals together in caring for mutual patients who have complex oral health needs. One exemplar is the creation of craniofacial teams. In 1962, the predecessor to the National Institute of Dental and Craniofacial Research funded the first multidisciplinary study of cleft palate, at the University of Pittsburgh Health Center (NIH, 2010), a team-based approach spearheaded since the 1930s by Dr. Herbert K. Cooper, an orthodontist in Lancaster, Pennsylvania (Long, 2009). Such an approach is now the standard of care for the management of children with cleft palate. However, there are no robust data on the impact of interprofessional training leading to interprofessional practice or on improving oral health outcomes.

REGULATING THE DENTAL WORKFORCE

Regulation of the health care workforce occurs at several levels. The primary role of the federal government is to protect consumers and promote fair competition. The bulk of activity to regulate the health professions occurs at the state level. In spite of national standards for education, each state develops its own statute for each health care profession, which establishes requirements for who may enter a profession, what competency requirements must be satisfied for licensure, and what services the professional may provide. Finally, the private sector can be involved in the healthcare workforce in that they often offer voluntary certification that may be required to practice in some states. For professions and occupations without licensure requirements, certification is one source of information and assurance of quality for consumers.

The Role of the Federal Government

The Federal Trade Commission (FTC) is charged by Congress to prevent "unfair methods of competition in or affecting commerce, and unfair or deceptive acts or practices in or affecting commerce,"[12] including the enforcement of antitrust laws and other basic consumer protection laws.

[12] 15 U.S.C. §45.

The FTC and the Department of Justice (DOJ) advocate against the actions of professions that limit or prevent competition for the delivery of health care services by another profession (e.g., scope of practice laws or licensure restrictions) without providing countervailing consumer benefit (Chiarello, 2009).

As the FTC often does not have institutional expertise in specific professions, it provides guidance but leaves ultimate decision making to legislators and others to determine proper constraints on competition. The FTC suggests a four-part test for legislators to use in assessing their regulations (Chiarello, 2009). First is whether the regulation restricts competition. This often applies in the health care professions, since scope of practice laws by definition limit who can perform a particular service. Second is whether the restriction benefits consumers in a way that would not exist without the regulation. This often relates to consumer safety in that the restriction might prevent incompetent individuals from providing services. Third is consideration of the costs versus benefits to the consumer. That is, would the consumer gain more if restrictions were removed, such as through increased provider access. Finally, is the consideration of whether there is a less restrictive way to achieve the same goal. For example, is foreclosing competition to a certain group of professionals less or more restrictive than changing the competency requirements of that profession?

Some have argued that health care practice is not consistent with the economic principles of competition in which rivals compete to satisfy the demands of well-informed consumers (Feinstein, 2009; FTC and DOJ, 2004). There are several ways in which economic principles of market forces fail in health care. First, consumers are not particularly well informed—either as to the quality of care they receive or, in the case of insured individuals, to the true cost of services (FTC and DOJ, 2004). Also, health care professionals do not necessarily benefit financially for providing higher-quality care. Finally, market principles of competition do not help individuals who cannot pay for the demanded services (FTC and DOJ, 2004).

In the 1980s and 1990s, the FTC advocated on behalf of consumers in a number of states on legislation or regulation regarding scope of practice or supervision, advertising restrictions, or other anticompetitive behavior. In recent years, the FTC has been involved in two notable cases directly related to oral health. In 2000, the South Carolina legislature changed supervision requirements for dental hygienists to allow the delivery of preventive services in school settings without the direct presence of a dentist (FTC, 2010, 2011). The following year, the South Carolina Board of Dentistry enacted an emergency regulation to reinstate the supervision requirement, and in 2003, the legislature amended the law to reflect the regulation. The FTC subsequently brought an antitrust action against the board for reasons of unfair competition that would lead to the loss of preventive services for thousands of children (Chiarello, 2009). More recently, the FTC became involved in actions surrounding in-school dental clinics. A 2009 state bill (HB 687) supported by the Louisiana Dental Association sought to make it illegal for anyone to provide school-based oral health care for a fee (FTC, 2009; Moller, 2010). In a May 2009 statement to the Louisiana house of representatives, the FTC noted the evidence base in favor of school-based dental programs and the lack of evidence for harm, and stated that "HB 687 restricts competition among dentists and does not appear to provide any countervailing benefits" (FTC, 2009).

The Role of States

Like other health care professions, dental professions are regulated on a state-by-state basis through statutes and regulation promulgated, interpreted, and enforced by boards of dentistry or dental examiners, or committees of those boards. A discussion by Safriet on scope of practice legislation and regulation for health professions describes the complexities of affecting change in the legislative arena to increase access to services (Safriet, 2002). At one level, she argues, laws and regulations are structured to protect the public, address patients' rights, provide accountability, encourage quality, and promote equitable access. At another level, laws and regulations establish professional autonomy or professional control of another group and help to control competition, support market share, and preserve financial gain. In 2007, Dower and colleagues noted that decisions on scope of practice often lack robust evidence bases, and that strong lobbying groups play a significant role in shaping legislation (Dower et al., 2007). The authors noted that independent committees are increasingly being used to review proposed expansions in scope of practice.

Scope of Practice and the Health Care Professions

Professional battles and controversy over expanding a profession's scope of practice are not new to the health care professions or unique to oral health care (Carson-Smith and Minarik, 2007; Daly, 2006; Huijbregts, 2007; RCHWS, 2003; Wing et al., 2004). The delegation of job responsibilites has been seen across the spectrum of the health care workforce as lesser trained workers take on increasingly complex duties. Nurse practitioners, for example, are largely seen as well-accepted members of the health care team, and there is a growing evidence base that attests to the quality of their care as compared to physicians (Lenz et al., 2004; Mundinger et al., 2000; Schulman et al., 1995; Sox, 1979; Wilson et al., 2005). In spite of this, their initial development was resisted, and extension of their scopes of practice remains a sensitive issue (Gardner, 2010; Hayes,

1985; Nelson, 2006; Office of Technology Assessment, 1986; Schachtel, 1978; Sharp, 1996; Sorrel, 2010; Sullivan and Rohlfsen, 2007). Professional tensions typically center around the quality of care (e.g., safety) provided by individuals with less training, but in many cases, evidence has not supported this. For example, advanced practice nurses are often involved in high-risk procedures such as childbirth and the administration of anesthesia, yet the evidence base continues to grow that the quality of their care is similar to that of physicians (Dulisse and Cromwell, 2010; MacDorman and Singh, 1998; Oakley et al., 1996; Rosenblatt et al., 1997). These examples may not track perfectly to serve as a comparison for some of the newer models of dental professionals (discussed later in this chapter) as PAs and NPs often have many more years of postsecondary education and training in comparison to some of these models (ADA, 2011a). However, they provide some insight for the development and use of multiple provider types. For decades, many have called for states to standardize entry-to-practice requirements (in part to improve the ability of professionals to move from state to state) and for state practice acts to be based on competence (Altschuler, 1994; Christian et al., 2007; Dower et al., 2007; Finocchio et al., 1995; Safriet, 1994). Several previous IOM reports have supported the idea of expanding scope of practice in alignment with professional competencies. In a 2008 IOM study of the health care workforce for older adults, the committee stated

> health care providers of all levels of education and training will need to assume additional responsibilities—or relinquish some responsibilities that they already have—to help ensure that all members of the health care workforce are used at their highest level of competence. (IOM, 2008)

In a 2010 IOM study of the nursing workforce, the committee recommended "Advanced practice registered nurses should be able to practice to the full extent of their education and training" (IOM, 2010). Specifically, that committee recommended that the FTC and the DOJ "Review existing and proposed state regulations concerning advanced practice registered nurses to identify those that have anticompetitive effects without contributing to the health and safety of the public" (IOM, 2010).

Structure of State Dental Boards

Dentists represent the overwhelming majority of members on state dental boards; it is common for the highest-level professional to be overrepresented on professional boards. Over 20 years ago, the IOM criticized the makeup of state health professions' licensing boards, especially in regards to the allied health professions, stating

> Licensing boards should draw at least half of their membership from outside the licensed occupation; members should be drawn from the public as well as from a variety of areas of expertise such as health administration, economics, consumer affairs, education, and health services research. (IOM, 1989)

Boards of dentistry typically regulate the dental hygiene profession, but as of August 2010, 17 states had either established dental hygiene advisory committees to the state dental board or enabled varying degrees of self-regulation for dental hygienists (ADHA, 2010a). This is similar to physician assistants; physician assistants are largely regulated by state boards of medicine, but several states have developed advisory committees or boards of physician assistants (AAPA, 2011). When one class of professionals is regulated by a different group of professionals, it is difficult to effect change in scope of practice to reflect the natural evolution of a profession (Dower et al., 2007; FTC and DOJ, 2004; Nolan et al., 2003). As a result of the current regulatory configurations in oral health, there is often tension between dentists and dental hygienists over requirements for practice in the profession (e.g., education, professional liability) and expansion in permissions or scope.

The primary purpose of a state dental board, like other health professional boards, is specifically to protect the interests of the public. However in a recent survey, 52 percent of dentists thought that the primary purpose of the state dental board was to protect the interest of dentists, and 32 percent thought they protected the interests of *both* dentists and the general public (Malcmacher, 2011).

Dental Scope of Practice, Supervision, and Ownership

Scope of practice laws and regulations in oral health generally distinguish between preventive and restorative procedures as proxies for the divide between services considered to be within the exclusive scope of dentists and those that are permitted or may be delegated to other dental professionals. While provision of preventive care and education by nondentists is generally accepted in the United States, some cite concerns for quality of care when considering permitting nondentists to provide restorative services (ADA, 2011a; AGD, 2008; GDA, 2010). Variations in permissible practice among the states are broad, especially for dental hygienists and dental assistants (ADAA/DANB Alliance, 2005; HRSA, 2004). Laws and rules governing dental professionals are often proscriptive describing explicit parameters on

- Particular tasks that can or cannot be performed,
- The exact settings in which particular services can be provided, and
- The conditions under which allied professionals may work (e.g., levels of requisite supervision, mandates for preauthorization by dentists).

State boards not only manage and interpret state dental practice acts, but they also promulgate rules to address practical issues including how many dental professionals may be supervised by a dentist, whether dental hygienists are permitted to supervise dental assistants, and who can own a dental practice or employ dental professionals (known as corporate practice rules). Both the ADA and the Academy of General Dentistry support legislation that restricts the ownership and operation of dental practices to dentists licensed in that state (ADA, 2010d; AGD, 2011). As in medicine, where physicians are given significant latitude to delegate to other health professions, in dentistry, dentists have the autonomy to delegate tasks at their professional discretion.

Impact on Access to Care

While restricting scope of practice is generally attributed to protecting consumers from unsafe or untrained professionals, data suggest that restrictive licensure laws in oral health are not tied to better health outcomes or supported by scientific evidence; in fact, stringent laws have been tied to increased consumer costs, which may restrict an individual's ability to access care (IOM, 1989; Kleiner and Kudrle, 2000; Shepard, 1978). Licensure laws also affect wages and employment opportunities. Studies show that more restrictive laws lead to increased income for dentists, while less restriction leads to decreased income and employment growth for dentists and greater income and employment opportunities for dental hygienists (Kleiner and Kudrle, 2000; Kleiner and Park, 2010; Shepard, 1978; Wanchek, 2010).

The Role of the Private Sector

Certification is a voluntary process by which a private organization imposes a certain level of standards, either through testing or some other method, in order to become "certified." Certification is often used as a measure of competence, especially in professions that do not have a formal licensure. The Dental Assisting National Board estimates that almost 12 percent of dental assistants in the United States are certified dental assistants (CDAs) (ADAA/DANB Alliance, 2005). The CDA credential is a nationally recognized credential offered by the Dental Assisting National

Board. Certification as a dental assistant requires passage of a three-part written examination in the areas of radiation health and safety, infection control, and general chairside assisting. More than 32,000 dental assistants have CDA certification (DANB, 2010). Currently 28 states recognize or require CDA certification to perform expanded duties, and a total of 37 states plus the District of Columbia recognize or require one or more components of the full CDA exam for particular expanded functions (e.g., Radiation Health and Safety Exam, Infection Control Exam) (DANB, 2010).

Dental technicians can voluntarily become certified dental technicians by the National Board for Certification in Dental Laboratory Technology, an independent board established by the National Association of Dental Laboratories (BLS, 2010e). Three states (Kentucky, South Carolina, and Texas) require this certification. Certification exists for the manufacture of crowns and bridges, ceramics, partial dentures, complete dentures, and orthodontic appliances. In Florida, dental laboratories must register with the state, and at least one technician must meet requirements for continuing education (18 hours every 2 years) (BLS, 2010e).

INNOVATIONS IN THE ORAL HEALTH CARE WORKFORCE

The following sections provide descriptions of an array of workforce innovations being used to improve access to oral health care. These examples include improving the diversity of the workforce, enhancing the education of health care professionals, encouraging the participation of nondental health care professionals, expanding the roles of existing dental professionals, and developing new types of dental professionals. In some cases, these innovations are too new to have robust outcomes data for impact on access to care or oral health status, especially in the long term, and therefore the committee does not intend to imply that it is recommending these approaches. In addition, these examples are not exhaustive of all of the strategies being used across the nation. Instead, they serve to illustrate the wide variety of ideas and opportunities for improving how the oral health care workforce is recruited, educated, trained, and used in order to improve access to care for vulnerable and underserved populations.

Innovations in Recruitment

Bridge and pipeline programs are two strategies used to promote awareness, increase enrollment, and foster retention of students from URM, lower-income, and rural populations into the oral health professions. In the literature, *bridge* and *pipeline* are sometimes used interchangeably. Technically, *bridge programs* are interventions that focus on prebaccalaureate (e.g., elementary school students through high school graduates), and *pipeline programs* are interventions that focus on undergraduate and pre-professional program populations. Key features of both types of programs include outreach to URM, lower-income, and rural students (sometimes as early as elementary school), community-based education opportunities, mentoring, and financial aid.

Bridge Programs

Bridge programs have a long history in specific health professions (e.g., medicine, nursing, and dentistry) (Awé and Bauman, 2010; Brooks et al., 2002; Kim et al., 2009; Lewis, 1996). For example, through its Bridge to Dentistry program, the Baylor College of Dentistry collaborated with local school districts, colleges and universities, community organizations, dental clinics, and community dentists to provide outreach, enrichment, and mentoring opportunities. Enrollment of URM students increased by 325 percent and subsequently, the school retained 91 percent of its URM students (Brooks, 2005; Brooks et al., 2002). More recently, the University of Minnesota School of Dentistry initiated the Building Bridges program with funding from HRSA's Health Careers Opportunity Program.[13] In partnership with the local school district, the university, and community-based organizations, the school of dentistry recruits middle school, high school, and college students from URM communities to participate in weekend and summer enrichment programs with community-based education experiences and mentoring.

Pipeline Education Programs

The pipeline strategy has been used in a variety of health professions (e.g., medicine, nursing, and dentistry) (Brunson et al., 2010; Cantor et al., 1998; Formicola et al., 2010; Grumbach and Chen, 2006; Hesser et al., 1996; Rackley et al., 2003; Thomson et al., 2010). In 2009, HRSA's Bureau of Health Professions and the Office of Minority Health conducted a review of studies and evaluations of diversity-oriented pipeline programs and concluded that

> These studies consistently indicate that pipeline interventions are associated with positive outcomes for racial/ethnic minority and disadvantaged students on several meaningful metrics, including academic performance and the likelihood of enrolling in a health professions school. (HHS, 2009)

---

[13] For more information, visit http://www.dentistry.umn.edu/programs_admissions/BuildingBridges/home.html.

Yet, there is scant research on which specific program components and approaches yield the greatest results and few studies that document the long-term effectiveness of pipeline programs (Thomson et al., 2010). As one recent study suggests, it may be necessary to track program participants for as many as 10 to 15 years to accurately assess the impact of pipeline programs (Winkleby, 2007).

The Dental Pipeline Program

Between 2001 and 2010, the Robert Wood Johnson Foundation (RWJF), in collaboration with the California Endowment and the W.K. Kellogg Foundation, supported the *Pipeline, Profession, and Practice: Community-Based Dental Education* initiative with two primary goals:

1. Increase the time that senior dental students spend in community clinics and private practices providing care to underserved populations.
2. Increase enrollment of low-income and URM students in dental school (Bailit and Formicola, 2010).

An initial round of funding provided an average of $1.3 million to 15 dental schools for program development and implementation (Chard et al., 2009). A second round of funding included 14 additional dental schools (Bailit and Formicola, 2010). Program profiles, including activities, accomplishments, and community partners, can be found on the RWJF project website.[14] Two recent supplemental issues of the *Journal of Dental Education* were devoted to the dental pipeline program. The first included an extensive evaluation of the program (Leviton, 2009a,b). The second described specific strategies for successful implementation of pipeline programs (Lavizzo-Mourey, 2010). In addition to these journals, there is a substantial literature related to dental pipeline programs (Andersen et al., 2005; Markel et al., 2008; Price et al., 2007; Thind et al., 2008; Veal et al., 2004). The following are some key findings:

- There was a 54 percent increase in the first year enrollment of URM students in the first phase of the program (compared to 16 percent in nonpipeline schools during the same time period) (Andersen et al., 2009; Formicola et al., 2010).
- Over the course of the program, pipeline schools increased the time senior students spent in community sites from an average of 10 days to 50 days (Formicola et al., 2010).

---

[14] See http://www.dentalpipeline.org.

- Based on the number of patients served by pipeline programs, one study estimated, "If all dental schools assigned senior students and pediatric and general dentistry residents to community clinics and private practices for 70 days per year, about 2 million more low-income patients would receive care" (Formicola et al., 2009).

A review of effective outreach and recruitment programs found that a number of strategies appear to have been especially effective, including summer enrichment programs, mentoring, and regional/collaborative outreach efforts (Brunson et al., 2010). Partnerships with affiliated medical schools and scholarship or loan programs were also noted as important elements of effective programs (Brunson et al., 2010).

However, the successes of the pipeline program represent small gains in national enrollment among URM students, and results were variable across schools (Brunson et al., 2010). Moreover, it has yet to be determined whether these programs will have a long-term impact on increasing diversity in the dental profession. Evidence suggests that pipeline programs require both a sustained commitment by participating schools and sufficient resources to maintain momentum (Brunson et al., 2010; Thind et al., 2009).

Innovations in Dental Education

As discussed previously, most dental schools are now moving toward adding community-based education to their curricula for both educational and financial reasons. In particular, community-based dental education has been associated with students' improved confidence and willingness to care for vulnerable and underserved populations. The Pipeline, Profession, and Practice program described above gives one example of an innovation to move dental education into community settings. Below, several schools of dentistry are highlighted as examples of other innovations in dental education.

The Arizona School of Dentistry & Oral Health

The Arizona School of Dentistry & Oral Health focuses on training dental students to become community-based educational leaders for populations in need. In that regard, the school officials look to recruit students with diverse backgrounds who show commitment to serving communities in need.For example, one of the main criteria of admission is the documented demonstration of previous community service (ASDOH, 2011). In their fourth year, students spend half of their time outside the school including sites such as community health settings and Indian Health Service clinics. About one-quarter of graduating classes went to work in community health centers (Dillenberg, 2009; Hood, 2009). Finally, every student graduates with a certificate in public health, which is a requirement for graduation.

East Carolina University School of Dental Medicine

The East Carolina University School of Dental Medicine was developed with capital funding from the North Carolina general assembly in response to the state's significant access disparities (Chadwick and Hupp, 2008). Scheduled to start admitting predoctoral students in 2011, the school seeks to build its educational program with a focus on primary care for rural and undeserved populations. To this end, the school will build up to 10 service learning centers in underserved and rural areas of North Carolina that will operate to train dental students and residents while acting as a safety net provider for underserved populations in the state. Senior dental students will spend up to 24 weeks in these centers providing care and learning how to work in a delivery system that functions more like a private practice than a traditional dental school clinic. The centers will include faculty, general and pediatric dentistry residents, dental hygienists, dental assistants, and senior dental students (Bailit and D'Adamo, 2010; Chadwick and Hupp, 2008). Features include

1. Senior students will treat at least six to seven patients per day;
2. Faculty will practice as they supervise residents and students;
3. Residents will have some responsibility for supervising students; and
4. Centers will be operated by a professional management team.

When fully operational, the centers are expected to average 150,000 or more visits annually (Bailit, 2010). It is important to emphasize that the clinical education strategy is feasible because of the availability of an enhanced Medicaid reimbursement rate (discussed further in Chapter 5).

West Virginia University School of Dentistry

The educational program at West Virginia University requires dental students to work in a rural practice for a 6-week rotation in their senior year. During these rotations, the dental students are housed with other health professions students and have formal interprofessional activities (Hood, 2009). In addition, students must perform 100 hours of approved community service over the 4 years of school. In 2007, 58 percent of graduates began practice in underserved areas of West Virginia (Hood, 2009).

Innovations in Nondental Education

Innovation in Medical School Education

The University of Washington Medical School created and has started to implement a comprehensive oral health curriculum for medical students; results show students have more confidence in identification of oral disease, and attitudes toward oral health care improved (Mouradian, 2010; Mouradian et al., 2005, 2006). The goals and competencies in oral health developed for this program are listed in Table 3-6.

Innovation in Graduate Medical Education

In 2005, the Society of Teachers of Family Medicine released *Smiles for Life*, a national oral health curriculum for improving the oral health training in family medicine residency programs (Douglass et al., 2007, 2009a; STFM, 2011b). This curriculum was developed with materials developed by dentists, physicians, and educators and within 2 years was adopted by most family medicine residency programs (STFM, 2011b). In 2008, a second edition was released in which the curriculum was expanded to reach all primary care providers, including physician assistants and nurse practitioners (STFM, 2011b). Finally, in June 2010, a third edition was released that added interactive, online learning modules for individual practitioners (STFM, 2011b). As of 2008, about two-thirds of family medicine residency directors reported using *Smiles for Life* materials in their residency programs (Douglass et al., 2009a).

The *Smiles for Life* curriculum consists of seven 45-minute modules and has been approved for continuing education credit by the American Academy of Family Physicians (STFM, 2011a). These modules address the nature, prevalence, and consequences of oral disease throughout the life cycle; the clinician role in preventing oral diseases and promoting oral health; basic risk assessment and examination; patient counseling; and the needs of special populations. *Smiles for Life* also provides online learning for primary care providers to apply fluoride varnish in their offices (STFM, 2011c). Completion of this module is required by many states as a prerequisite for reimbursement.

Innovation in Nursing Education

In 2005, New York University created a unique partnership in which a college of nursing was located within the college of dentistry. As part of the interdisciplinary educational model, pediatric nurse practitioner students work alongside dental students to provide care in school clinics and

TABLE 3-6
Oral Health Goals and Competencies for Medical Students

Goals for Student at Graduation	Competencies
Public Health	
Has dental public health knowledge, believes oral health is important, and that physicians have a role in oral health	Can describe which patients are at increased risk for oral diseases (low socioeconomic status/minority status, patients with special needs/disabilities, living in rural or underserved areas)
	Can describe barriers to access/utilization of dental services (lack of insurance or providers, cultural, geographic issues, etc.)
	Can describe importance and safety of public water fluoridation
	Can describe roles physicians can play in identification/prevention of oral disease
Dental Caries	
Has knowledge in caries prevention and can screen for caries and collaborate with dentists	Can describe caries process and sequelae
	Can screen for caries on exam
	Can assess risk factors for caries (i.e., socioeconomic status, diet, hygiene, lack of fluoride, caries in mother or siblings of children at risk, medicines with sugar or xerostomia, lack of access to dental care)
	Can counsel about caries process and prevention including diet/feeding, fluoride, oral hygiene (especially brushing with fluoridated toothpaste)
	Can counsel mothers about transmission of cariogenic bacteria to infants and need for maternal oral health care
	Can recommend regular dental care; refer to dentists appropriately

continued

TABLE 3-6 *Continued*

Goals for Student at Graduation	Competencies
Periodontal Disease	
Has knowledge in periodontal disease prevention and recognition, and can collaborate with dentists	Can describe periodontal disease, sequelae
	Can screen for periodontal disease
	Can counsel about periodontal disease prevention (smoking/tobacco, oral hygiene, including brushing and flossing, role of medications in treating, or promoting periodontal disease)
	Can recommend regular dental care and refer to dentists appropriately
	Can counsel patients about systemic importance of periodontal disease (e.g., can affect diabetic control; possible linkages with prematurity/low birth weight, heart disease)
	Can counsel pregnant patients about pregnancy gingivitis and the need for regular dental care
Oral Cancer	
Has knowledge of oral cancer risk factors and can screen for oral cancer and counsel patients	Can screen for oral malignancy on exam
	Can assess risk factors for malignancy (smoking, tobacco/alcohol use)
	Can counsel patients about prevention strategies (prevention/cessation of smoking, tobacco, and alcohol use)
Oral-Systemic Health Interactions	
Has understanding of important oral-systemic interactions and can monitor for these	Can monitor impact of oral health on nutrition (especially in infants/elderly and special populations)
	Can monitor oral impact of medications, including erosion, caries, and periodontal disease
	Can assess/treat oral conditions associated with AIDS, chemotherapy

SOURCE: Adapted from Mouradian et al., 2005.

Head Start programs (Garcia et al., 2010; Hallas and Shelley, 2009). This allows the pediatric nurse practitioner students to learn about caries risk assessment and how to apply fluoride varnish while the dental students can become more familiar with the role of the advanced practice nurse in oral health. Both sets of students also learn key skills in team-based care, including how to care for systemic oral health diseases.

Innovations That Enhance the Use of Nondental Professionals

One strategy for improving access to preventive services for oral health, especially for children, has been to expand the use of nondental health care professionals (Douglass et al., 2009b; Hallas, 2010; Hallas and Shelley, 2009; Okunseri et al., 2009). Nondental health care professionals can incorporate oral health into their routine exams and wellness visits with basic risk assessments, oral exams, anticipatory guidance, and the provision of basic preventive services (Cantrell, 2009; Morrow et al., 2008; Riter et al., 2008). For example, fluoride varnish is increasingly being applied by nondental health care professionals and in community-based settings (AAP, 2011b; ASTDD, 2007).

One barrier to engaging nondental health care professionals is their inability to be reimbursed for some services through traditional medical insurance. Health insurance plans do not routinely cover oral health care. State Medicaid programs do provide coverage under the Early and Periodic Screening and Diagnostic Treatment benefit for children and adolescents receiving routine oral health care, but in the past, state Medicaid programs often did not allow nondental health care professionals to be reimbursed for preventive care in oral health. However, this is changing. In 2008, 25 state Medicaid programs reimbursed primary care providers for preventive services in oral health (Cantrell, 2008). In 2009, 34 states did so, and as of 2011, 40 states reimbursed for this care (AAP, 2011a; Cantrell, 2009). The types of services typically reimbursed include oral examination, screening, and risk assessment; anticipatory guidance and caregiver education; and application of fluoride varnish (Cantrell, 2009). Other barriers to engaging nondental health care professionals in preventive care can include the lack of appreciation of the importance of oral health, lack of confidence in their skills, skepticism on the efficacy of preventive services, and inadequate time in the patient visit (Lewis et al., 2000; Rozier et al., 2003).

State-Based Initiatives

Several individual state-based initiatives have arisen to help improve nondental health care professionals' involvement in providing basic preventive services for oral health. North Carolina's Into the Mouths of Babes program targets children from birth to age 3 (Rozier et al., 2003, 2010). The project aims to improve practitioners' oral health knowledge, incorporate caregiver counseling and fluoride varnish application into primary care practices, and increase screenings and dental referrals for children with oral diseases or are at risk for diseases (Close et al., 2010). In 2009, the North Carolina Department of Health and Human Services reported a 10-fold increase in the number of preventive procedures since the inception of the program (NC Department of Health and Human Services, 2009).

Another state-based example is Washington's Access to Baby and Child Dentistry (ABCD) program. Like Into the Mouths of Babes, ABCD is a collaborative effort to engage primary care providers in oral health care and includes training in oral health screening and fluoride varnish application, referral plans, and reimbursement for services rendered (Riter et al., 2008; Shirk, 2010). The University of Washington trains dentists to work with young children, local health departments enroll children and link them to dentists, case managers work with families to help them meet their appointments, and the state increased payment rates. Evaluations of the ABCD program show mixed results: the percentage of Medicaid children receiving dental care has increased and untreated dental decay has decreased among all children, but decay has increased among low-income children aged 3–5 (Shirk, 2010).

Innovations That Expand the Duties of Existing Professionals

Efforts to define scopes of practice for new and existing dental professionals have been plagued by a decades-long, contentious history (Dunning, 1958; Edelstein, 2010; Fales, 1958; Hammons and Jamison, 1967, 1968; Hammons et al., 1971; Nash, 2009; Nash and Willard, 2010). This section will look generally at expanding the functions of existing dental professionals. The creation of new types of dental professionals (either from existing professionals or de novo) is discussed subsequently.

Dental Assistants

As described earlier in this chapter, EFDAs may perform some limited restoration functions under the supervision of a dentist (Skillman et al., 2010). Studies of expanded functions for dental assistants in the United States began in the 1960s and showed that certain procedures could be effectively taught to dental assistants and that the quality of the procedures performed by the EFDAs was equivalent to that of dentists, as determined through measures of technical excellence (by the independent examination of dentists) (Abramowitz, 1972; Abramowitz and Berg, 1973). Both the U.S. Army Dental Command and the Indian Health Service (IHS) have programs to train and employ EFDAs (IHS, 2011; Luciano et al., 2006). As discussed previously, many states have allowed dental assistants to perform expanded duties under a variety of titles. For example, the Kansas legislature enabled a new category of oral health worker called scaling dental assistants who are allowed to perform dental hygiene services, including coronal scaling and polishing, after 90 hours of training (Mitchell et al., 2006).

Dental Hygienists

In the 1970s, several projects examined the effects of teaching both preventive and restorative procedures to dental hygienists. The Forsyth experiment (named for Massachusetts' Forsyth Dental Center), conducted between 1972 and 1974, focused on training dental hygienists in restorative care (Lobene and Kerr, 1979). The demonstration project was curtailed in 1974 because of litigation by the state dental board contending that permitting dental hygienists to drill teeth was a violation of the state dental practice act. However, evaluation research during that time showed that the clinical services provided were comparable in quality to dentists (based on existing measures of quality) (Lobene and Kerr, 1979). Examination of independent dental hygienists in a demonstration project in the 1990s again showed the high quality and consumer satisfaction associated with their care (Freed et al., 1997). In this case, quality was determined by practice structure (e.g., availability of appointments within 15 working days, infection control); process (e.g., documentation of follow-up to significant findings); and technical excellence (e.g., periodontal evaluation, calculus removal, quality of X-rays).

As of 2007, 47 percent of dental hygienists had the ability to perform some form of expanded function (ADHA, 2009b). As of June 2010, 32 states permit some form of direct access to dental hygienists in some circumstances (ADHA, 2010b). This means dental hygienists may perform dental hygiene assessment and provide dental hygiene services without the prior authorization or presence of a dentist, and maintain a provider–patient relationship.

As noted earlier in this chapter, as of 2010, 15 states had enabled direct reimbursement to dental hygienists through state Medicaid programs (ADHA, 2010c). There is no guarantee that independent practice will result in these professionals primarily serving vulnerable and underserved populations, as they may face similar financial challenges to caring for these patients as dentists do. For example, a study of the 17 independent practices of 20 dental hygienists in Colorado found the practices were located in areas also served by dentists and prophylaxis fees were generally the same as neighboring dentists (Brown et al., 2005). The authors concluded that the practices had not had a notable effect on access to care in Colorado.

However, a study of the 287 registered dental hygienists in alternative practice (RDHAPs) in California showed that RDHAPs primarily provide care to vulnerable and underserved patients in a variety of nontraditional settings (Mertz and Glassman, 2011). Notably, 68 percent of the RDHAP patients in residential facilities, 82 percent of the homebound patients, and 79 percent of the nursing home patients reported having no other source of dental care. In addition, 69 percent of RDHAP patients are medically compromised, 52 percent are physically disabled, and only 11 percent of RDHAP patients have private dental coverage. Only 14 percent of RDHAPs have an independent office-based practice, and 82 percent report also working in a traditional dental hygiene position.

As the role of dental hygienists expands, further consideration will be needed for the educational preparation of these professionals. If dental hygienists take on additional duties, care for patients with more complex health care needs, or practice in nontraditional settings, consideration will be needed for whether the basic dental hygiene educational program is adequate, or if dental hygienists with expanded duties also need advanced education and training, perhaps in the form of postgraduate education. Also, consideration will be needed for legal liability.

Innovations in Developing New Dental Professionals

Several new types of dental professionals have been proposed by stakeholders, ranging from entry-level workers to more highly educated and clinically trained professionals. While many of these models are based on expanding the duties of existing dental professionals, they are distinguished from the previous examples in that they have separate pathways for education and licensure or certification. These efforts have been controversial with some arguing for their potential ability to increase access, especially for vulnerable and underserved populations, and others voicing concerns for the quality of care provided by these practitioners and the creation of a two-tiered oral health care system (ADA, 2007; AGD, 2008; Edelstein, 2010; National Dental Association, 2010; Pew Center on the States and National Academy for State Health Policy, 2009). However, due to quality measurement and assessment challenges in oral health (see Chapter 2), there is limited ability to assess the quality of care provided by *any* dental professionals, which therefore makes comparison of care even more challenging. Further, more research will be needed to determine how these new professionals could be reimbursed, as well as how career ladders might be developed from the existing professions. The ACA authorized the secretary to award grants for demonstration programs to train or employ alternative dental health care providers in order to increase access for rural and underserved populations. However, Congress' FY 2011 budget explicitly prohibited the funding of these programs (ADA, 2011b).

The Dental Health Aide Therapist (DHAT) in Alaska

Most of the attention regarding new dental professionals centers on the DHAT model. Since the early 20th century, New Zealand and Australia have used professionals called dental therapists or dental nurses. Since then, this model has spread to over 40 countries around the world (APHA, 2006; Nash et al., 2008). Recently, the IHS gained some experience in training and deploying dental therapists to deliver basic dental care in remote tribal areas (Bolin, 2008; Fiset, 2005; Wetterhall et al., 2010). In 2003, the Alaska Native Tribal Health Consortium, in collaboration with tribal health organizations, began to send students for training in the 2-year New Zealand program under the authority of the federal Community Health Aide Program for Alaska Natives (DENTEX, 2010; GAO, 2010; Wetterhall et al., 2010). After training, each therapist had to complete a clinical preceptorship under direct supervision of a dentist for 3 months or 400 hours (whichever was longer) (GAO, 2010). By 2010, 10 DHATs were practicing in Alaskan villages working under remote consultative supervision of a dentist (Wetterhall et al., 2010).

International evidence speaks to the safety and quality of care (based on available measures) provided by dental therapists as compared to dentists and about their acceptance by the populations served (Ambrose et al., 1976; Gallagher and Wright, 2003; Ministry of Health Malaysia, 2005; Nash et al., 2008; Riordan et al., 1991; Sun et al., 2010). While the models used around the world operate in different economic and social climates, they provide insight toward the development of other similar models. The American Association of Public Health has expressed its support of the DHAT program (APHA, 2006). While assessments to date of DHATs in Alaska have focused on only five sites, data show that DHATs are performing within their scope of practice, patients are satisfied with their care, and there is no significant difference between the quality of the treatment provided by the DHATs as compared with dentists (Bader et al., 2011; Bolin, 2008; Wetterhall et al., 2010). The authors of these recent assessments note that quality was evaluated based on available qualitative measures and quantitative measures, including direct observation of technical excellence; blinded evaluations of technical excellence; performance of oral hygiene instruction; consultation with supervising dentists; chart reviews for procedures performed and any resultant complications; and community surveys of satisfaction.

Other New Dental Professionals

Several other models of new professionals are in existence or fairly well-established in their development and testing. These efforts are described briefly in Table 3-7.

Existing Professionals vs. New Professionals

Proposals for new types of oral health professionals beg the questions of practicality and efficiency. Is creating a new class of oral health provider justified considering the concomitant need to then create and fund new education programs, establish certification and licensing structures, and enable payment mechanisms? Is it more expedient to expand the scope of practice for already existing oral health professionals or build upon their skills and knowledge through enhancement of existing education and accreditation mechanisms? Can the competencies of dental hygienists and dental assistants be expanded to safely meet the need for oral health services? Might new models of care provision rather than new classes of oral health care professionals be designed to address the pervasive access issues?

There is likely not a single definitive answer to any of these questions. Multiple professional models and different professional collaborations are needed to address the myriad needs of disparate demographics, depressed economies, distinct cultural backgrounds, and challenging geography, all of which affect the provision of oral health services and the engagement of the populations to be served. Retraining and repositioning existing personnel, producing new types or classes of oral health care professionals, reconfiguring provision of services using models of interprofessional care (including the use of nondental health care professionals), and creating new and multiple points of entry to oral health services would all help address concerns about emerging demand and the enduring need for oral health care.

FINDINGS AND CONCLUSIONS

The committee noted the following findings and conclusions:

- Most dentists practice in the traditional private practice setting.
- Diversity among dental professionals has not increased substantially and does not represent the diversity of the general population.
- Diversity of the workforce plays an important role in the care of underserved and vulnerable populations.
- Efforts to increase the diversity of the dental workforce have been successful but represent only small gains.

TABLE 3-7
Selected Models of New Dental Professionals

	Advanced Dental Hygiene Practitioner (ADHP)	Community Dental Health Coordinator (CDHC)	Minnesota Dental Therapist (DT)	Minnesota Advanced Dental Therapist (ADT)	Registered Dental Hygienist in Alternative Practice (RDHAP)
Developed by	American Dental Hygienists' Association	American Dental Association	Minnesota legislature (authorized in 2009)	Minnesota legislature (authorized in 2009)	Southern California Dental Hygienists' Association (1970s)
Stage of Development	Competencies finalized in 2008; educational program began in 2009	Curriculum complete Pilots began at UCLA, the University of Oklahoma Dental School, and Temple University in 2009 ADA plans evaluation by 2013	Two educational programs at University of Minnesota School of Dentistry basic DT training (bachelor's and master's) Graduates anticipated to enter workforce in 2011	Metropolitan State University offers 2-year master's of science Graduates anticipated to enter workforce in 2011; as of June 2010, neither certification requirements nor payment arrange-ments had been finalized	Two programs currently available: West Los Angeles College and the University of the Pacific Arthur A. Dugoni School of Dentistry Currently, 287 RDHAPs actively licensed

continued

TABLE 3-7 *Continued*

	Advanced Dental Hygiene Practitioner (ADHP)	Community Dental Health Coordinator (CDHC)	Minnesota Dental Therapist (DT)	Minnesota Advanced Dental Therapist (ADT)	Registered Dental Hygienist in Alternative Practice (RDHAP)
Basic Description	Primary dental care providers who assess risk, educate, provide preventive and basic restorative care, and refer patients for complex care; works under remote consultative supervision; uses telehealth	Community health workers (recruited from the communities they intend to serve) to provide limited preventive and palliative care Focus is risk assessment, education, care coordination, health promotion, and behavioral change	Performs a range of preventive and basic restorative procedures under remote consultative supervision and intermediate restorative care under on-site supervision	Performs a range of preventive and restorative care (basic and intermediate) under remote consultative supervision; develop treatment plans with authorization of consulting dentist	Practices in underserved settings. Provides all services allowed by dental hygiene license, but independently. Must have dentist of record on file for referral, consultation, and emergency care. After 18 months of care, physician or dentist must provide written prescription for continued care, which is valid for 2 years
Education and Training	Master's degree (program available to those with bachelor's degrees currently licensed in dental hygiene)	12 months of training and 6-month internship	Bachelor's degree	Master's degree	In-person and distance education programs for dental hygienists with baccalaureate degrees already licensed in dental hygiene
Certification or Licensure	Licensed as a dental hygienist first Envisioned to be licensed and regulated at the state level	Envisioned to be certified; no formal licensure	Pass competency and licensure exam	Licensed as DTs, have a master's degree in advanced dental therapy, complete 2,000 of clinical practice, and pass certification exam for advanced practice	State licensure

SOURCES: Edelstein, 2010; GAO, 2010; Mertz and Glassman, 2011; Pew Center on the States and National Academy for State Health Policy, 2009.

- Geographic maldistribution of the workforce occurs, in part, due to the inability to sustain practices in underserved communities.
- Cost of education may be a barrier for many students to either enter the dental professions or to pursue advanced education.
- Community-based training experiences with vulnerable and underserved populations increase dental professionals' comfort and intent to care for these populations.
- Overall, the nondental health care workforce (e.g., nurses, pharmacists, physician assistants, physicians) does not receive adequate education and training in basic oral health issues.
- Many nondental health care professionals demonstrate a willingness to participate in oral health care.
- Oral health care needs to become an integrated part of primary health care.
- State boards of dentistry regulate the profession of dental hygiene.
- Regulation of dental professionals has been characterized by polarization of the professions over scope of practice issues.
- Data suggest that restrictive licensure laws in oral health are not tied to better health outcomes or supported by scientific evidence, and may drive up costs for the patient.
- Early experiences with new types of dental professionals do not raise concerns for the quality of care provided based on the available measures of quality.
- More research is needed on the effective and efficient utilization of the existing health care workforce.
- No single workforce model will likely serve the needs of all vulnerable and underserved populations.
- More research is needed on the impact of new workforce models on access to care.

REFERENCES

AAMC (American Association of Medical Colleges). 2008. *Contemporary issues in medicine: Oral health education for medical and dental students*. Washington, DC: American Association of Medical Colleges.

AAP (American Academy of Pediatrics). 2011a. *Caries prevention services reimbursement table*. http://www.aap.org/commpeds/dochs/oralhealth/pdf/Caries-Prevention-Chart.pdf (accessed May 25, 2011).

AAP. 2011b. *Oral health risk assessment: Training for pediatricians and other child health professionals*. http://www.aap.org/oralhealth/cme/page46.htm (accessed March 15, 2011).

AAP. 2011c. *Protecting all children's teeth: A pediatric oral health training program*. http://www.aap.org/oralhealth/pact/index.cfm (accessed January 6, 2011).

AAPA (American Academy of Physician Assistants). 2010. *American Academy of Physician Assistants 2010-2012 strategic plan*. http://www.aapa.org/about-aapa/strategic-planning (accessed March 12, 2011).

AAPA. 2011. *Physician assistant state and territorial regulatory authorities.* http://www.aapa.org/education-and-certification/certification/515-physician-assistant-state-and-territorial-regulatory-authorities (accessed May 29, 2011).

AAPHD (American Association of Public Health Dentistry). 2004. *History of the American Association of Public Health Dentistry.* http://www.aaphd.org/default.asp?page=history.htm (accessed March 12, 2011).

ABP (American Board of Pediatrics). 2009. *General pediatrics certification examination: Content outline.* Chapel Hill, NC: American Board of Pediatrics.

Abramowitz, J. 1972. The implementation of a program for utilizing auxiliaries: The experience of the Indian Health Service. *Journal of Public Health Dentistry* 32(3):142-148.

Abramowitz, J., and L. E. Berg. 1973. A four-year study of the utilization of dental assistants with expanded functions. *Journal of the American Dental Association* 87(3):623-635.

ACGME (Accreditation Council for Graduate Medical Education). 2007a. *ACGME program requirements for graduate medical education in family medicine.* Chicago, IL: Accreditation Council for Graduate Medical Education.

ACGME. 2007b. *ACGME program requirements for graduate medical education in pediatrics.* Chicago, IL: Accreditation Council for Graduate Medical Education.

ACGME. 2008a. *ACGME program requirements for graduate medical education in obstetrics and gynecology.* Chicago, IL: Accreditation Council for Graduate Medical Education.

ACGME. 2008b. *ACGME program requirements for graduate medical education in sleep medicine.* Chicago, IL: Accreditation Council for Graduate Medical Education.

ACGME. 2009a. *ACGME program requirements for graduate medical education in geriatric medicine.* Chicago, IL: Accreditation Council for Graduate Medical Education.

ACGME. 2009b. *ACGME program requirements for graduate medical education in internal medicine.* Chicago, IL: Accreditation Council for Graduate Medical Education.

Ackermann, R. J., and K. A. Kemle. 1998. The effect of a physician assistant on the hospitalization of nursing home residents. *Journal of the American Geriatrics Society* 46(5):610-614.

ADA (American Dental Association). 1998. *1996 dentist profile survey.* Chicago, IL: American Dental Association.

ADA. 2001. *Future of dentistry.* Chicago, IL: American Dental Association.

ADA. 2002. *2000/01 Survey of Allied Dental Education.* Chicago, IL: American Dental Assocation.

ADA. 2007. *American Indian and Alaska Native oral health access summit: Summary report.* Santa Ana Pueblo, NM: American Dental Association.

ADA. 2009a. *2008-09 survey of allied dental education.* Chicago, IL: American Dental Association.

ADA. 2009b. *2008 survey of dental practice: Characteristics of dentists in private practice and their patients.* Chicago, IL: American Dental Association.

ADA. 2009c. *2008 survey of dental practice: Income from the private practice of dentistry.* Chicago, IL: American Dental Association.

ADA. 2009d. *Distribution of dentists in the United States by region and state, 2007.* Chicago, IL: American Dental Association.

ADA. 2010a. *2008-09 survey of dental education: Academic programs, enrollment, and graduates—volume 1.* Chicago, IL: American Dental Association.

ADA. 2010b. *2008-2009 survey of advanced dental education.* Chicago, IL: American Dental Association.

ADA. 2010c. *Accreditation standards for dental education programs.* http://www.ada.org/sections/educationAndCareers/pdfs/predoc.pdf (accessed May 18, 2011).

ADA. 2010d. *Current policies: Adopted 1954-2009.* Chicago, IL: American Dental Association.

ADA. 2011a. *Breaking down barriers to oral health for all Americans: The role of workforce.* Chicago, IL. American Dental Association.

ADA. 2011b. *Congress nixes funding for alternative provider pilot programs in FY 2011 budget.* http://www.ada.org/advocacy.aspx (accessed May 29, 2011).

ADAA/DANB Alliance. 2005. *Addressing a uniform national model for the dental assisting profession.* Chicago, IL: Dental Assisting National Board.

ADEA (American Dental Education Association). 2010. ADEA competencies for entry into the allied dental professions: As approved by the 2010 ADEA house of delegates. *Journal of Dental Education* 74(7):769-115.

ADEA. 2011a (unpublished). *Letter to the committee on an oral health initiative.* American Dental Education Association.

ADEA. 2011b. *Predoctoral dental education programs.* http://www.adea.org/about_adea/who_we_are/adeainstitutionalmembers/Pages/PredoctoralDentalEducationPrograms.aspx (accessed March 14, 2011).

ADHA (American Dental Hygienists' Association). 2006. *Dental hygiene education program director survey.* Chicago, IL: American Dental Hygienists' Association.

ADHA. 2009a. *2009 dental hygiene job market & employment survey.* http://www.adha.org/downloads/Job_employment_survey_2009_exec_sum.pdf (accessed November 30, 2010).

ADHA. 2009b. *Survey of dental hygienists in the United States: 2007.* American Dental Hygienists' Association.

ADHA. 2010a. *Dental hygiene participation in regulation.* http://www.adha.org/governmental_affairs/downloads/Self_Regulation_States.pdf (accessed March 12, 2011).

ADHA. 2010b. *Direct access in some settings outside the dental office.* http://www.adha.org/governmental_affairs/downloads/Direct_Access_Map.pdf (accessed February 26, 2010).

ADHA. 2010c. *States which directly reimburse dental hygienists for services under the Medicaid program.* http://www.adha.org/governmental_affairs/downloads/medicaid.pdf (accessed April 11, 2011).

Advisory Committee on Training in Primary Care Medicine and Dentistry. 2010. *8th annual report to the secretary of the U.S. Department of Health and Human Services and to the U.S. Congress: The redesign of primary care with implications for training.* Rockville, MD: U.S. Department of Health and Human Services.

AGD (Academy of General Dentistry). 2008. *White paper on increasing access to and utilization of oral health care services.* Chicago, IL: Academy of General Dentistry.

AGD. 2011. *Dental practice ownership trends.* http://www.agd.org/education/transcriptnews/Default.asp?PubID=47&IssID=659&ArtID=2737 (accessed March 16, 2011).

AHRQ (Agency for Healthcare Research and Quality). 2010. *National healthcare disparities report.* Rockville, MD: U.S. Department of Health and Human Services.

Allison, R. A., and R. J. Manski. 2007. The supply of dentists and access to care in rural Kansas. *Journal of Rural Health* 23(3):198-206.

Altschuler, M. 1994. The Dental Health Care Professionals Nonresidence Licensing Act: Will it effectuate the final decay of discrimination against out-of-state dentists? *Rutgers Law Journal* 26:187-223.

AMA (American Medical Association). 2011a. *Education & careers: Requirements for becoming a physician.* http://www.ama-assn.org/ama/pub/education-careers/becoming-physician.page? (accessed June 2, 2011).

AMA. 2011b. *Medical student debt.* http://www.ama-assn.org/ama/pub/about-ama/our-people/member-groups-sections/medical-student-section/advocacy-policy/medical-student-debt/background.shtml (accessed March 9, 2011).

Ambrose, E. R., A. B. Hord, and W. J. Simpson. 1976. *A quality evaluation of specific dental services provided by the Saskatchewan dental plan: Final report.* Saskatchewan Dental Plan.

ANA (American Nurses Association). 2011a. *More about RNs and advanced practice RNs.* http://www.nursingworld.org/EspeciallyForYou/StudentNurses/RNsAPNs.aspx (accessed March 15, 2011).

ANA. 2011b. *Who we are.* http://nursingworld.org/FunctionalMenuCategories/AboutANA/WhoWeAre.aspx (accessed March 15, 2011).

Ananaba, N., S. Malcheff, D. Briskie, and M. R. Inglehart. 2010. Infant oral health examinations: attitudes and professional behavior of general and pediatric dentists in Michigan and pediatric dentists in the U.S. *The Journal of the Michigan Dental Association* 92(12):38-43.

Andersen, R. M., P. L. Davidson, K. A. Atchison, E. Hewlett, J. R. Freed, J. A. Friedman, A. Thind, J. J. Gutierrez, T. T. Nakazono, and D. C. Carreon. 2005. Pipeline, profession, and practice program: Evaluating change in dental education. *Journal of Dental Education* 69(2):239-248.

Andersen, R. M., P. L. Davidson, K. A. Atchison, J. J. Crall, J.-A. Friedman, E. R. Hewlett, and A. Thind. 2009. Summary and implications of the dental pipeline program evaluation. *Journal of Dental Education* 73(Supp. 2):S319-S330.

Andersen, R. M., D. C. Carreon, P. L. Davidson, T. T. Nakazono, S. Shahedi, and J. J. Gutierrez. 2010. Who will serve? Assessing recruitment of underrepresented minority and low-income dental students to increase access to dental care. *Journal of Dental Education* 74(6):579-592.

Anderson, J. R. 2010. *HRSA oral health programs.* Paper presented at 2010 Dental Management Coalition, Annapolis, MD.

AOA (American Osteopathic Association). 2011. *What is a DO?* http://www.osteopathic.org/osteopathic-health/about-dos/what-is-a-do/Pages/default.aspx (accessed June 2, 2011).

APHA (American Public Health Association). 2006. *Policy statement database: Support for the Alaska dental health aide therapist and other innovative programs for underserved populations.* http://www.apha.org/advocacy/policy/policysearch/default.htm?id=1328 (accessed March 16, 2011).

APMA (American Podiatric Medical Association). 2011. *About podiatry.* http://www.apma.org/MainMenu/AboutPodiatry.aspx (accessed May 29, 2011).

APPAP (Association of Postgraduate PA Programs). 2008. *APPAP programs by specialty* (accessed January 2, 2008).

ARC-PA (Accreditation Review Commission on Education for the Physician Assistant). 2010. *Accreditation standards for physician assistant education: 4th edition.* Johns Creek, GA: Accreditation Review Commission on Education for the Physician Assistant.

ASDOH (Arizona School of Dentistry & Oral Health). 2011. *Doctor of dental medicine: Admission requirements.* http://www.atsu.edu/asdoh/programs/dental_medicine/admission_requirements.htm (accessed May 22, 2011).

Ast, D. B. 1952. What the physician should know about the current status of dental caries prophylaxis. *New York State Journal of Medicine* 52(1):57-62.

ASTDD (Association of State and Territorial Dental Directors). 2007. *Fluoride varnish: An evidence-based approach.* http://www.astdd.org/docs/Sept2007FINALFlvarnishpaper.pdf (accessed March 15, 2011).

ASTDD. 2011. *About ASTDD.* http://www.astdd.org/about-us/ (accessed March 12, 2011).

Atchison, K. A., R. S. Mito, D. J. Rosenberg, K. H. Lefever, S. Lin, and R. Engelhardt. 2002. PGD training and its impact on general dentist practice patterns. *Journal of Dental Education* 66(12):1348-1357.

Atchison, K. A., A. Thind, T. T. Nakazono, D. Wong, J. J. Gutierrez, D. C. Carreon, and R. M. Andersen. 2009. Community-based clinical dental education: Effects of the pipeline program. *Journal of Dental Education* 73(Supp. 2):S269-S282.

Awé, C., and J. Bauman. 2010. Theoretical and conceptual framework for a high school pathways to pharmacy program. *American Journal of Pharmaceutical Education* 74(8).

Babamoto, K. S., K. A. Sey, A. J. Camilleri, V. J. Karlan, J. Catalasan, and D. E. Morisky. 2009. Improving diabetes care and health measures among Hispanics using community health workers: Results from a randomized controlled trial. *Health Education and Behavior* 36(1):113-126.

Bader, J. D., J. Y. Lee, D. A. Shugars, B. B. Burrus, and S. Wetterhall. 2011. Clinical technical performance of dental therapists in Alaska. *Journal of the American Dental Association* 142(3):322-329.

Bailit, H. 1999. Community-based clinical education programs. Major findings and recommendations. *Journal of Dental Education* 63(12):981-989.

Bailit, H. L. 2010. Financial impact of community-based dental education. *Journal of Dental Education* 74(10 Suppl.):S33-S41.

Bailit, H., and J. D'Adamo. 2010 (unpublished). Report to the oral health access committee: State case studies: Improving access to dental care for the underserved.

Bailit, H., and A. Formicola. 2010. Preface: About the dental pipeline program. *Journal of Dental Education* 7(10):S5-S6.

Bailit, H. L., T. J. Beazoglou, A. J. Formicola, and L. Tedesco. 2007. Financing clinical dental education. *Journal of Dental Education* 71(3):322-330.

Ballweg, R., J. Berg, T. DeRouen, L. Fiset, W. Mouradian, and M. J. Somerman. 2011. Expanding dental education partnerships beyond the four walls. *Journal of Dental Education* 75(3):300-309.

Baum, K. D., and S. Axtell. 2005. Trends in North American medical education. *Keio Journal of Medicine* 54(1):22-28.

Baumeister, S. E., P. L. Davidson, D. C. Carreon, T. T. Nakazono, J. J. Gutierrez, and R. M. Andersen. 2007. What influences dental students to serve special care patients? *Special Care in Dentistry* 27(1):15-22.

Bender, I. B., and S. Seltzer. 1963. Dental procedures of interest to the physician in the management of patients with cardiovascular disease. *American Heart Journal* 66(5):679-684.

Berg, P., and D. Coniglio. 2006. Oral health in children: Overlooked and undertreated. *Journal of the American Academy of Physician Assistants* 19(4):40.

Berg, R., R. L. Call, K. Maguire, D. B. Berkey, B. A. Karshmer, B. Guyton, and K. Tawara-Jones. 2010. Impact of the University of Colorado's advanced clinical training and service (ACTS) program on dental students' clinical experience and cognitive skills, 1994-2006. *Journal of Dental Education* 74(4):423-433.

Bigler, J. A. 1951. The physician and oral health in children. *Missouri Medicine* 48(12):966-970.

BLS (Bureau of Labor Statistics). 2009a. *Occupational outlook handbook, 2010-11 edition, pharmacists*. http://www.bls.gov/oco/ocos079.htm (accessed December 28, 2010).

BLS. 2009b. *Occupational outlook handbook, 2010-11 edition, physician assistants*. http://www.bls.gov/oco/ocos081.htm (accessed December 28, 2010).

BLS. 2009c. *Occupational outlook handbook, 2010-11 edition, physicians and surgeons*. http://www.bls.gov/oco/ocos074.htm#training (accessed June 2, 2011).

BLS. 2009d. *Occupational outlook handbook, 2010-11 edition, podiatrists*. http://www.bls.gov/oco/ocos075.htm (accessed May 29, 2011).

BLS. 2010a. *Employment projections: Fastest growing occupations*. http://www.bls.gov/emp/ep_table_103.htm (accessed December 28, 2010).

BLS. 2010b. *Occupational outlook handbook 2010-11 edition, dental assistants*. http://www.bls.gov/oco/ocos163.htm (accessed December 28, 2010).

BLS. 2010c. *Occupational outlook handbook, 2010-11 edition, dental hygienists*. http://www.bls.gov/oco/ocos097.htm (accessed December 28, 2010).

BLS. 2010d. *Occupational outlook handbook, 2010-11 edition, dentists*. http://www.bls.gov/oco/ocos072.htm (accessed January 5, 2011).

BLS. 2010e. *Occupational outlook handbook, 2010-11 edition, medical, dental, and ophthalmic laboratory technicians* (accessed January 6, 2011).

Blue, A., B. F. Brandt, and M. H. Schmitt. 2010. American interprofessional health collaborative: Historical roots and organizational beginnings. *Journal of Allied Health* 39(Supp. 1):204-209.

Bolin, K. A. 2008. Assessment of treatment provided by dental health aide therapists in Alaska. *Journal of the American Dental Association* 139(11):1530-1535.

Bolin, K. 2010. *Survey of health center oral health providers: Dental salaries, provider satisfaction, and recruitment and retention strategies*. Denver, CO: National Network for Oral Health Access.

Bresch, J. 2010. *Critical importance of HHS to dental education and training*. Presentation at meeting of the Committee on an Oral Health Initiative, June 28, Washington, DC.

Brickhouse, T. H., J. H. Unkel, I. Kancitis, A. M. Best, and R. D. Davis. 2008. Infant oral health care: A survey of general dentists, pediatric dentists, and pediatricians in Virginia. *Pediatric Dentistry* 30(2):147-153.

Brooks, E. S. 2005. Bridge to dentistry: Charting a path to serving the underserved. *Texas Dental Journal* 122(5):436-442.

Brooks, E. S., T. C. Gravely, S. A. Hornback, L. C. Cunningham, A. L. McCann, and J. L. Long. 2002. Bridge to dentistry: One dental school's approach to improving its enrollment of underrepresented minorities. *Journal of the American College of Dentists* 69(1):23-30.

Brown, L. J. 2001. Dental work force strategies during a period of change and uncertainty. *Journal of Dental Education* 65(12):1404-1416.

Brown, L. J., K. S. Wagner, and B. Johns. 2000. Racial/ethnic variations of practicing dentists. *Journal of the American Dental Association* 131(12):1750-1754.

Brown, L. J., D. R. House, and K. D. Nash. 2005. *The economic aspects of unsupervised private hygiene practice and its impact on access to care*. Chicago, IL: American Dental Association.

Brownstein, J. N., L. R. Bone, C. R. Dennison, M. N. Hill, M. T. Kim, and D. M. Levine. 2005. Community health workers as interventionists in the prevention and control of heart disease and stroke. *American Journal of Preventive Medicine* 29(5 Supp. 1):128-133.

Brugna, R. A., J. F. Cawley, and M. D. Baker. 2007. Physician assistants in geriatric medicine. *Clinical Geriatrics* 15(10):22-29.

Brunson, W. D., D. L. Jackson, J. C. Sinkford, and R. W. Valachovic. 2010. Components of effective outreach and recruitment programs for underrepresented minority and low-income dental students. *Journal of Dental Education* 74(Supp. 10):S74-86.

Buelow, J. R., C. Rathsack, D. Downs, K. Jorgensen, J. R. Karges, and D. Nelson. 2008. Building interdisciplinary teamwork among allied health students through live clinical case simulations. *Journal of Allied Health* 37(2).

Cantor, J. C., L. Bergeisen, and L. C. Baker. 1998. Effect of an intensive educational program for minority college students and recent graduates on the probability of acceptance to medical school. *Journal of the American Medical Association* 280(9):772-776.

Cantrell, C. 2008. *The role of physicians in children's oral health*. Portland, ME: National Association for State Health Policy.

Cantrell, C. 2009. *Engaging primary care medical providers in children's oral health*. Portland, ME: National Academy for State Health Policy.

Carreon, D., P. Davidson, R. Andersen, and T. Nakazono. 2011. Altruism in dental students. *Journal of Healthcare for the Poor and Underserved* 22(1):56-70.

Carson-Smith, W. Y., and P. A. Minarik. 2007. Advanced practice nurses: A new skirmish in the continuing battle over scope of practice. *Clinical Nurse Specialist* 21(1):52-54.

Casamassimo, P. S., N. S. Seale, and K. Ruehs. 2004. General dentists' perceptions of educational and treatment issues affecting access to care for children with special health care needs. *Journal of Dental Education* 68(1):23-28.

Caspary, G., D. M. Krol, S. Boulter, M. A. Keels, and G. Romano-Clarke. 2008. Perceptions of oral health training and attitudes toward performing oral health screenings among graduating pediatric residents. *Pediatrics* 122(2):e465-e471.

CDC (Centers for Disease Control and Prevention). 2011. *Epidemic intelligence service*. http://www.cdc.gov/eis/index.html (accessed January 7, 2011).

Chadwick, D., and J. Hupp. 2008. East Carolina University School of Dentistry: Impact on access disparities. *The Journal of the American College of Dentists* 75(4):35-41.

Chalmers, J. M. 1996. Factors influencing nurses' aides' provision of oral care for nursing facility residents. *Special Care in Dentistry* 16(2):71-79.

Chard, D. J., H. Bailit, I. Bau, and G. Zamora. 2009. The dental pipeline program's impact on access disparities and student diversity. *Journal of the American Dental Association* 140(3):346-353.

Chiarello, G. P. 2009. *Regulating the professions: The intersection of competition and consumer protection policies*. Paper presented at the IOM workshop "The U.S. Oral Health Workforce in the Coming Decade," Washington, DC.

Christian, S., C. Dower, and E. O'Neil. 2007. *Overview of nurse practitioner scopes of practice in the United States—discussion*. San Francisco, CA: Center for the Health Professions.

Chu, M., L. E. Sweis, A. H. Guay, and R. J. Manski. 2007. The dental care of U.S. children: Access, use and referrals by nondentist providers, 2003. *Journal of the American Dental Association* 138(10):1324-1331.

Clemmens, D. A., and A. R. Kerr. 2008. Improving oral health in women: Nurses' call to action. *MCN The American Journal of Maternal/Child Nursing* 33(1):10-14.

Close, K., R. G. Rozier, L. P. Zeldin, and A. R. Gilbert. 2010. Barriers to the adoption and implementation of preventive dental services in primary medical care. *Pediatrics* 125(3):509-517.

Cohen, L. A., A. J. Bonito, D. R. Akin, R. J. Manski, M. D. Macek, R. R. Edwards, and L. J. Cornelius. 2009. Role of pharmacists in consulting with the underserved regarding toothache pain. *Journal of the American Pharmacists Association* 49(1):38-42.

Coleman, P., and N. M. Watson. 2006. Oral care provided by certified nursing assistants in nursing homes. *Journal of the American Geriatrics Society* 54(1):138-143.

Cooper, H., C. Carlisle, T. Gibbs, and C. Watkins. 2001. Developing an evidence base for interdisciplinary learning: A systematic review. *Journal of Advanced Nursing* 35(2):228-237.

Daly, R. 2006. Physician coalition prepares for scope-of-practice battles. *Psychiatric News* 41(3):10.

DANB (Dental Assisting National Board). 2007. *Dental assisting job titles in the U.S.* http://www.dentalassisting.org/PDFs/JobTitles.pdf (accessed March 15, 2011).

DANB. 2010. *2010 DANB national exam applications and candidate guide*. http://www.danb.org/PDFs/2010CDA.pdf (accessed November 3, 2010).

Danielsen, R., J. Dillenberg, and C. Bay. 2006. Oral health competencies for physician assistants and nurse practitioners. *Journal of Physician Assistant Education* 17(4):12-16.

DeCastro, J. E., D. Bolger, and C. A. Feldman. 2005. Clinical competence of graduates of community-based and traditional curricula. *Journal of Dental Education* 69(12):1324-1331.

Dehaitem, M. J., K. Ridley, W. E. Kerschbaum, and M. R. Inglehart. 2008. Dental hygiene education about patients with special needs: A survey of U.S. programs. *Journal of Dental Education* 72(9):1010-1019.

Dela Cruz, G. G., R. G. Rozier, and G. Slade. 2004. Dental screening and referral of young children by pediatric primary care providers. *Pediatrics* 114(5).

DENTEX. 2010. *Dental health aide training program.* http://depts.washington.edu/dentexak/mission.html (accessed September 19, 2011).

Dillenberg, J. 2009. *Meeting oral health workforce/access needs through an innovative educational model.* Paper presented at the IOM workshop "The U.S. Oral Health Workforce in the Coming Decade," Washington, DC.

Dixon, S., W. Dunn, and J. Fancher. 2002. Perceived initial clinical competencies of dentists at the start and completion of US Air Force advanced education in general dentistry residency programs. *Military Medicine* 167(6):470-473.

Dodds, J., W. Vann, J. Lee, A. Rosenberg, K. Rounds, M. Roth, M. Wells, E. Evens, and L. H. Margolis. 2010. The UNC-CH MCH leadership training consortium: Building the capacity to develop interdisciplinary MCH leaders. *Maternal and Child Health Journal* 14(4):642-648.

Douglass, A. B., W. Gonsalves, R. Maier, H. Silk, N. Stevens, J. Tysinger, and A. S. Wrightson. 2007. Smiles for Life: A national oral health curriculum for family medicine. A model for curriculum development by STFM groups. *Family Medicine* 39(2):88-90.

Douglass, A. B., M. Deutchman, J. Douglass, W. Gonsalves, R. Maier, H. Silk, J. Tysinger, and A. S. Wrightson. 2009a. Incorporation of a national oral health curriculum into family medicine residency programs. *Family Medicine* 41(3):159-160.

Douglass, A. B., J. M. Douglass, and D. M. Krol. 2009b. Educating pediatricians and family physicians in children's oral health. *Academic Pediatrics* 9(6):452-456.

Dower, C., S. Christian, and E. O'Neil. 2007. *Promising scope of practice modules for the health professions.* San Francisco, CA: Center for the Health Professions.

Duke University. 2011. *Resources for educators.* http://pa.mc.duke.edu/Our-Educators/ (accessed March 14, 2011).

Dulisse, B., and J. Cromwell. 2010. No harm found when nurse anesthetists work without supervision by physicians. *Health Affairs* 29(8):1469-1475.

Dunning, H. S. 1941. Medico-dental cooperation in the field of oral and physical diagnosis. *American Journal of Orthodontics and Oral Surgery* 27(7):347-349.

Dunning, J. M. 1958. Extending the field for dental auxiliary personnel in the United States. *American Journal of Public Health* 48(8):1059-1064.

Dyer, J. A. 2003. Multidisciplinary, interdisciplinary, and transdisciplinary: Educational models and nursing education. *Nursing Education Perspectives* 24(4):186-188.

Edelstein, B. L. 2010. *Training new dental health providers in the U.S.* Battle Creek, MI: W.K. Kellogg Foundation.

Edelstein, B., D. Krol, P. Ingargiola, and A. De Biasi. 2003. *Assessing pediatric dentistry Title VII training program success.* Washington, DC: American Academy of Pediatric Dentistry Foundation.

Everett, C. M., J. R. Schumacher, A. Wright, and M. A. Smith. 2009. Physician assistants and nurse practitioners as a usual source of care. *Journal of Rural Health* 25(4):407-414.

Fales, M. H. 1958. The potential role of the dental hygienist in public health programs. *American Journal of Public Health* 48(8):1054-1058.

Feinstein, R. A. 2009 July 16. *The importance of competition and antitrust enforcement to lower-cost, higher-quality health care.* Paper presented at Hearing of the Subcommittee on Consumer Protection, Product Safety, and Insurance; Committee on Commerce, Science & Transportation; U.S. Senate, Washington, DC.

Ferullo, A., H. Silk, and J. A. Savageau. 2011. A national survey of oral health curriculum in all U.S. allopathic and osteopathic medical schools. *Academic Medicine* 86(2):252-258.

Finocchio, L. J., C. M. Dower, T. McMahon, C. M. Gragnola, and Taskforce on Health Care Workforce Regulation. 1995. *Reforming health care workforce regulation: Policy considerations for the 21st century.* San Francisco, CA: Pew Health Professions Commission.

Fiset, L. 2005. *A report on quality assessment of primary care provided by dental therapists to Alaska Natives.* Seattle, WA: University of Washington School of Dentistry.

Formicola, A. J., H. Bailit, T. Beazoglou, and L. A. Tedesco. 2005. The Macy study: A framework for consensus. *Journal of Dental Education* 69(11):1183-1085.

Formicola, A. J., R. Myers, J. F. Hasler, M. Peterson, W. Dodge, H. L. Bailit, T. J. Beazoglou, and L. A. Tedesco. 2008. Evolution of dental school clinics as patient care delivery centers. *Journal of Dental Education* 72(2 Supp.):110-127.

Formicola, A., H. Bailit, K. D'Abreu, J. Stavisky, I. Bau, G. Zamora, and H. Treadwell. 2009. The dental pipeline program's impact on access disparities and student diversity. *Journal of the American Dental Association* 140(3):346-353.

Formicola, A. J., K. C. D'Abreu, and L. A. Tedesco. 2010. Underrepresented minority dental student recruitment and enrollment programs: An overview from the dental pipeline program. *Journal of Dental Education* 74(Supp. 10):S67-S73.

Freed, J. R., D. A. Perry, and J. E. Kushman. 1997. Aspects of quality of dental hygiene care in supervised and unsupervised practices. *Journal of Public Health Dentistry* 57(2):68-75.

FTC (Federal Trade Commission). 2009. FTC staff comment. Paper read at Louisiana House of Representatives, Baton Rouge, LA.

FTC. 2010. *Overview of FTC antitrust actions in health care services and products.* Washington, DC: Federal Trade Commission.

FTC. 2011. *Opinion and order of the commission: Docket no. 9311.* http://www.ftc.gov/os/adjpro/d9311/040728commissionopinion.pdf (accessed January 10, 2011).

FTC and DOJ (Department of Justice). 2004. *Improving health care: A dose of competition.* Washington, DC: Federal Trade Commission and Department of Justice.

Fulmer, T., K. Hyer, E. Flaherty, M. Mezey, N. Whitelaw, M. Orry Jacobs, R. Luchi, J. C. Hansen, D. A. Evans, C. Cassel, E. Kotthoff-Burrell, R. Kane, and E. Pfeiffer. 2005. Geriatric interdisciplinary team training program: Evaluation results. *Journal of Aging and Health* 17(4):443-470.

Gallagher, J. L., and D. A. Wright. 2003. General dental practitioners' knowledge of and attitudes towards the employment of dental therapists in general practice. *British Dental Journal* 194(1):37-41.

GAO (Government Accountability Office). 2006. *Health professional shortage areas: Problems remain with primary care shortage area designation system.* Washington, DC: U.S. General Accounting Office.

GAO. 2010. *Efforts under way to improve children's access to dental services, but sustained attention needed to address ongoing concerns.* Washington, DC: U.S. Government Accountability Office.

Garcia, R. I., R. E. Inge, L. Niessen, and D. P. DePaola. 2010. Envisioning success: The future of the oral health care delivery system in the United States. *Journal of Public Health Dentistry* 70(Supp. 1):S58-S65.

Gardner, D. 2010. Expanding scope of practice: Inter-professional collaboration or conflict? *Nursing Economics* 28(4):264-266.

Garrison Jr., R. S. 1991. General practice residency programs: Benefits to residents and patients. *Journal of Dental Education* 55(8):534-536; discussion 537.

Gatlin, L. J., S. L. Handelman, C. Meyerowitz, E. Solomon, B. Iranpour, and R. Weaver. 1993. Practice characteristics of graduates of postdoctoral general dentistry programs. *Journal of Dental Education* 57(11):798-803.

GDA (Georgia Dental Association). 2010. *White paper on Georgia's oral health status, access to and utilization of oral health care services.* Atlanta, GA: Georgia Dental Association.

Gies, W. J. 1926. *Dental education in the United States and Canada.* New York: Carnegie Foundation for the Advancement of Teaching.

Gladstone, R., and W. M. Garcia. 2007. *Dental hygiene: Reflecting on our past, preparing for our future.* http://findarticles.com/p/articles/mi_m1ANQ/is_9_21/ai_n25015055/ (accessed April 11, 2011).

Glassman, P., and C. Meyerowitz. 1999. Postdoctoral education in dentistry: Preparing dental practitioners to meet the oral health needs of America in the 21st century. *Journal of Dental Education* 63(8):615-625.

Green, A. R., J. R. Betancourt, E. R. Park, J. A. Greer, E. J. Donahue, and J. S. Weissman. 2008. Providing culturally competent care: Residents in HRSA Title VII-funded residency programs feel better prepared. *Academic Medicine* 83(11):1071-1079.

Grumbach, K., and E. Chen. 2006. Effectiveness of University of California postbaccalaureate premedical programs in increasing medical school matriculation for minority and disadvantaged students. *Journal of the American Medical Association* 296(9):1079-1085.

Grumbach, K., L. G. Hart, E. Mertz, J. Coffman, and L. Palazzo. 2003. Who is caring for the underserved? A comparison of primary care physicians and nonphysician clinicians in California and Washington. *Annals of Family Medicine* 1(2):97-104.

Habibian, M., L. Elizondo, and R. Mulligan. 2010. Dental students' attitudes toward homeless people while providing oral health care. *Journal of Dental Education* 74(11):1190-1196.

Haden, N. K., F. A. Catalanotto, C. J. Alexander, H. Bailit, A. Battrell, J. Broussard Jr., J. Buchanan, C. W. Douglass, C. E. Fox 3rd, P. Glassman, R. I. Lugo, M. George, C. Meyerowitz, E. R. Scott 2nd, N. Yaple, J. Bresch, Z. Gutman-Betts, G. G. Luke, M. Moss, J. C. Sinkford, R. G. Weaver, and R. W. Valachovic. 2003. Improving the oral health status of all Americans: Roles and responsibilities of academic dental institutions: The report of the ADEA president's commission. *Journal of Dental Education* 67(5):563-583.

Haden, N. K., W. D. Hendricson, D. K. Kassebaum, R. R. Ranney, G. Weinstein, E. L. Anderson, and R. W. Valachovic. 2010. Curriculum change in dental education, 2003-09. *Journal of Dental Education* 74(5):539-557.

Hall, P., and L. Weaver. 2001. Interdisciplinary education and teamwork: A long and winding road. *Medical Education* 35(9):867-875.

Hallas, D. 2010. Take action to influence children's oral health. *Nurse Practitioner* 35(2):6.

Hallas, D., and D. Shelley. 2009. Role of pediatric nurse practitioners in oral health care. *Academic Pediatrics* 9(6):462-466.

Hammick, M., D. Freeth, I. Koppel, S. Reeves, and H. Barr. 2007. A best evidence systematic review of interprofessional education: BEME guide no. 9. *Medical Teacher* 29(8):735-751.

Hammons, P. E., and H. C. Jamison. 1967. Expanded functions for dental auxiliaries. *Journal of the American Dental Association* 75(3):658-672.

Hammons, P. E., and H. C. Jamison. 1968. New duties for dental auxiliaries—the Alabama experience. *American Journal of Public Health and the Nation's Health* 58(5):882-886.

Hammons, P. E., H. C. Jamison, and L. L. Wilson. 1971. Quality of service provided by dental therapists in an experimental program at the University of Alabama. *Journal of the American Dental Association* 82(5):1060-1066.

Harper, D. C., and J. Johnson. 1998. The new generation of nurse practitioners: Is more enough? *Health Affairs* 17(5):158-164.

Hart-Hester, S., and C. Thomas. 2003. Access to health care professionals in rural Mississippi. *Southern Medical Journal* 96(2):149-154.

Hayes, E. 1985. The nurse practitioner: History, current conflicts, and future survival. *Journal of the American College Health Association* 34(3):144-147.

Hesser, A., Pond E, Lewis L, and A. B. 1996. Evaluation of a supplementary retention program for African-American baccalaureate nursing students. *Journal of Nursing Education* 35(7):304-309.

HHS (Department of Health and Human Services). 2003. *Advisory committee on training in primary care medicine and dentistry: Training culturally competent primary care professionals to provide high quality healthcare for all Americans: The essential role of Title VII, section 747, in the elimination of healthcare disparities.* Rockville, MD: U.S. Department of Health and Human Services.

HHS. 2009. *Pipeline programs to improve racial and ethnic diversity in the health professions: An inventory of federal programs, assessment of evaluation approaches, and critical review of the research literature.* Rockville, MD: U.S. Department of Health and Human Services.

HHS. 2010. *Advisory committee on training in primary care medicine and dentistry: The redesign of primary care with implications for training.* Rockville, MD: U.S. Department of Health and Human Services.

Hillenbrand, H. 1981. The necessity for trained advanced dental professionals. *Journal of Dental Education* 45(2):76.

Holtzman, J. S., and H. Seirawan. 2009. Impact of community-based oral health experiences on dental students' attitudes towards caring for the underserved. *Journal of Dental Education* 73(3):303-310.

Hood, J. G. 2009. Service-learning in dental education: Meeting needs and challenges. *Journal of Dental Education* 73(4):454-463.

Hooker, R. S., and L. E. Berlin. 2002. Trends in the supply of physician assistants and nurse practitioners in the United States. *Health Affairs* 21(5):174-181.

Hooker, R. S., D. J. Cipher, and E. Sekscenski. 2005. Patient satisfaction with physician assistant, nurse practitioner, and physician care: A national survey of Medicare beneficiaries. *Journal of Clinical Outcomes Management* 12(2):88-92.

Howe, J. L., and D. W. Sherman. 2006. Interdisciplinary educational approaches to promote team-based geriatrics and palliative care. *Gerontology and Geriatrics Education* 26(3):1-16.

HRSA (Health Resources and Services Administration). 2000. *The public health workforce: Enumeration 2000.* ftp://ftp.hrsa.gov//bhpr/nationalcenter/phworkforce2000.pdf (accessed March 16, 2011).

HRSA. 2004. *The professional practice environment of dental hygienists in the fifty states and the District of Columbia, 2001.* http://bhpr.hrsa.gov/healthworkforce/reports/hygienists/dh1.htm (accessed January 10, 2011).

HRSA. 2005. *Financing dental education: Public policy interests, issues and strategic considerations.* Washington, DC: U.S. Department of Health and Human Services.

HRSA. 2006. *The rationale for diversity in the health professions: A review of the evidence.* Rockville, MD: Department of Health and Human Services.

HRSA. 2010a. *Health professions: Public health.* http://bhpr.hrsa.gov/grants/public.htm (accessed December 22, 2010).

HRSA. 2010b. *NHSC loan repayment.* http://nhsc.hrsa.gov/loanrepayment/ (accessed December 22, 2010).

HRSA. 2010c. *Shortage designation: HPSAs, MUAs & MUPs.* http://bhpr.hrsa.gov/shortage/index.htm (accessed March 14, 2011).

HRSA. 2011a. *Dental HPSA designation criteria.* http://bhpr.hrsa.gov/shortage/hpsas/designationcriteria/dentalhpsacriteria.html (accessed October 11, 2011).

HRSA. 2011b. *Designated health professional shortage areas (HPSA) statistics.* http://ersrs.hrsa.gov/ReportServer?/HGDW_Reports/BCD_HPSA/BCD_HPSA_SCR50_Smry&rs:Format=HTML3.2 (accessed March 14, 2011).

HRSA. 2011c. *HRSA data warehouse: Map gallery.* http://datawarehouse.hrsa.gov/exportedmaps/HPSAs/HGDWMapGallery_BHPR_HPSAs_DC.pdf (accessed June 22, 2011).

Huijbregts, P. A. 2007. Chiropractic legal challenges to the physical therapy scope of practice: Anybody else taking the ethical high ground? *Journal of Manual and Manipulative Therapy* 15(2):69-80.

Iglehart, J. K. 2010. Health reform, primary care, and graduate medical education. *New England Journal of Medicine* 363(6):584-590.

IHS (Indian Health Service). 2011. Indian health manual, part 3, chapter 2, dental. http://www.ihs.gov/ihm/index.cfm?module=dsp_ihm_pc_p3c2 (accessed February 28, 2011).

IOM (Institute of Medicine). 1989. *Allied health services: Avoiding crises.* Washington, DC: National Academy Press.

IOM. 1995. *Dental education at the crossroads: Challenges and change.* Washington, DC: National Academy Press.

IOM. 1996. *Primary care: America's health in a new era.* Washington, DC: National Academy Press.

IOM. 2003. *Unequal treatment: Confronting racial and ethnic disparities in health care.* Washington, DC: The National Academies Press.

IOM. 2004. *In the nation's compelling interest: Ensuring diversity in the health-care workforce.* Washington, DC: The National Academies Press.

IOM. 2008. *Retooling for an aging America: Building the health care workforce.* Washington, DC: The National Academies Press.

IOM. 2010. *The future of nursing: Leading change, advancing health.* Washington, DC: The National Academies Press.

Jablonski, R. 2010. *Nursing education and research (geriatrics).* Paper presented at the meeting of the Committee on an Oral Health Initiative, Washington, DC.

Jablonski, R. A., C. L. Munro, M. J. Grap, C. M. Schubert, M. Ligon, and P. Spigelmyer. 2009. Mouth care in nursing homes: Knowledge, beliefs, and practices of nursing assistants. *Geriatric Nursing* 30(2):99-107.

Jacques, P. F., C. Snow, M. Dowdle, N. Riley, K. Mao, and W. C. Gonsalves. 2010. Oral health curricula in physician assistant programs: A survey of physician assistant program directors. *Journal of Physician Assistant Education* 21(2):22-30.

Johnson, B. R., P. M. Loomer, S. C. Siegel, E. S. Pilcher, J. E. Leigh, M. J. Gillespie, R. K. Simmons, and S. P. Turner. 2007. Strategic partnerships between academic dental institutions and communities: Addressing disparities in oral health care. *Journal of the American Dental Association* 138(10):1366-1371.

Johnson, D. W. 1969. Dental manpower resources in the United States. *American Journal of Public Health and the Nation's Health* 59(4):689-693.

Jones, P. E., and J. F. Cawley. 1994. Physician assistants and health system reform: Clinical capabilities, practice activities, and potential roles. *Journal of the American Medical Association* 271(16):1266-1272.

Kaiser Family Foundation. 2011. *Professionally active dentists per 10,000 civilian population, 2007.* http://www.statehealthfacts.org/comparemapdetail.jsp?ind=966&cat=8&sub=104&yr=18&typ=3 (accessed October 14, 2011).

Kennedy, J. E., and L. A. Tedesco. 1999. The predoctoral curriculum in an era of required postgraduate dental education; or if only it were true. *Journal of Dental Education* 63(8):648-653.

Kim, M. J., K. Holm, P. Gerard, B. McElmurry, M. Foreman, S. Poslusny, and C. Dallas. 2009. Bridges to the doctorate: Mentored transition to successful completion of doctoral study for underrepresented minorities in nursing science. *Nursing Outlook* 57(3):166-171.

Kleiner, M. M., and R. T. Kudrle. 2000. Does regulation affect economic outcomes? The case of dentistry. *Journal of Law and Economics* 43(2):547-582.

Kleiner, M. M., and K. W. Park. 2010. *Battles among licensed occupations: Analyzing government regulations on labor market outcomes for dentists and hygienists*. Cambridge, MA: National Bureau of Economic Research.

Kressin, N., M. Nunn, H. Singh, M. Orner, L. Pbert, C. Hayes, C. Culler, S. Glicken, S. Palfrey, and P. Geltman. 2009. Pediatric clinicians can help reduce rates of early childhood caries: Effects of a practice-based intervention. *Medical Care* 47(11):1121-1128.

Krol, D. M. 2004. Educating pediatricians on children's oral health: Past, present, and future. *Pediatrics* 113(5):e487-e492.

Krol, D. M. 2010. Children's oral health and the role of the pediatrician. *Current Opinion in Pediatrics* 22(6):804-808.

Lam, H. T. C., T. Ward, T. G. O'Toole, P. E. Arola, and B. K. Chang. 2009. Impact of infrastructure on graduate dental education and dental clinic productivity. *Journal of Dental Education* 73(2):184-191.

Lavizzo-Mourey, R. 2010. Foreword. *Journal of Dental Education* 74(Supp. 10):S7-S8.

Lefever, K. H., K. A. Atchison, K. R. McCauley, R. D. Mito, and R. Engelhardt. 2003. Views of practicing dentists regarding a mandatory fifth year of training. *Journal of Dental Education* 67(3):317-327.

Lenz, E. R., M. O. Mundinger, R. L. Kane, S. C. Hopkins, and S. X. Lin. 2004. Primary care outcomes in patients treated by nurse practitioners or physicians: Two-year follow-up. *Medical Care Research and Review* 61(3):332-351.

Lerner, S., D. Magrane, and E. Friedman. 2009. Teaching teamwork in medical education. *Mount Sinai Journal of Medicine* 76(4):318-329.

Leviton, L. C. 2009a. Evaluating the dental pipeline program: Recruiting minorities and promoting community-based dental education. *Journal of Dental Education* 73(Supp. 2):S5-S7.

Leviton, L C. 2009b. Foreword. *Journal of Dental Education* 73(Supp. 2):S5-S7.

Lewin, S., S. Munabi-Babigumira, C. Glenton, K. Daniels, X. Bosch-Capblanch, B. E. van Wyk, J. Odgaard-Jensen, M. Johansen, G. N. Aja, M. Zwarenstein, and I. B. Scheel. 2010. Lay health workers in primary and community health care for maternal and child health and the management of infectious diseases. *Cochrane Database of Systematic Reviews* (3):CD004015.

Lewis, C. L. 1996. A state university's model program to increase the number of its disadvantaged students who matriculate into health professions schools. *Academic Medicine* 71(10):1050-1057.

Lewis, C. W., D. C. Grossman, P. K. Domoto, and R. A. Deyo. 2000. The role of the pediatrician in the oral health of children: A national survey. *Pediatrics* 106(6):e84.

Lewis, C. W., S. Boulter, M. A., Keels, D. M. Krol, W. E. Mouradian, K. G. O'Connor, and R. B. Quinonez. 2009. Oral health and pediatricians: Results of a national survey. *Academic Pediatrics* 9(6):457-461.

Lobene, R. R., and A. Kerr. 1979. *The Forsyth experiment: An alternative system for dental care*. Cambridge, MA: Harvard University Press.

Long, R. E. 2009. Improving outcomes for the patient with cleft lip and palate: The team concept and 70 years of experience in cleft care. *Journal of Lancaster General Hospital* 4(2).

Luciano, W. J., L. G. Rothfuss, and A. S. von Gonten. 2006. The expanded function dental assistant training program. *Army Medical Department Journal* January-March 2006:16-20.

MacDorman, M. F., and G. K. Singh. 1998. Midwifery care, social and medical risk factors, and birth outcomes in the USA. *Journal of Epidemiology and Community Health* 52(5):310-317.

Machen, J. B. 2008. Will we allow dentistry to be left behind? Principles underlying dental education and practice. *Journal of Dental Education* 72(Supp. 2):S10-S13.

Macleod, I., G. Bell, and A. Lorimer. 2003. A role for pharmacists in cancer detection. *Pharmaceutical Journal* 270(7240):367.

Malcheff, S., T. C. Pink, W. Sohn, M. R. Inglehart, and D. Briskie. 2009. Infant oral health examinations: Pediatric dentists' professional behavior and attitudes. *Pediatric Dentistry* 31(3):202-209.

Malcmacher, L. 2011. What does your state dental board do? *Dental Economics* 101(1).

Markel, G., M. Woolfolk, and M. R. Inglehart. 2008. Feeding the pipeline: Academic skills training for predental students. *Journal of Dental Education* 72(6):653-661.

Mascarenhas, A. K., and M. Henshaw. 2010. Infrastructure for a community-based dental education program: Students and clinics. *Journal of Dental Education* 74(10 Supp.):S17-S24.

McAndrew, M. 2010. Community-based dental education and the importance of faculty development. *Journal of Dental Education* 74(9):980-985.

McDonough, D. 2007. *What's new in ADAA demographics.* http://findarticles.com/p/articles/mi_m0MKX/is_1_76/ai_n18645509/ (accessed March 9, 2011).

McKinnon, A., and D. Jorgenson. 2009. Pharmacist and physician collaborative prescribing: For medication renewals within a primary health centre. *Canadian Family Physician* 55(12):e86-e91.

McQuistan, M. R., R. A. Kuthy, F. Qian, K. J. Riniker-Pins, and K. E. Heller. 2010. Dentists' treatment of underserved populations following participation in community-based clinical rotations as dental students. *Journal of Public Health Dentistry* 70(4):276-284.

McWhorter, A. G., N. Sue Scale, and S. A. King. 2001. Infant oral health education in U.S. dental school curricula. *Pediatric Dentistry* 23(5):403-409.

Mertz, E., and P. Glassman. 2011. Alternative practice dental hygiene in California: Past, present, and future. *CDA Journal* 39(1).

Mertz, E. A., and K. Grumbach. 2001. Identifying communities with low dentist supply in California. *Journal of Public Health Dentistry* 61(3):172-177.

Mezey, M., S. G. Burger, H. G. Bloom, A. Bonner, M. Bourbonniere, B. Bowers, J. B. Burl, E. Capezuti, D. Carter, J. Dimant, S. A. Jerro, S. C. Reinhard, and M. Ter Maat. 2005. Experts recommend strategies for strengthening the use of advanced practice nurses in nursing homes. *Journal of the American Geriatrics Society* 53(10):1790-1797.

Ministry of Health Malaysia. 2005. *Oral healthcare in Malaysia.* http://ohd.moh.gov.my/uploads/oral_healthcare_in_malaysia_05.pdf (accessed April 30, 2009).

Misra, S., R. H. Harvey, D. Stokols, K. H. Pine, J. Fuqua, S. M. Shokair, and J. M. Whiteley. 2009. Evaluating an interdisciplinary undergraduate training program in health promotion research. *American Journal of Preventive Medicine* 36(4):358-365.

Mitchell, D. A., and S. L. Lassiter. 2006. Addressing health care disparities and increasing workforce diversity: The next step for the dental, medical, and public health professions. *American Journal of Public Health.* 96(12):2093-2097.

Mitchell, T. V., R. Peters, C. C. Gadbury-Amyot, P. R. Overman, and L. Stover. 2006. Access to care and the allied oral health care workforce in Kansas: Perceptions of Kansas dental hygienists and scaling dental assistants. *Journal of Dental Education* 70(3):263-278.

Moller, J. 2010. Mobile dental clinic rules endorsed by legislative committee. *Times-Picayune*, August 10. http://www.nola.com/politics/index.ssf/2010/08/mobile_dental_clinic_rules_end.html (accessed April 11, 2011).

Morgan, M. A., J. Crall, R. L. Goldenberg, and J. Schulkin. 2009. Oral health during pregnancy. *Journal of Maternal-Fetal and Neonatal Medicine* 22(9):733-739.

Morris, A. L., J. F. Hasler, and J. E. Mulvihill. 1982. Resolved: That a fifth year of dental education be a requirement. Remarks for the affirmative. *Journal of Dental Education* 46(6):327-331.

Morrow, J. W., M. A. Keels, K. J. Hale, H. F. Thomas, M. J. Davis, C. S. Czerepak, P. A. Weiss, J. Crall, D. Krol, J. Lee, M. W. Ng, R. Quinonez, J. Stigers, and A. Stolic. 2008. Preventive oral health intervention for pediatricians. *Pediatrics* 122(6):1387-1394.

Mouradian, W. E. 2010. *Wanted . . . physicians who understand oral health*. Paper presented at meeting of the Committee on an Oral Health Initiative, Washington, DC.

Mouradian, W. E., J. H. Berg, and M. J. Somerman. 2003. Addressing disparities through dental-medical collaborations, part 1. The role of cultural competency in health disparities: Training of primary care medical practitioners in children's oral health. *Journal of Dental Education* 67(8):860-868.

Mouradian, W. E., A. Reeves, S. Kim, R. Evans, D. Schaad, S. G. Marshall, and R. Slayton. 2005. An oral health curriculum for medical students at the University of Washington. *Academic Medicine* 80(5):434-442.

Mouradian, W. E., A. Reeves, S. Kim, C. Lewis, A. Keerbs, R. L. Slayton, D. Gupta, R. Oskouian, D. Schaad, and T. Kalet. 2006. A new oral health elective for medical students at the University of Washington. *Teaching and Learning in Medicine* 18(4):336-342.

Mouradian, W., C. N. Bertolami, L. Tedesco, C. Aschenbrener, S. J. Crandall, R. M. Epstein, M. Da Fonseca, N. K. Haden, A. Ruffin, J. J. Sciubba, S. Silverton, and R. P. Strauss. 2008. Curriculum and clinical training in oral health for physicians and dentists: Report of panel 2 of the Macy study. *Journal of Dental Education* 72(Supp. 2):73-85.

Mundinger, M. O., R. L. Kane, E. R. Lenz, A. M. Totten, W. Y. Tsai, P. D. Cleary, W. T. Friedewald, A. L. Siu, and M. L. Shelanski. 2000. Primary care outcomes in patients treated by nurse practitioners or physicians: A randomized trial. *Journal of the American Medical Association* 283(1):59-68.

Nash, D. A. 2009. Adding dental therapists to the health care team to improve access to oral health care for children. *Academic Pediatrics* 9(6):446-451.

Nash, D. A., and W. R. Willard. 2010. On why the dental therapists' "movement" in the United States should focus on children—not adults. *Journal of Public Health Dentistry* 70(4):259-261.

Nash, D. A., J. W. Friedman, T. B. Kardos, R. L. Kardos, E. Schwarz, J. Satur, D. G. Berg, J. Nasruddin, E. G. Mumghamba, E. S. Davenport, and R. Nagel. 2008. Dental therapists: A global perspective. *International Dental Journal* 58(2):61-70.

National Dental Association. 2010. *The National Dental Association comments on access to care and mid-level providers for underserved communities*. http://www.dentistryiq.com/index/display/article-display/0456395037/articles/dentisryiq/hygiene-department/2010/11/NDA_position_paper_on_mid-level_providers.html (accessed March 16, 2011).

National Denturist Association. 2011. *Affiliates*. http://www.nationaldenturist.com/affiliates.html (accessed March 9, 2011).

National Task Force on Quality Nurse Practitioner Education. 2008. *Criteria for evaluation of nurse practitioner programs*. Washington, DC: National Organization of Nurse Practitioner Faculties.

NC Department of Health and Human Services. 2009. *2008-2009 annual report: North Carolina oral health section*. http://www.ncdhhs.gov/dph/oralhealth/library/includes/08-09%20OHS%20Annual%20Report.pdf (accessed March 15, 2011).

Nelson, R. 2006. Protecting patients or turf? The AMA aims to limit nonphysician health care professionals. *American Journal of Nursing* 106(8):25-26.

Neumann, L. M. 2004. Trends in dental and allied dental education. *Journal of the American Dental Association* 135(9):1253-1259.

Ng, M., P. Glassman, and J. Crall. 2008. The impact of Title VII on general and pediatric dental education and training. *Academic Medicine* 83(11):1039.

Nickens, H. W. 1992. The rationale for minority-targeted programs in medicine in the 1990s. *Journal of the American Medical Association* 267(17).

NIH (National Institutes of Health). 2010. *The NIH almanac: National Institute of Dental and Craniofacial Research*. http://www.nih.gov/about/almanac/organization/NIDCR.htm (accessed November 1, 2010).

Nolan, L., B. Kamoie, J. Harvey, L. Vaquerano, S. Blake, S. Chawla, J. Levi, and S. Rosenbaum. 2003. *The effects of state dental practice laws allowing alternative models of preventive oral health care delivery to low-income children*. Washington, DC: Center for Health Services Research and Policy, School of Public Health and Health Services, The George Washington University.

Oakley, D., M. E. Murray, T. Murtland, R. Hayashi, H. F. Andersen, F. Mayes, and J. Rooks. 1996. Comparisons of outcomes of maternity care by obstetricians and certified nurse-midwives. *Obstetrics and Gynecology* 88(5):823-829.

O'Brien, M. J., C. H. Halbert, R. Bixby, S. Pimentel, and J. A. Shea. 2010. Community health worker intervention to decrease cervical cancer disparities in Hispanic women. *Journal of General Internal Medicine* 25(11):1186-1192.

Office of Technology Assessment. 1986. *Nurse practitioners, physician assistants, and certified nurse-midwives: A policy analysis (Health technology case study 37)*. Washington, DC: U.S. Government Printing Office.

Okunseri, C., A. Szabo, S. Jackson, N. Pajewski, and R. Garcia. 2009. Increased children's access to fluoride varnish treatment by involving medical care providers: Effect of a Medicaid policy change. *Health Services Research* 44(4):1144-1156.

Okwuje, I., E. Anderson, and R. W. Valachovic. 2009. Annual ADEA survey of dental school seniors: 2008 graduating class. *Journal of Dental Education* 73(8):1009-1032.

Okwuje, I., E. Anderson, and R. W. Valachovic. 2010. Annual ADEA survey of dental school seniors: 2009 graduating class. *Journal of Dental Education* 74(9):1024-1045.

O'Leary, K. J., D. B. Wayne, C. Haviley, M. E. Slade, J. Lee, and M. V. Williams. 2010. Improving teamwork: Impact of structured interdisciplinary rounds on a medical teaching unit. *Journal of General Internal Medicine* 25(8):826-832.

Oregon State Denturist Association. 2011. *About denturism*. http://www.ordenturist.org/about_denturism.htm (accessed March 9, 2011).

Orlans, J., E. Mertz, and K. Grumbach. 2002. *Dental health professional shortage area methodology: A critical review.* San Francisco, CA: UCSF Center for the Health Professions.

Pew Center on the States and National Academy for State Health Policy. 2009. *Help wanted: A policy maker's guide to new dental providers*. Washington, DC: Pew Center on the States, National Academy for State Health Policy.

PHI. 2010. *Facts 3: Who are direct care workers?* http://www.directcareclearinghouse.org/download/PHI%20FactSheet3_singles.pdf (accessed September 27, 2010).

Pierce, K. M., R. G. Rozier, and W. F. Vann. 2002. Accuracy of pediatric primary care providers' screening and referral for early childhood caries. *Pediatrics* 109(5):e82.

Price, S. S., W. D. Brunson, D. A. Mitchell, C. J. Alexander, and D. L. Jackson. 2007. Increasing the enrollment of underrepresented minority dental students: Experiences from the dental pipeline program. *Journal of Dental Education* 71(3):339-347.

Pyle, M., S. C. Andrieu, D. G. Chadwick, J. E. Chmar, J. R. Cole, M. C. George, G. N. Glickman, J. F. Glover, J. S. Goldberg, N. K. Haden, W. D. Hendricson, C. Meyerowitz, L. Neumann, L. A. Tedesco, R. W. Valachovic, R. G. Weaver, R. L. Winder, S. K. Young, and K. L. Kalkwarf. 2006. The case for change in dental education. *Journal of Dental Education* 70(9):921-924.

Quijano, A., A. J. Shah, A. I. Schwarcz, E. Lalla, and R. J. Ostfeld. 2010. Knowledge and orientations of internal medicine trainees toward periodontal disease. *Journal of Periodontology* 81(3):359-363.

Rackley, B., J. Wheat, C. Moore, R. Garner, and B. Harrell. 2003. The southern rural access program and Alabama's rural health leaders pipeline: A partnership to develop needed minority health care professionals. *Journal of Rural Health* 19(5):354-360.

Rauh, S. J. 1917. The present status of and necessity for mouth hygiene. *American Journal of Public Health* 7:631-636.

RCHWS (Regional Center for Health Workforce Studies). 2003. *Changes in the scope of practice and the supply of non-physician clinicians in Texas*. San Antonio, TX: Regional Center for Health Workforce Studies, Center for Health Economics and Policy, The University of Texas Health Science Center at San Antonio.

Reeves, S., M. Zwarenstein, J. Goldman, H. Barr, D. Freeth, M. Hammick, and I. Koppel. 2008. Interprofessional education: Effects on professional practice and health care outcomes. *Cochrane Database of Systematic Reviews* (1): CD002213.

Reeves, S., M. Zwarenstein, J. Goldman, H. Barr, D. Freeth, I. Koppel, and M. Hammick. 2010. The effectiveness of interprofessional education: Key findings from a new systematic review. *Journal of Interprofessional Care* 24(3):230-241.

Remington, T. L., M. A. Foulk, and B. C. Williams. 2006. Evaluation of evidence for interprofessional education. *American Journal of Pharmaceutical Education* 70(3).

Reynolds, P. P. 2008. A legislative history of federal assistance for health professions training in primary care medicine and dentistry in the United States, 1963-2008. *Academic Medicine* 83(11):1004-1014

Riordan, P. J., I. Espelid, and A. B. Tveit. 1991. Radiographic interpretation and treatment decisions among dental therapists and dentists in Western Australia. *Community Dentistry and Oral Epidemiology* 19(5):268-271.

Riter, D., R. Maier, and D. C. Grossman. 2008. Grantwatch report: Delivering preventive oral health services in pediatric primary care: A case study. *Health Affairs* 27(6):1728-1732.

Rosenblatt, R. A., S. A. Dobie, L. G. Hart, R. Schneeweiss, D. Gould, T. R. Raine, T. J. Benedetti, M. J. Pirani, and E. B. Perrin. 1997. Interspecialty differences in the obstetric care of low-risk women. *American Journal of Public Health* 87(3):344-351.

Rosenthal, E. L., J. N. Brownstein, C. H. Rush, G. R. Hirsch, A. M. Willaert, J. R. Scott, L. R. Holderby, and D. J. Fox. 2010. Community health workers: Part of the solution. *Health Affairs* 29(7):1338-1342.

Rozier, R. G., B. K. Sutton, J. W. Bawden, K. Haupt, G. D. Slade, and R. S. King. 2003. Prevention of early childhood caries in North Carolina medical practices: Implications for research and practice. *Journal of Dental Education* 67(8):876-885.

Rozier, R. G., S. C. Stearns, B. T. Pahel, R. B. Quinonez, and J. Park. 2010. How a North Carolina program boosted preventive oral health services for low-income children. *Health Affairs* 29(12):2278-2285.

Safriet, B. J. 1994. Impediments to progress in health care workforce policy: License and practice laws. *Inquiry* 31(3):310-317.

Safriet, B. J. 2002. Closing the gap between *can* and *may* in health-care providers' scopes of practice: A primer for policymakers. *Yale Journal on Regulation* 19(2):301-334.

Salama, F., and A. Kebriaei. 2010. Oral care for infants: A survey of Nebraska general dentists. *General Dentistry* 58(3):182-187.

Saman, D. M., O. Arevalo, and A. O. Johnson. 2010. The dental workforce in Kentucky: Current status and future needs. *Journal of Public Health Dentistry* 70(3):188-196.

Schachtel, B. P. 1978. The pediatric nurse practitioner: Origins and challenges. *Medical Care* 16(12):1019-1026.

Schulman, M., K. R. Lucchese, and A. C. Sullivan. 1995. Transition from house staff to nonphysicians as neonatal intensive care providers: Cost, impact on revenue, and quality of care. *American Journal of Perinatology* 12(6):442-446.

Sharp, N. 1996. Nurse practitioner reimbursement: History and politics. *Nurse Practitioner* 21(3):100, 103-104.

Shepard, L. 1978. Licensing restrictions and the cost of dental care. *Journal of Law and Economics* 21(1):187-201.

Shirk, C. 2010. *Oral health checkup: Progress in tough fiscal times?* Washington, DC: National Health Policy Forum.

Silk, H., S. O. G. Stille, R. Baldor, and E. Joseph. 2009. Implementation of STFM's "Smiles for Life" oral health curriculum in a medical school interclerkship. *Family Medicine* 41(7):487-491.

Siriphant, P., T. F. Drury, A. M. Horowitz, and R. M. Harris. 2001. Oral cancer knowledge and opinions among Maryland nurse practitioners. *Journal of Public Health Dentistry* 61(3):138-144.

Skillman, S. M., M. P. Doescher, W. E. Mouradian, and D. K. Brunson. 2010. The challenge to delivering oral health services in rural America. *Journal of Public Health Dentistry* 70(Supp. 1):S49-S57.

Snyder, M. E., A. J. Zillich, B. A. Primack, K. R. Rice, M. A. Somma McGivney, J. L. Pringle, and R. B. Smith. 2010. Exploring successful community pharmacist-physician collaborative working relationships using mixed methods. *Research in Social and Administrative Pharmacy* 6(4):307-321.

Sorrel, A. M. 2010. Organized medicine pushes back on expansions of scope of practice. *American Medical News* 53(2).

Sowter, J. R., and D. K. Raynor. 1997. The management of oral health problems in community pharmacies. *Pharmaceutical Journal* 259(6957):308-310.

Sox Jr., H. C. 1979. Quality of patient care by nurse practitioners and physician's assistants: A ten-year perspective. *Annals of Internal Medicine* 91(3):459-468.

Spielman, A. I., T. Fulmer, E. S. Eisenberg, and M. C. Alfano. 2005. Dentistry, nursing, and medicine: A comparison of core competencies. *Journal of Dental Education* 69(11): 1257-1271.

Statler, M. 2010. *Physician assistant leadership gather to address "hidden threat" in primary care at oral health summit.* http://paeaonline.org/index.php?ht=d/ContentDetails/i/112672 (accessed March 14, 2011).

STFM (Society of Teachers of Family Medicine). 2011a. *For educators: Downloadable modules.* http://www.smilesforlifeoralhealth.org/default.aspx?tut=555&pagekey=62948&s1=1223096 (accessed May 22, 2011).

STFM. 2011b. *Smiles for Life: A national oral health curriculum.* http://www.smilesforlife2.org (accessed May 22, 2011).

STFM. 2011c. *State varnish training information.* http://www.smilesforlifeoralhealth.org/default.aspx?tut=555&pagekey=62948&s1=1223096 (accessed May 22, 2011).

Strafford, K. E., C. Shellhaas, and, E. M. Hade. 2008. Provider and patient perceptions about dental care during pregnancy. *Journal of Maternal-Fetal and Neonatal Medicine* 21(1):63-71.

Strauss, R. P., M. B. Stein, J. Edwards, and K. C. Nies. 2010. The impact of community-based dental education on students. *Journal of Dental Education* 74(10 Supp.):S42-S55.

Sullivan, D., and L. Rohlfsen. 2007. Professional politics and the challenge of anesthesia availability in rural hospitals. *Research in the sociology of health care* 25:149-167.

Sullivan Commission. 2004. *Missing persons: Minorities in the health professions, a report of the Sullivan Commission on diversity in the healthcare workforce.* The Sullivan Commission.

Sun, N., G. Burnside, and R. Harris. 2010. Patient satisfaction with care by dental therapists. *British Dental Journal* 208(5):E9.

Tejani, A., J. Epstein, G. Gibson, and N. Le. 2002. A survey assessing the impact of a hospital-based general practice residency program on dentists and dental practice. *Special Care in Dentistry* 22(1):16-22.

Thierer, T., and C. Meyerowitz. 2005. Education of dentists in the treatment of patients with special needs. *Journal of the California Dental Association.* 33(9):723-729.

Thind, A., K. A. Atchison, R. M. Andersen, T. T. Nakazono, and J. J. Gutierrez. 2008. Reforming dental education: Faculty members' perceptions on the continuation of pipeline program changes. *Journal of Dental Education* 72(12):1472-1480.

Thind, A., K. A. Atchison, T. T. Nakazono, J. J. Gutierrez, D. C. Carreon, and J. Bai. 2009. Sustainability of dental school recruitment, curriculum, and community-based pipeline initiatives. *Journal of Dental Education* 73(Supp. 2):S297-S307.

Thistlethwaite, J., and M. Moran. 2010. Learning outcomes for interprofessional education (IPE): Literature review and synthesis. *Journal of Interprofessional Care* 24(5):503-513.

Thomson, W. A., P. Ferry, J. King, C. M. Wedig, and G. B. Villarreal. 2010. A baccalaureate-MD program for students from medically underserved communities: 15-year outcomes. *Academic Medicine* 85(4):668-674.

Todd, B. A., A. Resnick, R. Stuhlemmer, J. B. Morris, and J. Mullen. 2004. Challenges of the 80-hour resident work rules: Collaboration between surgeons and nonphysician practitioners. *Surgical Clinics of North America* 84(6):1573-1586.

Tomar, S. L. 2005. *Dental public health training: Time for new models?* Paper presented at the National Oral Health Conference, Pittsburgh, PA.

Tomar, S. L. 2006. An assessment of the dental public health infrastructure in the United States. *Journal of Public Health Dentistry* 66(1):5-16.

U.S. Census Bureau. 2010. *Table 1. Estimates of the resident population by selected age groups for the United States, states, and Puerto Rico: July 1, 2009 (SC-EST2009-01).* http://www.census.gov/popest/states/asrh/tables/SC-EST2009-01.xls (accessed March 14, 2011).

U.S. Department of Education. 2010. *College accreditation in the United States: Specialized accrediting agencies.* http://www2.ed.gov/admins/finaid/accred/accreditation_pg7.html#health (accessed December 22, 2010).

USMLE (U.S. Medical Licensing Examination). 2010a. *2011 step 2 clinical knowledge: Content description and general information.* Philadelphia, PA: Federation of State Medical Boards of the United States and National Board of Medical Examiners.

USMLE. 2010b. *2011 step 3: Content description and general information.* Philadelphia, PA: Federation of State Medical Boards of the United States and National Board of Medical Examiners.

Vainio, L., M. Krause, and M. R. Inglehart. 2011. Patients with special needs: Dental students' educational experiences, attitudes, and behavior. *Journal of Dental Education* 75(1):13-22.

Veal, K., M. Perry, J. Stavisky, and K. D. Herbert. 2004. The pathway to dentistry for minority students: From their perspective. *Journal of Dental Education* 68(9):938-946.

Viswanathan, M., J. L. Kraschnewski, B. Nishikawa, L. C. Morgan, A. A. Honeycutt, P. Thieda, K. N. Lohr, and D. E. Jonas. 2010. Outcomes and costs of community health worker interventions: A systematic review. *Medical Care* 48(9):792-808.

Walker, M. P., S. I. Duley, M. M. Beach, L. Deem, R. Pileggi, N. Samet, A. Segura, and J. N. Williams. 2008. Dental education economics: Challenges and innovative strategies. *Journal of Dental Education* 72(12):1440-1449.

Wall, T. P., and L. J. Brown. 2007. The urban and rural distribution of dentists, 2000. *Journal of the American Dental Association* 138(7):1003-1011.

Wanchek, T. 2010. Dental hygiene regulation and access to oral healthcare: Assessing the variation across the us states. *British Journal of Industrial Relations* 48(4):706-725.

Weil, T. N., and M. R. Inglehart. 2010. Dental education and dentists' attitudes and behavior concerning patients with autism. *Journal of Dental Education* 74(12):1294-1307.

Weinberg, M. A., and W. J. Maloney. 2007. Treatment of common oral lesions. *U.S. Pharmacist* 32(3):82-88.

Wendling, W. R. 2010. Private sector approaches to workforce enhancement. *Journal of Public Health Dentistry* 70(Supp. 1):S24-S31.

Wetterhall, S., J. D. Bader, B. B. Burrus, J. Y. Lee, and D. A. Shugars. 2010. *Evaluation of the dental health aide therapist workforce model in Alaska.* Research Triangle Park, NC: W.K. Kellogg Foundation, Rasmuson Foundation, Bethel Community Services Foundation.

Whitley, E. M., R. M. Everhart, and R. A. Wright. 2006. Measuring return on investment of outreach by community health workers. *Journal of Health Care for the Poor and Underserved* 17(1 Supp.):6-15.

WICHE (Western Interstate Commission for Higher Education). 2011. *Professional student exchange program (PSEP).* http://wiche.edu/psep (accessed January 11, 2011).

Wilder, R., C. Robinson, H. L. Jared, S. Lieff, and K. Boggess. 2007. Obstetricians' knowledge and practice behaviors concerning periodontal health and preterm delivery and low birth weight. *Journal of Dental Hygiene* 81(4):81.

Wilder, R. S., J. A. O'Donnell, J. M. Barry, D. M. Galli, F. F. Hakim, L. J. Holyfield, and M. R. Robbins. 2008. Is dentistry at risk? A case for interprofessional education. *Journal of Dental Education* 72(11):1231-1237.

Williams, B. C., T. L. Remington, M. A. Foulk, and A. L. Whall. 2006. Teaching interdisciplinary geriatrics ambulatory care: A case study. *Gerontology and Geriatrics Education* 26(3):29-45.

Wilson, I. B., B. E. Landon, L. R. Hirschhorn, K. McInnes, L. Ding, P. V. Marsden, and P. D. Cleary. 2005. Quality of HIV care provided by nurse practitioners, physician assistants, and physicians. *Annals of Internal Medicine* 143(10):729-736, I772.

Wing, P., M. H. Langelier, E. S. Salsberg, and R. S. Hooker. 2004. The changing professional practice of physician assistants: 1992 to 2000. *JAAPA: Official Journal of the American Academy of Physician Assistants* 17(1):37-40, 42, 45.

Winkleby, M. A. 2007. The Stanford medical youth science program: 18 years of a biomedical program for low-income high school students. *Academic Medicine* 82(2):139-145.

Yeager, A. L. 2001. Where will the genome lead us? Dentistry in the 21st century. *Journal of the American Dental Association* 132(6):801-807.

Young, W. O. 1958. Dental manpower and the public's health: The role of the state health agency. *American Journal of Public Health* 48(1):46-50.

4

Settings of Oral Health Care

The oral health care system is bifurcated with its two parts functioning in almost complete separation; in general, they use different financing systems, serve different population groups, and provide care in different settings. In the private delivery system, care is typically provided in small, private dental offices and financed primarily through employer-based or privately purchased dental coverage and out-of-pocket payments. The safety net, in contrast, is made up of a diverse and fragmented group of providers in various settings. It is financed primarily through Medicaid and the Children's Health Insurance Program (CHIP), other government programs, private grants, and out-of-pocket payments. (Financing will be discussed more specifically in Chapter 5.) The safety net has an important role providing care to the underserved, but it is limited in its capacity. As discussed in Chapter 3, the nondental health care workforce is becoming increasingly involved in the provision of oral health care. While primary care settings (including private medical offices) should also be seen as settings of care for oral health, this chapter will focus primarily on settings for care provided by dental professionals.

This chapter gives an overview to the delivery of care in both private practices and safety net settings, including descriptions of their patients, staffing, challenges, and successes. The capacity of the system to care for vulnerable and underserved populations will be addressed, as well as particular non-financial challenges. Finally, the chapter concludes with descriptions of innovations occurring across the country to change how and where oral health services are provided in order to meet the needs of vulnerable and underserved populations.

PRIVATE DELIVERY SYSTEMS

Most dental services are provided in private dental practices owned and staffed by a single dentist. Approximately 92 percent of professionally active dentists work in this private practice model (ADA, 2009a). (See Box 3-1 in Chapter 3 for a description of types of dentists.) About 60 percent of private practice dentists are solo dentists (Wendling, 2010). Thirteen percent of private practice dentists are employees, and 3 percent function as independent contractors (ADA, 2009d). Private practices tend to be located in areas that have the population to support them; thus, there are more practices located in urban areas than rural areas, and more practices are located in high-income than low-income areas (ADA, 2009a; Solomon, 2007; Wall and Brown, 2007).

Staffing

Independent dentists usually employ one or more individuals in the private practice setting, with an average of 4.8 total staff members per dentist (ADA, 2009b). On average, the independent dentist employs 1.3 dental hygienists per dentist and 1.8 chairside assistants per dentist. Nearly 90 percent of independent dentists employ at least one full-time person, and 68 percent employ at least one person who only works part-time. The majority of these dentists employ chairside assistants (94 percent of dentists), secretaries/receptionists (91 percent), and dental hygienists (68 percent). Some independent dentists employ office managers (31 percent), financial coordinators (16 percent), and other personnel such as sterilization assistants and laboratory technicians. However, dental assistants often perform many of these duties.

Workload

Independent dentists work about 47.5 weeks annually and 35.9 hours per week. These dentists spend about 90 percent of their work hours treating patients (ADA, 2009a). In a survey by the American Dental Association (ADA) of the perceived workload of independent dentists, about 20 percent stated they were "not busy enough, could have treated more patients" (ADA, 2009a). Independent general practitioners have an average of 1,871 active patients[1] (for single dentist practices) (ADA, 2009a). Independent general practitioners spend about 51 minutes per patient, and their patients have about 3.3 visits per year. Independent specialists spend slightly less time per patient (42 minutes), and the typical patient visits

[1] Active patients are commonly defined as those treated within the previous 2 years.

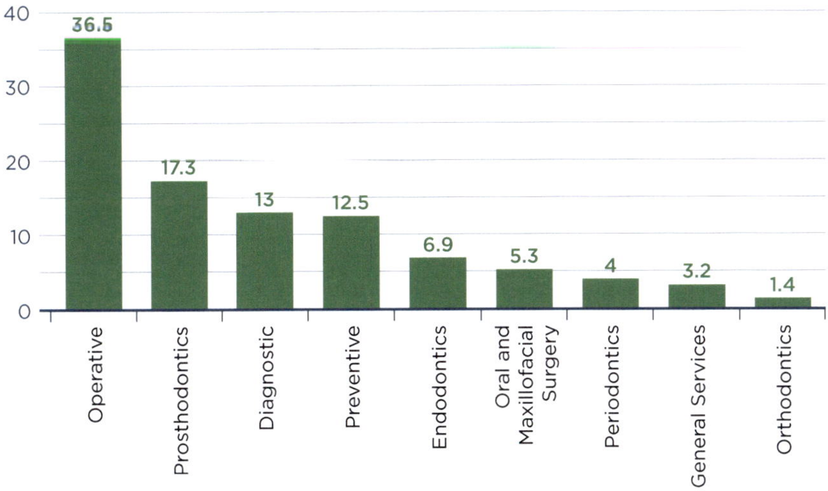

FIGURE 4-1
Percentage distribution of time spent by independent general practitioners in private practice, 2007.

SOURCE: ADA, 2009a.

more frequently (five times per year). Independent general practitioners only spend about one-quarter of their time on diagnosis or prevention (see Figure 4-1). Both new and existing patients wait about a week for a new appointment (a decrease of one full day from 2003). Independent dentists see a little over five walk-in or emergency patients each week. In 2007, independent dentists had about 81 weekly scheduled visits (including dental hygiene appointments).

In the private practices of independent dentists, dental hygienists work, on average, almost 47 weeks per year and 24 hours per week (ADA, 2009b). Dental hygienists see about 25 patients per week. Chairside assistants work almost 48 weeks per year and 32 hours per week.

Patient Population

The patients of independent general practitioners are spread relatively evenly across the age spectrum (see Figure 4-2). Specialists see a significantly greater proportion of patients aged 17 years or less, likely due to the practice profiles of orthodontists and pediatric dentists (ADA, 2009a).

Slightly more than half (55 percent) of independent dentists' patients are female, and nearly two-thirds (63 percent) have private insurance (ADA, 2009a). Only 7 percent of the patients of independent dentists re-

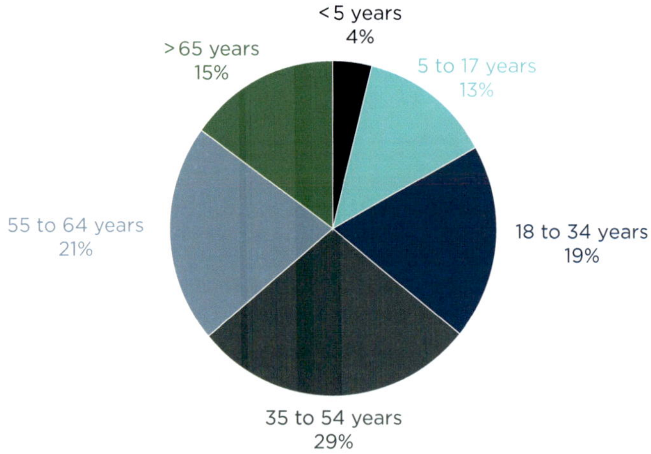

FIGURE 4-2
Age breakdown for patients of independent general practitioners in private practice, 2007.

NOTE: Does not total 100 percent due to rounding.
SOURCE: ADA, 2009a.

ceive public assistance for their dental coverage; the remaining 30 percent of patients are not covered by any dental insurance. Nearly two-thirds of all independent dentists (63.3 percent) and slightly more than half of all new independent dentists (57.5 percent) do not have any patients covered by public sources.

Expenses and Income

In 2007, the average gross billings per owner from the primary private practice for all independent dentists was approximately \$774,000 (or about \$656,000 per dentist in the practice and \$500 per active patient), of which approximately 94 percent was collected[2] (ADA, 2009c). Independent dentists in incorporated practices tend to have higher gross billings per owner than those in unincorporated practices. Independent dentists primarily receive payment from private insurance and direct patient payment (see Figure 4-3). Specialists tend to receive less payment from private insurance and more from direct patient payment.

[2] Gross billings are the total amount of fees charged. Calculations are made on a per owner basis assuming equal contribution by all partners. Gross billings are only reported for independent dentists who own their private practice.

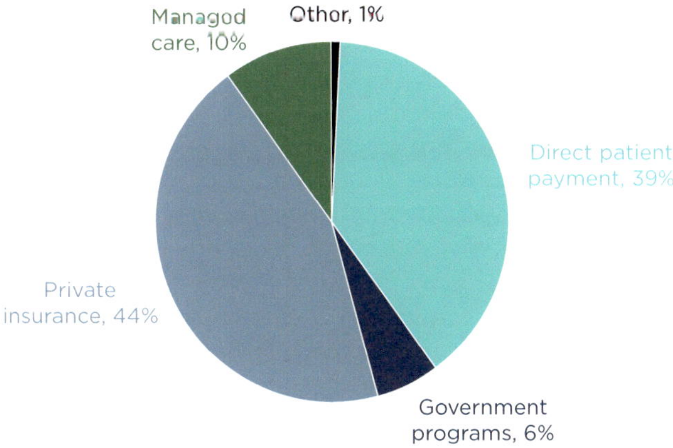

FIGURE 4-3
Sources of gross billings, all independent dentists, 2007.

SOURCE: ADA, 2009c.

In 2007, practice expenses (excluding the salaries of owners, but including the salaries of other employees) accounted for 59 percent of gross billings from the primary private practice of all independent dentists (ADA, 2009c). As discussed in Chapter 3, the salaries of private practice dentists vary depending on employment situation and type of practice. For all independent practitioners, net income does not vary greatly by number of years since graduation. However, this does not take the number of hours worked into account. Between 2003 and 2007, the net income of independent dentists increased about 1 percent annually (when adjusted for inflation) (ADA, 2009c). Between 1982 and 2000, dentists' real income grew without change to their workload (essentially, the number of patients seen per day and the number of weeks worked per year remained relatively constant) (Guay, 2005). This increase in productivity is, in part, due to the increased use of dental hygienists and dental assistants (Brown, 2005; Guay, 2005). (The capacity and efficiency of the oral health care system is discussed further later in this chapter.)

Demand for dental care may vary with the economic climate of the country (Guay, 2005; Wendling, 2010). For example, the recent recession was identified as a key factor contributing to 2009 having the slowest rate of growth in health spending (4 percent) in the last 50 years (Martin et al., 2011). Notably, expenditures on dental services had a negative rate of growth (–0.1 percent) in 2009, down from a positive rate of growth of 5.1 percent in 2008.

THE ORAL HEALTH SAFETY NET

Underserved and vulnerable populations often cannot access the private dental system due to geographic, monetary, or other barriers, and so they rely on the safety net. While the term *safety net* may give the impression of an organized group of providers available to serve anyone who cannot access the private system, the dental safety net is composed of unrelated entities that both individually and collectively have very limited capacity. Generally, the safety net is composed of an array of providers, including (but not limited to) Federally Qualified Health Centers (FQHCs), FQHC look-alikes, non-FQHC community health centers, dental schools, school-based clinics, state and local health departments, and not-for-profit and public hospitals. Each type of provider offers some type of dental care, but the extent of the services provided and the number of patients served varies widely. Even with this variety of options, the safety net still does not meet the needs of all who are left out of the private system, often because of a lack of capacity of these providers or a perceived lack of affordable options by individuals (Bailit et al., 2006; Haley et al., 2008; Kenney et al., 2009; Mertz and O'Neil, 2002). The following sections give brief overviews of several types of providers and programs typically considered as part of the safety net.

Federally Qualified Health Centers

An FQHC is any health center that receives a grant established by section 330 of the Public Health Service Act.[3] FQHCs must be located in or serve a medically underserved area or medically underserved population, provide both primary health care services as well as supportive services (e.g., education, transportation, translation services), and see patients regardless of their ability to pay for those services. FQHCs are governed by community boards that have a fiduciary responsibility for the center, and more than half of the board members must be patients of the health center and represent the population served. The statute that established FQHCs specifically identifies migratory and seasonal agricultural workers, the homeless, and residents of public housing as underserved populations. Thus, some FQHCs are referred to as Migrant Health Centers, Health Care for the Homeless Programs, and Public Housing Primary Health Care Centers. All of these programs fall under the umbrella term FQHC. FQHCs receive a number of additional benefits in addition to section 330 grants, including higher Medicare and Medicaid reimbursement rates, access to

[3] 42 U.S.C. §254b.

providers funded by the National Health Service Corps, and drug pricing discounts (HRSA, 2010).

FQHCs primarily provide care to underserved and vulnerable individuals. In 2009, 71 percent of patients served by FQHCs had income at or below 100 percent of the federal poverty level, 93 percent had income at or below 200 percent of the federal poverty level, 38 percent were uninsured, and 37 percent were insured by Medicaid. Table 4-1 illustrates the proportion of FQHC patients who come from vulnerable and underserved populations, as compared to their representation in the U.S. population as a whole.

The FQHC program is growing steadily. In 2009, the Health Resources and Services Administration (HRSA) funded 1,131 FQHCs, which are located in all 50 states, the District of Columbia, and Puerto Rico (HRSA, 2011b). That number is up from 914 FQHCs in 2004. Funding for FQHCs is also increasing. The American Recovery and Rehabilitation Act includes $2 billion for FQHCs (HHS, 2010a), and the health care reform bills includes $11 billion for a Community Health Centers Trust Fund that will allow FQHCs to expand access and make capital improvements, and $1.5 billion for a new National Health Service Corps Trust Fund.[4]

FQHCs are required to provide certain services—including preventive, but not comprehensive, dental services—either in the clinic or by referral. In 2008, 80 percent of the 1,080 FQHCs provided on-site dental services, and 88 percent provided dental services on site or by referral (Anderson, 2010; Cottam, 2010). This reflects significant progress towards the *Healthy People 2020* goal of 83 percent of health centers including an oral health component (HHS, 2010b). In 2009, FQHCs provided dental care to 3.4 million patients, in 8.4 million dental visits, which is nearly a three-fold increase over the number of patients and visits in 2000 (HRSA, 2011c; Ruddy, 2007). This care is not exclusively preventive; although FQHCs are not required to provide comprehensive oral health services, over 75 percent do so, and millions of patients received restorative and rehabilitative care through FQHCs in 2009 (Anderson, 2010; HRSA, 2011b). The expansion of dental services in FQHCs reflects a concerted commitment from HRSA. Since 2001, HRSA has invested $55 million in oral health service expansion grants (Anderson, 2010). In addition, a statutory change in the Children's Health Insurance Program Reauthorization Act allows FQHCs to expand their reach outside of their physical facilities.[5] FQHCs may now contract with private practice dentists to provide oral health services to FQHC

---

[4] *Patient Protection and Affordable Care Act*, Public Law 148, 111th Cong., 2nd sess. (March 23, 2010); *Health Care and Education Reconciliation Act of 2010*, Public Law 152, 111th Cong. 2nd sess. (March 30, 2010).

[5] *Children's Health Insurance Program Reauthorization Act of 2009*, Public Law 3, 111th Cong., 1st sess. (February 4, 2009), §501.

TABLE 4-1
Underserved and Vulnerable Populations Served in FQHCs as Compared to Their Representation in the U.S. Population, 2009

	Percentage of FQHC Population	Percentage of U.S. Population
Poverty		
At or below 100% of poverty	71	14
Medical insurance status		
Uninsured	38	17
Medicaid (Title XIX)	36	16
Private insurance	15	64
Race		
Asian/Pacific Islander	5	5
American Indian/Alaska Native	2	1
African American	27	13
White	62	72
Ethnicity		
Hispanic/Latino	35	16

NOTES: Percentages are of the FQHC population reporting a certain characteristic.
SOURCES: DeNavas-Walt et al., 2010; HRSA, 2011c; U.S. Census Bureau, 2010.

patients in the dentist's office. Previously, some states required the dentist to individually enroll in Medicaid before providing services for the FQHC (CMS, 2011b).

FQHCs employ over 8,000 full-time equivalent dental staff, including over 2,500 dentists and over 1,000 dental hygienists (HRSA, 2011e). FQHC executive directors report that they most commonly recruit dentists through the National Health Service Corps, although only 10.2 percent of FQHC dentists report receiving a NHSC scholarship, and an additional 19.4 percent report receiving NHSC loan repayment (Bolin, 2010). Even fewer dental hygienists report receiving funding from the NHSC. A large number of FQHC dentists previously worked in the private sector; 31.9 percent reported previously working as a private practice owner, partner, or associate, and 18.5 percent reported previously working as an employee dentist in a private practice (Bolin, 2010). Dentists and dental hygienists working at FQHCs report being generally satisfied with their work: 80.2

percent of dentists and 93.3 percent of dental hygienists intend to remain employed in a health center practice (Bolin, 2010). But more than 39 percent of health centers reported at least one dentist vacancy, and over 50 percent of those positions were vacant for more than 6 months (Bolin, 2010; Cottam, 2010).

With the rapid expansion of dental programs in FQHCs, there appears to be a lack of training and guidance for FQHC dentists. FQHC dental programs are unique within dentistry because they generally function within a general health clinic, may not be ultimately overseen by a dental professional, and charge per encounter, rather than per procedure. Therefore, specialized guidance may be necessary for the dental programs to thrive (Geiermann, 2010). Previously, HRSA offered training and technical assistance to FQHC dentists through its regional dental consultant program. That program has essentially been eliminated, with the retirement of the last consultant in 2009 (Geiermann, 2010). The number of dental public health professionals employed by HRSA has dwindled from a high of over 100 to under 20, most of whom are not able to provide technical assistance to FQHCs. Anecdotal reports indicate that current FQHC dentists do not have a reliable source of assistance (Geiermann, 2010). Indeed, the last oral health guidance to FQHCs was issued in March 1987 (Geiermann, 2010).

FQHC Look-Alikes

FQHC look-alikes were established by Congress to extend the concept of FQHCs (HRSA, 2003). Look-alikes must meet all of the statutory requirements of FQHCs—for example, they provide services to the medically underserved, operate as nonprofits, and be governed by a community board—but they do not receive grant funding under section 330 (HRSA, 2003). FQHCs look-alikes are eligible for many, but not all, of the benefits extended to FQHCs, such as increased Medicaid and Medicare payments and drug pricing discounts (HRSA, 2003). Very little data are available about the dental care provided at FQHC look-alikes because they are not required to submit detailed information to the Department of Health and Human Services about visits.

Community Health Centers

Many community health centers (CHCs) do not receive federal funding or subsidies and operate completely outside of the FQHC system. Some of those health centers are nonprofits, while some are supported or operated by state and local governments. There is no national database of CHCs, so very little information is available about the types of services they provide or the numbers of patients they serve. One study roughly estimated that they serve about 2.2 million dental patients each year (Bailit et al., 2006). CHCs generally have very limited funding. In 2001, for example, Illinois CHCs had an average annual budget of $182,000 (Byck et al., 2005).

Dental Schools and Residency Programs

Dental students gain experience treating patients in dental school-based clinics. The patients served in those clinics are generally low-income, so dental school clinics are considered part of the dental safety net (Bailit et al., 2006). Dental students provided about 2.9 million patient visits in 2001–2002, with an average of 13 visits per patient, meaning that dental students treated about 224,000 patients during the year (Bailit et al., 2006). The number of patient visits has remained relatively constant; in 2009, dental students had 2.9 million patient visits in dental school clinics and in community-based rotations (ADA, 2010).

The care provided in dental school clinics is affordable but time consuming for patients because clinics are organized as student teaching laboratories rather than patient-centered delivery systems (Bailit et al., 2007). *Dental Education at the Crossroads* recognized that the mixed missions of educating students and caring for patients lead to trade-offs in both efficiency and quality of care:

> Dental students must gain sufficient clinical experience in a variety of technical procedures to become competent entry-level practitioners, qualified to graduate and become licensed. A procedure-driven learning process does not necessarily translate into efficient, high-quality patient care, particularly when student care is further constrained by low budgets for clinical and administrative support. (IOM, 1995)

Some progress has been made toward increasing the efficiency and patient-centeredness of dental school clinics, but more can be done (Formicola et al., 2008).

In addition to on-site clinics at dental schools, dental students also provide care through community rotations in FQHCs and community health centers (ADA, 2010). Of the 2.9 million dental visits provided by dental students in 2009, approximately 450,000 were provided in the community (ADA, 2010), and a large proportion of those visits were in underserved communities (Atchison et al., 2009).

Residencies in dentistry, as in medicine, are an important source of care for underserved populations, including economically and socially disadvantaged populations and medically compromised patients (Mito et al., 2002). One recent study concluded that requiring 1 year of residency training would significantly expand the capacity of community hospitals (or dental schools) to care for the underserved (Bailit et al., 2006). By their estimates, approximately 1,800 additional dental school graduates would participate in a 1-year general dentistry residency program and an additional 887,000 patients would receive care each year.

School-Based Dental Clinics

School-based health centers (SBHCs) were developed to provide basic health care services, including dental care, in elementary and secondary schools. SBHCs are perhaps the most convenient care location for both children and parents because they eliminate the need for transportation, parent time off, and missed school. Children with access to a SBHC are more likely to have seen a dentist in the past year than similar students without access to a SBHC (Kaplan et al., 1999). In addition, children at high risk for dental caries who have access to a school-based dental sealant program are more than twice as likely to have sealants than children without access (Siegal and Detty, 2010). SBHCs are also associated with improved academic performance, increased use of primary care, reduced use of emergency rooms, and increased use of vaccines (Allison et al., 2007; Walker et al., 2010; Young et al., 2001).

While SBHCs offer significant potential to increase access to oral health care, only a small number of schools have SBHCs, and only a small percentage of those SBHCs offer dental services. Approximately 1,900 school-based health centers operate throughout the country (NASBHC, 2010). Table 4-2 summarizes the oral health services provided by SBHCs during the 2007–2008 school year. Many SBHCs offer simple preventive oral health care, such as oral health education and dental screenings, both on site and by referral, but fewer clinics offer more complex procedures. For example, 84 percent of SBHCs provide oral health education both on site and by referral, but that number drops to 57 percent for dental screenings, 20 percent for dental examinations by a dentist, and the ability of an SBHC to provide oral health services is limited by the number staff qualified to provide oral health services. Only 12.4 percent of SBHCs have a dental provider on staff (NASBHC, 2010). The dental capacity could potentially be expanded by using the new and emerging providers discussed in Chapter 3, as is now done with nurse practitioners and physician assistants in providing medical care in SBHCs. SBHCs have successfully worked in collaboration with public health departments (discussed below) to provide both screening and treatment services. Recognizing the potential for SBHCs to expand access to oral health care to underserved populations, HRSA recently announced a grant program to fund comprehensive oral health care services in SBHCs (HRSA, 2011d).

Although some concern has been raised about whether SBHCs have an adequate funding source (Silberberg and Cantor, 2008), the Patient

TABLE 4-2
Percentage of SBHCs Offering Selected Oral Health Services by Mode of Delivery, 2007–2008 School Year

	Onsite and referral (%)	By referral only (%)	Not provided or referred (%)
Oral health education	83.7	11.3	5.0
Dental screenings	56.7	37.0	6.3
Dental examination (by a dentist)	19.5	68.3	12.1
Dental sealants	25.1	61.2	13.7
Fluoride mouth rinse	21.3	57.6	21.1
Fluoride varnish	20.1	58.3	21.6
Fluoride supplements	14.9	61.2	24.0
Dental cleaning	22.6	65.4	12.1
General dental care (fillings, extractions)	10.3	75.8	13.9
Specialty dental care (orthodontics, root canal)	4.8	79.1	16.0

SOURCE: NASBHC, 2010.

Protection and Affordable Care Act established federal grant programs for the establishment and operation of SBHCs.[6] While the legislation does not require SBHCs to offer oral health care, it does require any SBHC that receives federal funding to offer referrals to, and follow-up for, oral health services.

Mobile Dental Clinics

Mobile dental clinics (e.g., mobile vans) have also been used to bring oral health services to underserved populations. A mobile dental clinic can be set up in a retrofitted recreational vehicle or bus using portable dental equipment (ASTDD, 2011c). A range of dental services can be provided in a mobile dental clinic, from preventive care including oral exams, radiographs, and sealant placement, to restorative and specialty care (Carr et al., 2008). Mobile dental clinics are often operated by other safety net provid-

[6] *Patient Protection and Affordable Care Act*, Public Law 148, 111th Cong., 2nd sess. (March 23, 2010).

ers, such as FQHCs, state and local health departments, and dental schools, in an effort to extend their reach. They are generally funded through a combination of grants, insurance payments, state and local agency funds, out-of-pocket payments, and volunteers (ASTDD, 2011b). Comprehensive data are not available on the number of mobile dental clinics in operation or on the number of patients they serve (ASTDD, 2011b).

Increasingly, mobile equipment is being used to provide care in settings such as nursing homes. Rather than requiring individuals to travel to a specific site of care (as may be difficult for older adults with physical limitations), this option allows oral health care professionals to provide care to patients where they live, work, and learn. The use of mobile equipment (apart from mobile vans) in alternative settings is discussed later in this chapter in the section on innovations.

Health Departments

Most states have established an oral health plan, whether as a part of the state's direct dental public health activities or as a part of a larger health plan (CDC, 2011c). Such plans are usually developed and overseen by oral health directors or dental directors under the umbrella of state departments of (public) health. The Association of State and Territorial Dental Directors lists membership in all 50 states (ASTDD, 2011a). The range of services and activities provided under the auspices of state public health dentistry, however, vary considerably, and range from assessment (e.g., gathering oral health data through surveillance activities), to policy development (e.g., related to access), to assurance (e.g., providing clinical preventive and treatment services, supporting community-level water fluoridation) (ASTDD, 2011d).

Oral health data gathered through state public health dental programs allow state and federal agencies to identify trends in oral diseases, oral health professional shortage areas, and to provide the basis for future planning. Examples of policy development through state-level dental public activities include mandating that all children in kindergarten, second, and sixth grades receive an annual dental examination in Illinois (Conis, 2009); requiring Medicaid recipients in Iowa to have a dental home and receive preventive dental care (Rodgers et al., 2010); and developing statewide oral health coalitions.

State-level dental public health programs provide both population and individual-level preventive, promotive, and restorative care. State public health dental programs, through county and city health departments, also provide fluoride varnish, mouth rinse, and fluoride tablets (ASTDD, 2011d). School-based dental sealant programs are available in at least a dozen states and often target high-poverty areas where there is little availability of oral health care. For example, in 2009–2010, under the auspices of the Tennessee Department of Health, school-based dental sealant programs targeted schools with 50 percent or higher rate of free and reduced lunch, reaching over 300 schools and providing sealants to almost 50,000 children (Tennessee Department of Health, 2010).

Through a combination of both state and local support (including Title V funds), local health departments (LHDs) also provide a variety of oral health services. In 2008–2009, 394 LHDs in 28 states had a dental program that provided restorative services (ASTDD, 2010). Overall, a survey of states found more than 2,700 community-based dental clinics for low-income populations (ASTDD, 2010). The level and intensity of such services, though, varies considerably by the size of the community served by the LHD; for example, only 20 percent of LHDs that serve populations of less than 25,000 offer oral health services, while 57 percent of LHDs serving populations of 500,000 or more offer oral health services (NACCHO, 2009). The provision of oral health care at the LHD level, however, is decreasing: in 1992–1993, 44 percent of LHDs provided some level of oral health services; this decreased to 31 percent in 2005 and 29 percent in 2008 (NACCHO, 2006, 2009) and is likely to decrease further with state and local budget deficits.

Funding for state and local dental public health services continues to be challenging. In 2011, the Centers for Disease Control and Prevention (CDC) provided $6.8 million to just 20 state oral health programs to support evidence-based prevention programs (e.g., community water fluoridation and school-based sealant programs), to provide surveillance of the oral disease burden, and to develop plans to improve oral health and address disparities (CDC, 2011a). This is an increase from $2.3 million in 2003 to support 12 programs (CDC, 2011b). These funds are used to

- Ensure program leadership and staff support.
- Monitor oral diseases and their risk factors.
- Develop a state oral health plan.
- Develop and work with state oral health coalitions and other partnerships.
- Develop and evaluate disease prevention programs, such as community water fluoridation and school-based dental sealant programs (CDC, 2010).

HRSA also supports states through grants (e.g., Title V) for innovative programs to address the needs of designated dental health professional shortage areas. In the past, states have used these funds to increase the availability of school, community, and mobile-based oral health care; to develop cultural competence curriculum for allied health professionals;

and to implement school-based sealant programs, among many others (HRSA, 2011a). In the past, HRSA has also supported local public health infrastructure by training state dental directors and other dental public health professionals and offering technical assistance to state and local health departments through the regional dental consultant program described above (Geiermann, 2010). As mentioned previously, as of 2009, all of the regional dental consultants had retired, and the program had ended (Geiermann, 2010).

Hospital Emergency Departments

People have increasingly turned to hospital emergency departments (EDs) for dental care (Ladrillo et al., 2006; Maiuro, 2009; Shesser, 2010). One hospital reported a 121 percent increase in ED visits for dental complaints between 1997 and 2001, compared to a 28 percent increase for nondental complaints (Ladrillo et al., 2006). In many counties in California, the rate of ED visits for preventable dental complaints exceeds the rate of visits for both asthma and diabetes (Maiuro, 2009). In a presentation to this committee, Dr. Robert Shesser shared data from The George Washington University ED showing that they had 1,700 ED visits related to oral health between 2006 and 2009, accounting for 0.66 percent of all ED visits (Shesser, 2010). The most common diagnoses included dental caries (683 visits), dental pain (452 cases), and dental abscesses (321 cases).

Patients may seek dental care in EDs because they do not have access to traditional dental care. For example, residents of dental health professional shortage areas are more likely to visit an ED for dental care than people who do not live in shortage areas (Okunseri et al., 2008). A study of five Minneapolis hospital systems showed that most ED dental visits were made during normal business hours, when patients might visit a dental office or clinic if they had access to one (Davis et al., 2010). In Wisconsin, African Americans, Native Americans, and Asian Americans, who are more likely than the general population to have unmet dental needs, were also more likely to seek dental treatment in an ED (Okunseri et al., 2008).

Dental coverage appears to be a predictor of use of EDs for dental care (Cohen et al., 2002; Davis et al., 2010). In the Minneapolis study, most ED dental visits were paid by Medicaid or out-of-pocket (Davis et al., 2010). And when Maryland eliminated Medicaid dental coverage for adults, the rate of Medicaid ED claims for dental visits increased 12 percent (Cohen et al., 2002). In Washington state, dental disorders are the most common diagnosis in the ED for uninsured patients and the sixth most common for patients insured by Medicaid, but it is not in the top 25 diagnoses for patients with private insurance (Washington State Hospital Association, 2010).

EDs are not well suited to treat oral health problems; few have the equipment or staff necessary to diagnose and treat dental disease. Likely as a result, ED dental visits are more likely than nondental ED visits to result in a prescription for antibiotics or pain medication, and a referral to a another provider (Lewis et al., 2003). This method of care increases costs, because insurance must pay for both an unnecessary ED visit in addition to a follow-up dental appointment (Okunseri et al., 2008).

Volunteer Efforts

Private-sector efforts to supplement the safety net include the organization of volunteer events to provide free oral health care. These efforts are typically single-day events and provide temporary relief for some people, but they do not provide a regular source of care. As mentioned in Chapter 1, these include the Missions of Mercy (MOM) projects. MOM projects are often organized by state dental societies or private foundations and staffed by volunteer dental professionals to provide care on a first-come, first-served basis. At these events, thousands of individuals often wait in lines for many hours (Dickinson, 2010). As of March 2010, 44 MOM projects served approximately 35,000 patients in 20 states (Dickinson, 2010). This included over $17 million in dental services, including 60,255 extractions and 31,018 restorations.

In 2003, the ADA established the annual Give Kids a Smile Day, an annual program that includes regional 1-day events to provide educational, screening, preventive, and clinical (e.g., restorative) services to underserved children. In 2010, over 2,100 single-day events served 317,319 children and were staffed by 10,455 dentists and 37,724 other volunteers. Overall, 30 percent of children received educational services; 27 percent received screening services; 23 percent received clinical services; and 20 percent received preventive services (Warren, 2010).

Remote Area Medical, founded in 1985, is a nonprofit, charitable organization that provides free health care, dental care, eye care, veterinary services, and technical and educational assistance to remote populations around the world, but most typically in Appalachia (www.ramusa.org). Volunteers offer a range of health care services (often concurrently) at events which typically last 2 or 3 days at a single location. The extent of dental services offered expanded from emergency extractions only to the provision of restorative care, cleanings, and fluoride treatments. Since its inception, Remote Area Medical has hosted over 600 events (Remote Area Medical, 2011).

CAPACITY AND EFFICIENCY OF THE CURRENT SYSTEM

Several factors contribute to the capacity and efficiency of the oral health care system. In large part, assessments of the oral health care system have focused on the adequacy of the dental workforce. These assessments are usually based either on unmet need or demand for dental services (Guthrie et al., 2009). In 2005, Brown did a comprehensive assessment of the adequacy of the dental workforce (Brown, 2005). He noted a combination of "demand-generating and demand-reducing" forces contribute to such an assessment, including the growth of the population, the retirement rate of dentists, the proportion of the population that seeks care, the types of services needed, the state of the economy, and the development of new treatment modalities. For example, wider recognition of the impact of oral diseases, especially by nondental professionals, could cause a shift toward preventive care and then potentially decrease the need for restorative care. Tough economic times may lead to decreased utilization, especially when services are not covered, or when job loss leads to the loss of dental benefits. Wider adoption of health information technology could help streamline practices and improve efficiency.

Capacity also relates to the typical characteristics of a dental practice. Very few dentists work in large practices, and often are in solo practice. Most of the expansion in the capacity of the private practice has been due to increased use of other personnel, such as dental hygienists and dental assistants, which allows them to delegate some responsibilities (Beazoglou et al., 2009; Brown, 2005). The use of these professionals, changes in office hours, and the design of office space have been attributed to the near doubling of dentist productivity between 1960 and 2002 (Brown et al., 2005). Another consideration is the interval of recall for routine dental examinations and cleanings. While the standard of biannual visits to the dentist is commonly accepted, there is no evidentiary basis to support this interval (Bader, 2005; Beirne et al., 2007). In fact, research suggests that the interval might be better determined for each individual patient based on a combination of factors including risk for oral diseases and clinical judgment and expertise of the dental team (Anthonappa and King, 2008; Bader, 2005; Gibson and Moosajee, 2008; National Institute for Clinical Excellence, 2004; Patel et al., 2010). Reassessment of recall intervals for low-risk populations might improve the capacity of the oral health care system to provide more care for those at higher risk for oral disease.

Estimating Workforce Adequacy

Historically, estimating the adequacy of the workforce itself has been difficult. Similar to the findings of Brown in 2005, in 2009, Guthrie et al. (2009) noted that

> considering only unmet need without factoring in the role of economic, social, and cultural factors can lead to large miscalculations of the amount of dental care that will actually be used, which, in turn, can result in large miscalculations on workforce.

Between 1983 and 2001, estimates of the need for dentists fluctuated several times from predicting oversupply to undersupply (Brown, 2005). For example, between 1986 and 2001, seven dental schools closed, exacerbating concerns for future shortages (Guthrie et. al., 2009). Instead of simply estimating the number of individual dental professionals needed to deliver care to every American, more consideration is needed for the influences of supply and demand. Through several modeling exercises, Brown concluded that expanding the number of dentists would be costly and that a better approach to improving productivity would be for dentists to use more allied personnel (Brown, 2005). Brown did not consider expanding the scope of practice in his models. A recent economic modeling exercise to gauge the impact of the addition of several types of dental professionals (including dental therapists) to a private practitioner's office showed that

> By raising the number of patients served each day, allied providers can make it possible for most existing private practices to care for Medicaid-enrolled patients without sacrificing profitability. (Pew Center on the States, 2010)

Estimating the Capacity of the Safety Net

In 2006, Bailit and colleagues (2006) examined the capacity of the safety net to expand in order to care for, in their estimate, 33.3 million underserved individuals. (They assumed these expansions would occur within the current structure of the oral health care system.) Specifically, they looked to FQHCs, health centers, community hospitals, school-based clinics, and dental schools. Overall, they estimated that 7.4 million individuals were already being served in those sites of care, and that there was only capacity to add another 2.6 million patients. The authors, however, did note a lack of data for some of their assumptions. They did conclude that the three most important strategies for increasing the capacity of the safety net are to improve the productivity of FQHCs, require dental residency programs, and require dental student rotations in community-based care of underserved populations. They also concluded

> Even with an expanded safety net, the majority of underserved patients would continue to receive care in private practices. Thus, a long-term reduction in access-to-care and oral health disparities requires greater participation by the private practice community. (Bailit et al., 2006)

The safety net system has an important role providing care to the underserved, but it is very limited in size. Compared with other safety net providers, only FQHC dental clinics have a definable source of long-term funding. While the number and size of FQHCs are likely to expand, they do not have the capacity to care for all the unmet needs of vulnerable and underserved populations. While safety net providers are essential to the care of vulnerable and underserved populations, access disparities cannot be reduced unless more private-sector dentists provide care to these populations.

Future Trends

Several trends may influence the future capacity and efficiency of the oral health care system in the future, although the extent of these influences, especially on access to care for vulnerable and underserved populations, remains to be seen.

The Changing Gender Profile in Dentistry

As noted in Chapter 3, entering classes of dental students are approaching an even split between male and female students. Some data show that up to the age of 45, female dentists are more likely to work part time than male dentists (with not enough data existing for female dentists after age 45) (Brown, 2005). However, in a 2009 IOM workshop, Valachovic stated that male dentists tend to work many hours early in their careers and then start to diminish the number of hours they work later in their careers, while women tend to take time off early in their careers for family-related issues, but then increase their number of hours later in their careers (IOM, 2009). Further research and data will be needed in order to fully understand the impact of the changing gender profile of dentists both on the productivity of dentists in general as well as on access to care.

Retirement Rates

In 2008, the IOM noted that a challenge to the health care workforce in general is the aging of its members (IOM, 2008). As noted in Chapter 3, the demographic profiles of dentists and dental hygienists raise concerns about the proportions of those workforces that will reach retirement ages over the next decade. However, retirement rates will depend on many factors including the better health of older adults today which might lead to longer careers on either a full time or part-time basis (Guthrie et al., 2009). As the IOM suggested in 2008, older workers might be retained by the development of less physically demanding roles or more flexible work schedules (IOM, 2008). In addition, the economic downturn of recent years might lead to delays in planned retirement (Guthrie et al., 2009). Again, however, these changes in practice patterns have unknown effects on access to care for vulnerable and underserved populations.

New Dental Schools

Another factor to consider is the impact of the several new dental schools that are in various stages of planning and development. An assessment by Guthrie et al. (2009) estimated more than 8,000 additional graduates by 2022, but ultimately concluded that "the increase in dentists will not noticeably improve access to care for low-income and rural populations absent additional public funding to support demand for these populations and concurrent measures to effect even distribution of dentists throughout the country" (Guthrie et al., 2009).

While the number of dental schools is expanding, existing schools are having difficulty with attracting and retaining faculty (Chmar et al., 2008; Haden et al., 2000; McAndrew, 2010; Vanchit et al., 2011). Common reasons for being unable to fill faculty positions include lack of response to position announcements, unqualified candidates, and budgetary limits (Chmar et al., 2008). Among faculty who leave academics, approximately one-third do so for more lucrative careers in private practice (Chmar et al., 2008). The Patient Protection and Affordable Care Act[7] of 2010 (ACA) includes financial assistance to dentists who plan to teach or are teaching in general; pediatric or public health dentistry; and faculty loan repayment programs for general, pediatric, and public health dentists who agree to serve as full-time faculty. In addition, under Title VII, individuals from disadvantaged backgrounds who agree to serve as faculty for at least two years at dental and dental hygiene schools are eligible for the Faculty Loan Repayment Program.[8]

Overcoming Barriers in the System

The current oral health care system is not well designed to overcome barriers to caring for vulnerable and underserved populations. As was

[7] *Patient Protection and Affordable Care Act*, Public Law 148, 111th Cong., 2nd sess. (March 23, 2010).

[8] 42 U.S.C. §293b.

discussed in Chapter 2, literacy issues have a profound effect on the appreciation of oral health care and subsequent utilization of oral health services, and the current system is not well designed to promote education and literacy improvement efforts. Patient behaviors—missed appointments in particular—are frequently cited as barriers to provider participation in Medicaid and as obstacles to providing care to Medicaid patients, especially in the private system (Borchgrevink et al., 2008; CMS, 2011a; GAO, 2000). It is important to note, however, that there may be significant challenges to keeping scheduled appointments for many lower-income patients, aside from health literacy issues. For example, many lower-income individuals may experience difficulty taking time off from work for dental appointments (by design of office hours that are inconvenient for working adults and parents), arranging transportation to the dentist, or finding child care (GAO, 2000; Greenberg et al., 2008; Mofidi et al., 2002; Shirk, 2010). Because providers are prohibited from charging Medicaid for missed appointments, they are financially disadvantaged when patients miss appointments. Therefore, reducing the number of missed appointments can be an important part of efforts to improve provider participation in Medicaid. (Provider participation in Medicaid is discussed further in Chapter 5.)

Well-designed case management programs can address many of dentists' issues with Medicaid (ADA, 2004; Binkley et al., 2010; Greenberg et al., 2008). For example, a case management program in New York state took a multipronged approach to increasing Medicaid dental utilization in a rural county (Greenberg et al., 2008). The case manager recruited dentists through presentations, letters, phone calls, and mailings. To assist with billing concerns, the case manger arranged billing training for dental office support staff, tracked billing problems until they were resolved, and informed dental offices when patients lost or gained Medicaid coverage. The case manager addressed dentists' concerns about missed appointments by educating patients about the importance of oral health and the appropriate use of oral health care, helping patients select the dentist that was most convenient to their work or home, making appointments, and following up with patients when the dental office could not reach them or when they had missed appointments. During the course of the case management program, the number of dentists participating in the program went from 2 to 28, and the percentage of Medicaid-eligible patients receiving dental care increased from 9 percent to over 40 percent. Other, comparable case management programs (some of which also included a reimbursement rate increase) have had similar results (ADA, 2004; Binkley et al., 2010).

INNOVATIONS IN SETTINGS OF CARE

The following sections provide descriptions of an array of innovations being used to improve access to oral health care by delivering care in alternative settings or through the use of new modalities. In some cases, these innovations are too new to have robust outcomes data for impact on access to care or oral health status, especially in the long term, and therefore the committee does not intend to imply that it is recommending these approaches. In addition, these examples are not exhaustive of all of the strategies being used across the nation. Instead, the following section serves to illustrate the wide variety of ideas and opportunities for providing care in a variety of settings, partnering with existing programs, or developing new sites of care in order to improve access to care for vulnerable and underserved populations.

Virtual Care

The use of telehealth technologies is emerging as a strategy to provide dental services in underserved communities where significant barriers to receiving care in a traditional dental office setting exist (Glassman and Subar, 2010; Kopycka-Kedzierawski et al., 2007; Sanchez Dils et al., 2004). The University of the Pacific Arthur A. Dugoni School of Dentistry has initiated a 4-year demonstration program for providing basic oral health care services to disadvantaged populations in remote locations. Dental professionals (including registered dental hygienists, registered dental hygienists in alternative practice, and registered dental assistants) provide screening, preventive services, temporary restorations, and case management services to low-income and disabled patients in nursing homes, public schools, and residential homes for developmentally disabled individuals under the supervision of dentists linked to the remote locations electronically (e.g., via portable video camera). The professionals in the field electronically send diagnostic information (e.g., physical examination, history, photographs, X-rays) to dentists who review the materials, make diagnoses, and develop treatment plans. Then, the field-based professionals provide preventive services such as oral hygiene instruction, prophylaxes and fluoride varnish, temporary restorations, and refer patients needing dental services to dental clinics or private practices. In some cases, dentists come to the remote sites with portable equipment and provide services. At this time the project is operating in nine remote sites (University of the Pacific, 2011).

While telehealth-enabled delivery systems have the potential to expand the reach of dentists and allied dental personnel into community sites, there are a number of barriers that currently limit their spread. These include the fact that most state laws do not allow general supervision of allied dental personnel using telehealth technology (Center for Connected Health Policy, 2011). In addition, many private payers do not recognize the use of telehealth-delivered care (Whitten and Buis, 2007), although Medicare and many state Medicaid programs now pay for telehealth services (CMS, 2011c; Youngblade et al., 2005).

Extending the Reach of FQHCs

School-Based Care

In addition to formal SBHCs, school-based care systems have the potential to reduce access disparities and improve the oral health of children from low-income families. For example, in 2003, in response to low utilization rates of Medicaid and SCHIP-eligible children, an FQHC in central Connecticut initiated a school dental program in which dental hygienists provide screening and basic preventive services in schools using mobile equipment and temporary space (Bailit et al., 2010). The dental hygienists also identify children in need of more advanced care. As part of the hygienist's examination, children are placed into risk groups that determine the frequency and types of preventive services they receive. Another program feature is organized as educational modules for teachers, caregivers, and students.

Since 2003, several other state FQHCs have established similar programs that currently provide oral health care to low-income children in over 200 public schools and Head Start programs. The estimated number of children treated each year is over 10,000 and growing rapidly (Bailit et al., 2010). The FQHCs target schools with large numbers of Medicaid- and CHIP-eligible children, aged 3 to 18 years, but all low-income children are eligible to receive care. FQHCs consider these children FQHC patients and are reimbursed at their usual visit rate. While most children are enrolled in the Medicaid or CHIP programs, those without insurance are also eligible to receive care at a low fee.

A major challenge is making sure that children receive needed restorative care. The Connecticut program began using case managers to arrange for caregivers to bring children to FQHC clinics, where they were given priority in obtaining timely appointments. Only 40 percent of referred children actually received care with this approach (Bailit et al., 2010). To increase the completion of restorative care, FQHC dentists now follow the hygienists and provide restorative and other services in schools using portable equipment. Only a relatively small percentage of these students have behavioral, medical, and dental problems that cannot be treated by dentists using portable equipment. In these cases, a case manager works with caregivers to make sure that these children receive treatment.

The program has the full support of organized dentistry in Connecticut, and it is highly regarded by public school administrators and teachers. In time, Connecticut FQHCs are expected to develop the capacity to meet the needs of all interested schools (Bailit et al., 2010). This plan has many advantages including

- Minimal need, if any, for special grant funding, since in most states FQHC per-visit Medicaid reimbursement rates should be adequate to cover program costs;
- Effective use of dental professionals;
- Limited startup capital; elimination of caregiver transportation, time, and scheduling barriers to taking children to dental offices and clinics;
- Availability of FQHCs to patients who require a more advanced level of care; and
- Dental education to teachers, caregivers, and patients.

Multisite FQHCs

The Marshfield Clinic has been successful at reducing oral health disparities in rural Wisconsin through a targeted, multisite FQHC approach (Nycz, 2010). As of July 2010, Marshfield clinic operated seven dental clinics in rural Wisconsin; at that time, the number was projected to increase to nine by 2011, and they planned to operate 16 dental clinics throughout the state by 2016 (Nycz, 2010). At that time, Marshfield dental clinics will have the capacity to provide over 400,000 visits per year to 158,000 patients in nearly 400 operatories staffed by 91 dentists and 69 hygienists (Nycz, 2010).

Marshfield has a four-part strategy for reducing oral health disparities in their community: regionalizing care, integrating dentistry with medicine, treating all populations, and training its own workforce (Nycz, 2010). To efficiently reach a dispersed, rural population, Marshfield opened clinics in regional centers, often county seats. This strategy also allowed them to place multiple dentists in each center, which they suspected might improve dentist recruitment and retention. Marshfield integrated dental records into their medical records and vice versa, which prompts physicians to educate their patients about oral health and refer them to the dental clinics, and gives dentists full access to patients' medical records. In addition, each clinic is accessible to people with special health care needs, including wheelchair accessible operatories. Finally, Marshfield is in the process of establishing a dental school to train dentists specifically to work with underserved and vulnerable populations in rural areas (Kilsdonk, 2010; Nycz, 2010).

Three years after Marshfield opened its first dental clinic, the publicly insured population in the county where it is located accessed care at the same rates as those who have private coverage (Nycz, 2010). In addition, cost per visit has decreased over time because the burden of disease has decreased in the population (Nycz, 2010).

Building on Existing Community Services

Another strategy to increase access is for dental professionals to partner with existing community partners, as a delivery point for providing oral health care. Below, two such examples are given in which oral health care has been incorporated into larger programs.

Women, Infants, and Children Agencies

The primary mission of the Special Supplemental Nutrition Program for Women, Infants, and Children (WIC) is to promote healthy diets and feeding practices for women, infants, and children. To participate, caregivers are required to go to WIC offices for food vouchers and education on a quarterly or monthly basis. As an example, California has the nation's largest WIC program and serves 60 percent of all children born in California (Center for Oral Health, 2010). The WIC Early Intervention for Oral Health project builds on the existing nutrition program and adds a dental education, screening, prevention, and referral component. Partnerships between dental providers and California WIC programs are required to develop protocols for providing oral health care directly on site, in a mobile van, or an adjacent dental clinic; develop plans for parental education; track numbers seen; and provide case management for follow-up care (Center for Oral Health, 2010).

Head Start

In another example, the Head Start program, administered by the Office of Head Start of the Administration for Children and Families, is "a national program that promotes school readiness by enhancing the social and cognitive development of children through the provision of educational, health, nutritional, social and other services to enrolled children and families" (OHS, 2011). Head Start programs are required to determine whether a child has received age-appropriate preventive dental care within 90 days of the child entering the Head Start program.[9] If a child has not received appropriate care, the Head Start program must help the parents

[9] Code of Federal Regulations, Office of Human Development Services, Department of Health and Human Services, title 45, sec. 1304.20 (2009).

make arrangements for the child to receive it.[10] Appropriate care is determined by the state's Early and Periodic Screening, Diagnosis, and Treatment program and periodicity schedule. Head Start programs must also obtain or arrange for testing, examination, and treatment for children with known or suspected dental problems, and develop and implement a follow-up plan for any problems identified.

To foster access to oral health for children enrolled in Head Start, in 2006, the Office of Head Start invested $2 million in grants to 52 Head Start, Early Head Start, and Migrant/Seasonal Head Start programs for the Head Start Oral Health Initiative; grantees received supplemental funding for 4 additional years. While grantees reported successfully developing partnerships with community organizations and providers who would serve Head Start children, educating staff about the importance of oral health, and incorporating oral health education into the curriculum, they reported that they likely could not sustain much of the oral health programming when the grant funding ended (Del Grosso et al., 2008).

Requirements Tied to Public Education

Several states have introduced programs requiring a dental examination or oral health assessment prior to school entry, though the provisions of these programs differ across states. Even though the requirements have been legislated, many of the plans do not have enforcement or follow-up mechanisms in place. In addition, little data exist on the impact of these types of requirements. Examples include the following:

- Illinois will withhold student report cards if the requirement is unfulfilled (Conis, 2009).
- In 2008, Kentucky passed a law effective in the 2010–2011 school year requiring children to have a dental examination prior to enrolling in public school (Conis, 2009).
- New York requests parents to provide a dental certificate documenting an oral health exam at certain points during a child's school career (Conis, 2009).

Alternative Sites of Care

Portable Equipment

Patient-centered approaches to caring for vulnerable and underserved populations may require consideration for bringing oral health care to the

[10] Ibid.

sites that are more convenient for those populations. In particular, older adults and disabled individuals may be unable to travel to travel to dentists' offices. In these cases, portable equipment is increasingly being used to provide on-site, community-based care in settings such as nursing homes, group homes, schools, and Head Start centers.

For example, Apple Tree Dental (Apple Tree) is a private, nonprofit organization in Minnesota that has provided care to individuals with special health care needs across the life span in a variety of settings for over 25 years (Silow-Carroll and Alteras, 2004). The program has two dental clinic "hubs," but it provides most of its care through community-based mobile programs. Apple Tree contends advantages to mobile care include reduced anxiety for patients (due to the familiar environment), interdisciplinary care, and improved efficiency (e.g., reduction in transportation costs for each patient) (Silow-Carroll and Alteras, 2004). Apple Tree has been a source of community-based educational experiences for dental hygienists and dental assistants through partnerships with dental hygiene and dental assisting programs. Apple Tree also collects data on its patient population, which facilitates research on special care populations. In 2008, Apple Tree reported almost 60,000 patient encounters (Helgeson, 2009).

In another example, Dr. Greg Folse made a presentation to this committee regarding his work providing mobile oral health services for residents in 23 nursing facilities (Folse, 2010). Dr. Folse estimated that 61 percent of the dentate nursing home residents (or 45 percent of the total resident population) needed surgical interventions due to abscesses and/or severe gum disease. He further estimated that this meant that 1,062 existing patients were in need of surgical interventions and that an additional 371 new residents would need such care each year. In 2009, working part-time in these nursing homes and using portable equipment, Dr. Folse reported being able to treat 392 surgical cases, manage 3 cases of oral cancer, direct between 1 and 5 dental emergencies weekly (many of which were life threatening), and treat 262 denture patients. He also noted one death occurring as a result of oral disease. Dr. Folse also noted using portable dental equipment to care for children in Louisiana schools. He reported using 15 dentists and 18 expanded duty dental assistants to provide care in 275 schools. He stated that the benefits of using portable equipment included decrease in "no-show" patients, no late appointments, and no loss of time from work for parents. Disadvantages include difficulty with scheduling time during the school hours and obtaining parental consent. Dr. Folse noted that since 2001, his Louisiana school-based model had treated over 20,000 children in the school setting and included over 30,000 patient visits.

Retail Health Clinics

Retail health clinics have been rapidly developing as a new site of care for general health care (Hunter et al., 2009; Laws and Scott, 2008; Mullin, 2009; Pollack and Armstrong, 2009; Pollack et al., 2010; Rudavsky et al., 2009; Thygeson et al., 2008; Wang et al., 2010). Recently, retail dental clinics have been proposed as an alternative site of dental care (Scott, 2009, 2010). Much like retail health clinics, retail dental clinics would be located in pharmacies, grocery stores, and large retailers. The clinics would offer a limited menu of services at set prices, focus primarily on preventive and diagnostic care, and refer patients with more complex needs to dentists. Although no retail dental clinics currently exist, an economic model suggests that they could be viable if dental professionals could provide care without the presence of a dentist (Scott, 2009).

Dental Homes

While not a physical site of care, the dental home is an emerging strategy to increase access to consistent oral health care. A dental home is an ongoing relationship between a patient and a dentist (AAPD, 2010a). The dentist provides, among other things, regular comprehensive oral health assessment and care, individualized preventive care based on caries- and periodontal-risk assessments, education on proper nutrition and home care, and referrals to specialists when necessary (AAPD, 2010b). To date, dental homes have centered on providing care to children. However, the medical home model, on which dental homes are based, has been used with all populations to provide acute, chronic, and preventive medical services (Martin et al., 2004). Thus, there may be an opportunity to expand the dental home beyond the pediatric population.

One example of a dental home program is the Access to Baby and Child Dentistry (ABCD) program, operated across Washington state through a variety of public–private partnerships (ABCD, 2011; Donahue et al., 2005). Partners include local health departments, the Washington State Dental Society, local dental societies, the Washington Department of Health (WDOH), the Washington Department of Social and Health Services (WDSHS), the University of Washington School of Dentistry, the Washington Dental Service Foundation, private dentists, and other community partners. Local health departments typically manage the daily functions of ABCD programs. They work with the state and local dental professional organizations to encourage dentist participation. Dentists who participate in the program receive training and are paid an enhanced reimbursement rate. The health departments also actively recruit Medicaid-eligible children to the program through partnerships with community organizations such as WIC, Head

Start, and Early Head Start. In addition, the health departments provide case management services to ABCD families. The WDSHS, WDOH, University of Washington School of Dentistry, and Washington Dental Service Foundation oversee the program at the state level. The WDSHS oversees Medicaid financing in the state, and thus provides reimbursement to ABCD-certified dentists, and provides billing assistance, among other things. The WDSHS also contracts with the University of Washington Dental School to provide training and ongoing education to ABCD providers. The WDOH provides technical assistance and grants to local health departments. The Washington Dental Service Foundation provides start-up grants and ongoing technical assistance to local ABCD programs.

ABCD programs have significantly increased the rate of dental visits among children enrolled in Medicaid (Grembowski and Milgrom, 2000; Lewis et al., 2009; Milgrom et al., 1999), particularly among the youngest children (Kaakko et al., 2002). However, the evidence indicates that the programs may be more successful at encouraging parents to make a single dental appointment than develop an ongoing relationship with a dentist, which is a key component of a dental home (Kaakko et al., 2002; Milgrom et al., 1999). More long-term evaluations of the program need to be done to assess the program's ability to establish dental homes.

FINDINGS AND CONCLUSIONS

The committee noted the following findings and conclusions:

- Most oral health care in the United States is provided in the private practice setting by dentists, who employ dental hygienists and dental assistants.
- Most patients seen in the private practice setting either have dental insurance or pay out of pocket.
- Only a small portion of private-sector oral health care is supported by publicly funded programs such as Medicaid.
- An array of programs provides oral health care to underserved and vulnerable populations, including FQHCs, dental schools, and health departments.
- An oral health safety net exists in concept, but the components of this safety net are not necessarily connected or coordinated.
- No single setting of care will meet the various needs or overcome the multitude of barriers for vulnerable and underserved populations.
- More research is needed on the impact of individual site of care models in improving access to care.

- More research is needed on best practices for individual sites of carc.
- There is room for building the capacity of the safety net to care for vulnerable and underserved populations, but it will not be enough to care for all patients in need. Strategies to improve access to care for these populations will require the participation of dentists in the private practice setting.

REFERENCES

AAPD (American Academy of Pediatric Dentistry). 2010a. *Definition of dental home.* http://www.aapd.org/media/Policies_Guidelines/D_DentalHome.pdf (accessed May 23, 2011).

AAPD. 2010b. *Policy on the dental home.* http://www.aapd.org/media/Policies_Guidelines/P_DentalHome.pdf (accessed May 23, 2011).

ABCD (Access to Baby and Child Dentistry). 2011. *Partners & roles.* http://www.abcd-dental.org/part.html (accessed May 24, 2011).

ADA (American Dental Association). 2004. *State and community models for improving access to dental care for the underserved—a white paper.* Chicago, IL.

ADA. 2009a. *2008 survey of dental practice: Characteristics of dentists in private practice and their patients.* Chicago, IL: American Dental Association.

ADA. 2009b. *2008 survey of dental practice: Employment of dental practice personnel.* Chicago, IL: American Dental Association.

ADA. 2009c. *2008 survey of dental practice: Income from the private practice of dentistry.* Chicago, IL: American Dental Association.

ADA. 2009d. *Distribution of dentists in the United States by region and state, 2007.* Chicago, IL: American Dental Association.

ADA. 2010. *2008-09 survey of dental education: Academic programs, enrollment, and graduates—volume 1.* Chicago, IL: American Dental Association.

Allison, M. A., L. A. Crane, B. L. Beaty, A. J. Davidson, P. Melinkovich, and A. Kempe. 2007. School-based health centers: Improving access and quality of care for low-income adolescents. *Pediatrics* 120(4):e887-e894.

Anderson, J. R. 2010. *HRSA oral health programs.* Paper presented at 2010 Dental Management Coalition, June 27, Annapolis, MD.

Anthonappa, R., and N. King. 2008. Six-month recall dental appointments, for all children, are (un)justifiable. *Journal of Clinical Pediatric Dentistry* 33(1):1-8.

ASTDD (Association of State and Territorial Dental Directors). 2010. *Synopses of state dental public health programs: Data for FY 2008-2009.* Sparks, NV: Association of State and Territorial Dental Directors.

ASTDD. 2011a. *Membership roster.* http://www.astdd.org/membership-roster/ (accessed January 25, 2011).

ASTDD. 2011b. *Mobile and portable dental services in preschool and school settings: Complex issues.* Sparks, NV: Association of State and Territorial Dental Directors.

ASTDD. 2011c. *Mobile portable dental manual.* http://mobile-portabledentalmanual.com/index.html (accessed March 10, 2011).

ASTDD. 2011d. *State & territorial dental public health activities: A collection of descriptive summaries.* http://www.astdd.org/state-activities/ (accessed January 25, 2011).

Atchison, K., A. Thind, T. Nakazono, D. Wong, J. Gutierrez, D. Carreon, and R. Andersen. 2009. Community-based clinical dental education: Effects of the pipeline program. *Journal of Dental Education* 73(2):S269-S282.

Bader, J. 2005. Risk-based recall intervals recommended. *Evidence-based Dentistry* 6(1):2-4.

Bailit, H., T. Beazoglou, N. Demby, J. McFarland, P. Robinson, and R. Weaver. 2006. Dental safety net: Current capacity and potential for expansion. *Journal of the American Dental Association* 137(6):807-815.

Bailit, H. L., T. J. Beazoglou, A. J. Formicola, and L. Tedesco. 2007. Financing clinical dental education. *Journal of Dental Education* 71(3):322-330.

Bailit, H., J. D'Adamo, and T. Beazoglou. 2010 (unpublished). *Report to the Oral Health Access Committee: State case studies: Improving access to dental care for the underserved.*

Beazoglou, T., L. J. Brown, S. Ray, L. Chen, and V. Lazar. 2009. *An economic study of expanded duties of dental auxiliaries in Colorado.* Chicago, IL: American Dental Association.

Beirne, P. V., J. E. Clarkson, and H. V. Worthington. 2007. Recall intervals for oral health in primary care patients. *Cochrane Database of Systematic Reviews* (4):CD004346.

Binkley, C. J., B. Garrett, and K. W. Johnson. 2010. Increasing dental care utilization by Medicaid-eligible children: A dental care coordinator intervention. *Journal of Public Health Dentistry* 70(1):76-84.

Bolin, K. A. 2010. *Survey of health center oral health providers: Dental salaries, provider satisfaction, and recruitment and retention strategies.* Denver, CO: National Network for Oral Health Access.

Borchgrevink, A., A. Snyder, and S. Gehshan. 2008. *The effects of Medicaid reimbursement rates on access to dental care.* Washington, DC: National Academy for State Health Policy.

Brown, L. J. 2005. *Adequacy of current and future dental workforce: Theory and analysis.* Chicago, IL: American Dental Association.

Brown, L. J., D. R. House, and K. D. Nash. 2005. *The economic aspects of unsupervised private hygiene practice and its impact on access to care.* Chicago, IL: American Dental Association.

Byck, G. R., J. A. Cooksey, and H. Russinof. 2005. Safety-net dental clinics: A viable model for access to dental care. *Journal of the American Dental Association* 136(7):1013-1021.

Carr, B. R., U. Isong, and J. A. Weintraub. 2008. Identification and description of mobile dental programs—a brief communication. *Journal of Public Health Dentistry* 68(4):234-237.

CDC (Centers for Disease Control and Prevention). 2010. *Division of oral health: About us.* http://www.cdc.gov/oralhealth/about.htm (accessed November 24, 2010).

CDC. 2011a. *CDC-funded states.* http://www.cdc.gov/oralhealth/state_programs/cooperative_agreements/index.htm (accessed October 7, 2011).

CDC. 2011b. *CDC-previously funded states.* http://www.cdc.gov/OralHealth/state_programs/cooperative_agreements/previously_funded.htm (accessed October 7, 2011).

CDC. 2011c. *State health plans.* http://www.cdc.gov/OralHealth/state_programs/OH_plans/index.htm (accessed January 25, 2011).

Center for Connected Health Policy. 2011. *Advancing California's leadership in telehealth policy: A telehealth model statute & other policy recommendations.* Sacramento, CA: Center for Connected Health Policy.

Center for Oral Health. 2010. *WIC programs.* http://www.centerfororalhealth.org/programs/wic-programs (accessed January 31, 2011).

Chmar, J. E., R. G. Weaver, and R. W. Valachovic. 2008. Dental school vacant budgeted faculty positions, academic years 2005-06 and 2006-07. *Journal of Dental Education* 72(3):370-385.

CMS (Centers for Medicare and Medicaid Services). 2011a. *Innovative state practices for improving the provision of Medicaid dental services.* Baltimore, MD.

CMS. 2011b. *Recent developments in Medicaid and CHIP policy*. http://www.cms.gov/CMCSBulletins/downloads/CMCS-Info-Bulletin-March-2011-Final.pdf (accessed May 31, 2011).

CMS. 2011c. *Telehealth services: Rural health fact sheet series*. https://www.cms.gov/MLNProducts/downloads/TelehealthSrvcsfctsht.pdf (accessed May 27, 2011).

Cohen, L. A., R. J. Manski, L. S. Magder, and C. D. Mullins. 2002. Dental visits to hospital emergency departments by adults receiving Medicaid: Assessing their use. *Journal of the American Dental Association* 133(6):715-724.

Conis, E. 2009. Steps to improve oral health in Kentucky. *Health Policy Monitor*.

Cottam, W. W. 2010. *The NNOHA survey of health center dental salaries: Trends and analysis*. http://www.cdnetwork.org/NewCDN/LibraryView.aspx?ID=cdn565 (accessed March 8, 2011).

Davis, E. E., A. S. Deinard, and E. W. H. Maïga. 2010. Doctor, my tooth hurts: The costs of incomplete dental care in the emergency room. *Journal of Public Health Dentistry* 70(3):205-210.

Del Grosso, P., A. Brown, S. Silva, J. Henderson, N. Tein, and D. Paulsell. 2008. *Strategies for promoting prevention and improving oral health care delivery in Head Start: Findings from the oral health initiative evaluation*. Princeton, NJ: Mathematica Policy Research, Inc.

DeNavas-Walt, C., B. D. Proctor, and J. C. Smith. 2010. *Income, poverty, and health insurance coverage in the United States: 2009*. Washington, DC: U.S. Census Bureau.

Dickinson, T. D. 2010. *The MOM experience: Pathways to collaboration and conversation*. Paper presented at meeting of the Committee on Oral Health Access to Services, Washington, DC.

Donahue, G. J., N. Waddell, A. L. Plough, M. A. del Aguila, and T. E. Garland. 2005. The ABCDs of treating the most prevalent childhood disease. *American Journal of Public Health* 95(8):1322-1324.

Folse, G. 2010. *Outreach dentistry*. Paper presented at meeting of the Committee on Oral Health Access to Services, San Francisco, CA.

Formicola, A. J., R. Myers, J. F. Hasler, M. Peterson, W. Dodge, H. L. Bailit, T. J. Beazoglou, and L. A. Tedesco. 2008. Evolution of dental school clinics as patient care delivery centers. *Journal of Dental Education* 72(2 Supp.):110-127.

GAO (Government Accountability Office). 2000. *Factors contributing to low use of dental services by low-income populations*. Washington, DC: U.S. General Accounting Office.

Geiermann, S. L. 2010. *Expertise and technical assistance in health centers*. Presentation at meeting of the Committee on Oral Health Access to Services, San Francisco. July 27, 2010.

Gibson, C., and A. Moosajee. 2008. Selecting appropriate recall intervals for patients in general dental practice—an audit project to categorize patients according to risk. *Dental Update* 35(3):188-190, 193-194.

Glassman, P., and P. Subar. 2010. Creating and maintaining oral health for dependent people in institutional settings. *Journal of Public Health Dentistry* 70(Supp. 1):S40-S48.

Greenberg, B. J. S., J. V. Kumar, and H. Stevenson. 2008. Dental case management: Increasing access to oral health care for families and children with low incomes. *Journal of the American Dental Association* 139(8):1114-1121.

Grembowski, D., and P. M. Milgrom. 2000. Increasing access to dental care for Medicaid preschool children: The Access to Baby and Child Dentistry (ABCD) program. *Public Health Reports* 115(5):448-459.

Guay, A. H. 2005. Dental practice: Prices, production and profits. *Journal of the American Dental Association* 136(3):357-361.

Guthrie, D., R. W. Valachovic, and L. J. Brown. 2009. The impact of new dental schools on the dental workforce through 2022. *Journal of Dental Education* 73(12):1353-1360.

Haden, N. K., P. L. Beemsterboer, R. G. Weaver, and R. W. Valachovic. 2000. Dental school faculty shortages increase: An update on future dental school faculty. *Journal of Dental Education* 64(9):657-673.

Haley, J., G. Kenney, and J. Pelletier. 2008. *Access to affordable dental care: Gaps for low-income adults*. http://www.kff.org/medicaid/upload/7798.pdf (accessed May 18, 2011).

Helgeson, M. 2009. *Older adults and people with disabilities*. Paper presented at IOM workshop on the U.S. Oral Health Workforce in the Coming Decade, Washington, DC.

HHS (Department of Health and Human Services). 2010a. *Recovery Act (ARRA): Community health centers*. http://www.hhs.gov/recovery/hrsa/healthcentergrants.html (accessed February 3, 2010).

HHS. 2010b. Healthy People 2020*: Oral health objectives*. http://www.healthypeople.gov/2020/topicsobjectives2020/objectiveslist.aspx?topicid=32 (accessed December 27, 2010).

HRSA (Health Resources and Services Administration). 2003. *Program information notice 2003-21: Federally qualified health center look-alike guidelines and application*. Rockville, MD: U.S. Department of Health and Human Services.

HRSA. 2010. *The health center program: Benefits*. http://bphc.hrsa.gov/about/benefits.htm (accessed February 3, 2010).

HRSA. 2011a. *BHPR grants: Oral health workforce activities FY 2010 grantee abstracts*. http://bhpr.hrsa.gov/grants/10oralhealthabstracts.htm (accessed January 10, 2011).

HRSA. 2011b. *Health centers: 2009 at-a-glance*. http://www.hrsa.gov/data-statistics/health-center-data/NationalData/2009/2009datasnapshot.html (accessed March 1, 2011).

HRSA. 2011c. *Health centers: 2009 national total summary data*. http://bphc.hrsa.gov/healthcenterdatastatistics/nationaldata/2009/2009nattotsumdata.html (accessed August 9, 2011).

HRSA. 2011d. *School-based comprehensive oral health services grant program*. https://grants.hrsa.gov/webExternal/SFO.asp?ID=513FD7F0-C025-48E0-B6EC-AAFEFD528AA7 (accessed June 1, 2011).

HRSA. 2011e. *Staffing & utilization: National summary for 2009*. http://www.hrsa.gov/data-statistics/health-center-data/NationalData/2009/2009_national_staffing.html (accessed March 10, 2011).

Hunter, L. P., C. E. Weber, A. P. Morreale, and J. H. Wall. 2009. Patient satisfaction with retail health clinic care. *Journal of the American Academy of Nurse Practitioners* 21(10):565-570.

IOM (Institute of Medicine). 1995. *Dental education at the crossroads: Challenges and change*. Washington, DC: National Academy Press.

IOM. 2008. *Retooling for an aging America: Building the health care workforce*. Washington, DC: The National Academies Press.

IOM. 2009. *The U.S. oral health workforce in the coming decade: Workshop summary*. Washington, DC: The National Academies Press.

Kaakko, T., E. Skaret, T. Getz, P. Hujoel, D. Grembowski, C. S. Moore, and P. Mllgrom. 2002. An ABCD program to increase access to dental care for children enrolled in Medicaid in a rural county. *Journal of Public Health Dentistry* 62(1):45-50.

Kaplan, D. W., C. D. Brindis, S. L. Phibbs, P. Melinkovich, K. Naylor, and K. Ahlstrand. 1999. A comparison study of an elementary school-based health center. *Archives of Pediatrics and Adolescent Medicine* 153(3):235-243.

Kenney, G. M., J. M. Haley, and J. E. Pelletier. 2009. *Covering Kids & Families evaluation*. Washington, DC: Urban Institute.

Kilsdonk, G. J. 2010. *Family health center of Marshfield & Marshfield clinic's response to the surgeon general's report: Oral health in America*. Paper presented at the National Health Policy Forum, Washington, DC.

Kopycka-Kedzierawski, D. T., R. J. Billings, and K. M. McConnochie. 2007. Dental screening of preschool children using teledentistry: A feasibility study. *Pediatric Dentistry* 29:209-213.

Ladrillo, T. E., M. H. Hobdell, and A. C. Caviness. 2006. Increasing prevalence of emergency department visits for pediatric dental care, 1997-2001. *Journal of the American Dental Association* 137(3):379-385.

Laws, M., and M. K. Scott. 2008. The emergence of retail-based clinics in the United States: Early observations. *Health Affairs* 27(5):1293-1298.

Lewis, C., H. Lynch, and B. Johnston. 2003. Dental complaints in emergency departments: A national perspective. *Annals of Emergency Medicine* 42(1):93-99.

Lewis, C., E. Teeple, A. Robertson, and A. Williams. 2009. Preventive dental care for young, Medicaid-insured children in Washington State. *Pediatrics* 124(1):e120-e127.

Maiuro, L. S. 2009. *Emergency department visits for preventable dental conditions in California*. Oakland, CA: California HealthCare Foundation.

Martin, A., D. Lassman, L. Whittle, A. Catlin, J. Benson, C. Cowan, B. Dickensheets, M. Hartman, P. McDonnell, O. Nuccio, and B. Washington. 2011. Recession contributes to slowest annual rate of increase in health spending in five decades. *Health Affairs* 30(1):11-22.

Martin, J. C., R. F. Avant, M. A. Bowman, J. R. Bucholtz, J. R. Dickinson, K. L. Evans, L. A. Green, D. E. Henley, W. A. Jones, and S. C. Matheny. 2004. The future of family medicine: A collaborative project of the family medicine community. *Annals of Family Medicine* 2(Supp. 1):S3-S32.

McAndrew, M. 2010. Community-based dental education and the importance of faculty development. *Journal of Dental Education* 74(9):980-985.

Mertz, E., and E. O'Neil. 2002. The growing challenge of providing oral health care services to all Americans. *Health Affairs* 21(5):65-77.

Milgrom, P., P. Hujoel, D. Grembowski, and R. Fong. 1999. A community strategy for Medicaid child dental services. *Public Health Reports* 114(6):528-532.

Mito, R. S., K. A. Atchison, K. H. Lefever, S. Lin, and R. Engelhardt. 2002. Characteristics of civilian postdoctoral general dentistry programs. *Journal of Dental Education* 66(6):757-765.

Mofidi, M., R. G. Rozier, and R. S. King. 2002. Problems with access to dental care for Medicaid-insured children: What caregivers think. *American Journal of Public Health* 92(1):53-58.

Mullin, K. 2009. Considering retail health clinics. *Journal of Nursing Administration* 39(12): 531-536.

NACCHO (National Association of County & City Health Officials). 2006. *2005 national profile of local health departments*. Washington, DC: National Association of County & City Health Officials.

NACCHO. 2009. *2008 national profile of local health departments*. Washington, DC: National Association of County & City Health Officials.

NASBHC (National Assembly on School-Based Health Care). 2010. *Census 2007-08: School-based, school-linked and mobile health care survey*. Washington, DC: National Assembly on School-Based Health Care.

National Institute for Clinical Excellence. 2004. Dental recall: Recall interval between routine dental examinations. London, UK: National Institute for Clinical Excellence.

Nycz, G. 2010. *Solving oral health access: A regionalized, integrated, and rural dental system*. Paper presented at meeting of the Committee on Oral Health Access to Services, San Francisco, CA.

OHS (Office of Head Start). 2011. *About the Office of Head Start*. http://www.acf.hhs.gov/programs/ohs/about/index.html (accessed May 22, 2011).

Okunseri, C., N. M. Pajewski, D. C. Brousseau, S. Tomany-Korman, A. Snyder, and G. Flores. 2008. Racial and ethnic disparities in nontraumatic dental-condition visits to emergency departments and physician offices: A study of the Wisconsin Medicaid program. *Journal of the American Dental Association* 139(12):1657-1666.

Patel, S., R. C. Bay, and M. Glick. 2010. A systematic review of dental recall intervals and incidence of dental caries. *Journal of the American Dental Association* 141(5):527-539.

Pew Center on the States. 2010. *It takes a team: How new dental providers can benefit patients and practices*. Washington, DC: The Pew Charitable Trusts.

Pollack, C. E., and K. Armstrong. 2009. The geographic accessibility of retail clinics for underserved populations. *Archives of Internal Medicine* 169(10):945-949.

Pollack, C. E., C. Gidengil, and A. Mehrotra. 2010. The growth of retail clinics and the medical home: Two trends in concert or in conflict? *Health Affairs* 29(5):999-1003.

Remote Area Medical. 2011. *RAM expeditions*. http://www.ramusa.org/expeditions/expeditions.htm (accessed October 6, 2011).

Rodgers, T., B. Russell, and S. Meister. 2010. *Inside I-Smile 2009: An update on Iowa's dental home initiative for children*. Des Moines, IA: Iowa Department of Public Health, Oral Health Bureau.

Rudavsky, R., C. E. Pollack, and A. Mehrotra. 2009. The geographic distribution, ownership, prices, and scope of practice at retail clinics. *Annals of Internal Medicine* 151(5):315-320.

Ruddy, G. 2007. *Health centers' role in addressing the oral health needs of the medically underserved*. Washington, DC: National Association of Community Health Centers.

Sanchez Dils, E., C. Lefebvre, and K. Abeyta. 2004. Teledentistry in the United States: A new horizon of dental care. *International Journal of Dental Hygiene* 2:161-164.

Scott, M. K. 2009. *Retail dental clinics: A viable model for the underserved?* Oakland, CA: California HealthCare Foundation.

Scott, M. K. 2010. *Dental care in the express lane*. Paper presented at meeting of the Committee on Oral Health Access to Services, San Francisco, CA.

Shesser, R. 2010. *Oral health emergencies*. Paper presented at meeting of the Committee on Oral Health Access to Services, Washington, DC.

Shirk, C. 2010. *Oral health checkup: Progress in tough fiscal times?* Washington, DC: National Health Policy Forum.

Siegal, M. D., and A. M. R. Detty. 2010. Do school-based dental sealant programs reach higher risk children? *Journal of Public Health Dentistry* 70(3):181-187.

Silberberg, M., and J. C. Cantor. 2008. Making the case for school-based health: Where do we stand? *Journal of Health Politics Policy and Law* 33(1):3-37.

Silow-Carroll, S., and T. Alteras. 2004. *Community-based oral health programs: Lessons from three innovative models*. Battle Creek, MI: W. K. Kellogg Foundation.

Solomon, E. S. 2007. Demographic characteristics of general dental practice sites. *General Dentistry* 55(6):552-558.

Tennessee Department of Health. 2010. *School based dental prevention project*. http://health.state.tn.us/oralhealth/schoolbased.html (accessed January 25, 2011).

Thygeson, M., K. A. Van Vorst, M. V. Maciosek, and L. Solberg. 2008. Use and costs of care in retail clinics versus traditional care sites. *Health Affairs* 27(5):1283-1292.

University of the Pacific. 2011. *Virtual dental home demonstration project*. http://dental.pacific.edu/Community_Involvement/Pacific_Center_for_Special_Care_(PCSC)/Projects/Virtual_Dental_Home_Demonstration_Project.html (accessed January 31, 2011).

U.S. Census Bureau. 2010. *USA quickfacts from the U.S. Census Bureau.* http://quickfacts.census.gov/qfd/states/00000.html (accessed March 9, 2011).

Vanchit, J., M. Papageorge, L. Jahangiri, M. Wheater, D. Cappelli, R. Frazer, and W. Sohn. 2011. Recruitment, development, and retention of dental faculty in a changing environment. *Journal of Dental Education* 75(1):82-89.

Walker, S. C., S. E. U. Kerns, A. R. Lyon, E. J. Bruns, and T. J. Cosgrove. 2010. Impact of school-based health center use on academic outcomes. *Journal of Adolescent Health* 46(3):251-257.

Wall, T. P., and L. J. Brown. 2007. The urban and rural distribution of dentists, 2000. *Journal of the American Dental Association* 138(7):1003-1011.

Wang, M. C., G. Ryan, E. A. McGlynn, and A. Mehrotra. 2010. Why do patients seek care at retail clinics, and what alternatives did they consider? *American Journal of Medical Quality* 25(2):128-134.

Warren, M. 2010. *Statistical analysis and overview of the 2010 GKAS day data.* http://www.ada.org/sections/newsAndEvents/pdfs/gkas_statisticalanalysis.pdf (accessed March 16, 2011).

Washington State Hospital Association. 2010. *Emergency room use.* http://www.wsha.org/files/127/ERreport.pdf (accessed April 11, 2011).

Wendling, W. R. 2010. Private sector approaches to workforce enhancement. *Journal of Public Health Dentistry* 70(Supp. 1):S24-S31.

Whitten, P., and L. Buis. 2007. Private payer reimbursement for telemedicine services in the United States. *Telemedicine and e-Health* 13(1):15-24.

Young, T. L., S. L. D'Angelo, and J. Davis. 2001. Impact of a school-based health center on emergency department use by elementary school students. *Journal of School Health* 71(5):196-198.

Youngblade, L., T. Malasanos, E. Shenkman, S. Aydede, J. Nackashi, S. Tuli, B. Vogel, L. Curry, D. Wegenre, K. Lustig, and P. Sloyer. 2005. *Telemedicine for CSHCN: A state-by-state comparison of Medicaid reimbursement policies and Title V activities.* Institute for Child Health Policy, University of Florida, Telehealth Connections for Children and Youth.

5

Expenditures and Financing for Oral Health Care

Understanding how oral health services are financed in the United States is critical to the access question. Financing for oral health care greatly influences where and whether individuals receive care. At the individual level, dental coverage and socioeconomic factors play a significant role in access to oral health care. That is, individuals who have private dental coverage or can afford care, either through private insurance or through out-of-pocket expenditures, are generally able to obtain care. On the other hand, individuals who lack dental coverage, who have minimal dental coverage, and/or those of limited financial means experience significant barriers to care. Financing also has a powerful influence on providers' practice patterns. For example, low reimbursement by public programs, such as Medicaid and the Children's Health Insurance Program (CHIP), are often cited as a disincentive to providers' willingness to participate in these publicly funded programs. Finally, state and federal spending on oral health has a tremendous impact on what oral health services are available and to whom. This begins at the level of support for dental schools and continues in the form of subsidies for residency programs, reimbursement policies of public insurance programs, mandated benefits, and additional financial incentives. For example, the federal government makes considerable investments in improving the distribution of oral health care professionals in urban and rural areas while states are authorized under federal law to determine the rate of Medicaid reimbursement for oral health services provided.

This chapter provides an overview of the various sources and mechanisms of financing for oral health care in the United States and describes the influences that these expenditures have on access to oral health care among vulnerable and underserved populations.

OVERVIEW OF EXPENDITURES

Health care costs and spending have been rapidly increasing in the United States in recent years. In 2009, overall health expenditures were \$2.5 trillion, including the cost of hospital care, physician and dental services, home health care, nursing home services, prescription drugs, medical equipment and supplies, and public health direct services (CMS, 2010b). This translates to more than \$8,000 per person and accounted for 17.6 percent of the national gross domestic product (CMS, 2010b). Growth in national health expenditures is expected to increase by 6.1 percent between 2009 and 2019 (CMS, 2010c). In contrast, expenditures for dental services in the United States in 2009 were \$102.2 billion, approximately 5 percent of total spending on health care (CMS, 2010b). While medical and dental spending both have been rising, the growth in medical expenditures has far outpaced the growth in dental expenditures.

The reported national expenditure levels undercount the total spent on improving oral health. Estimates represent only the costs associated with direct services delivered by dentists in traditional practice settings. Spending on public health initiatives (e.g., water fluoridation and public education campaigns) and oral health services delivered in medical care settings are not included in estimates of overall expenditures. For example, there are approximately 3.6 million craniofacial cases (e.g., diabetes-related conditions, oral cancers, and injuries) treated in medical care settings each year, and the total costs for these treatments exceed several billion dollars (Snowden et al., 2003).

Average Annual Dental Expenses

In 2007, the average annual expense for individuals who had any dental expenses was \$643 (Rohde, 2010). Individual expenses varied by age, income, race and ethnicity, and insurance status (see Figure 5-1). Annual dental expenses also varied by source of insurance. The average annual dental expense for individuals with private dental insurance was \$662. Among individuals with public dental insurance (e.g., Medicaid or CHIP), the average annual dental expense was \$370 (AHRQ, 2009). Individuals with higher incomes had higher annual dental expenses. The average annual dental expense for "high-income" individuals (>400 percent of the federal poverty level [FPL]) was \$710. Among "poor" individuals (≤100 percent FPL), the average annual dental expense was \$428 (AHRQ, 2009). This difference in expenses may reflect the ability of individuals with higher

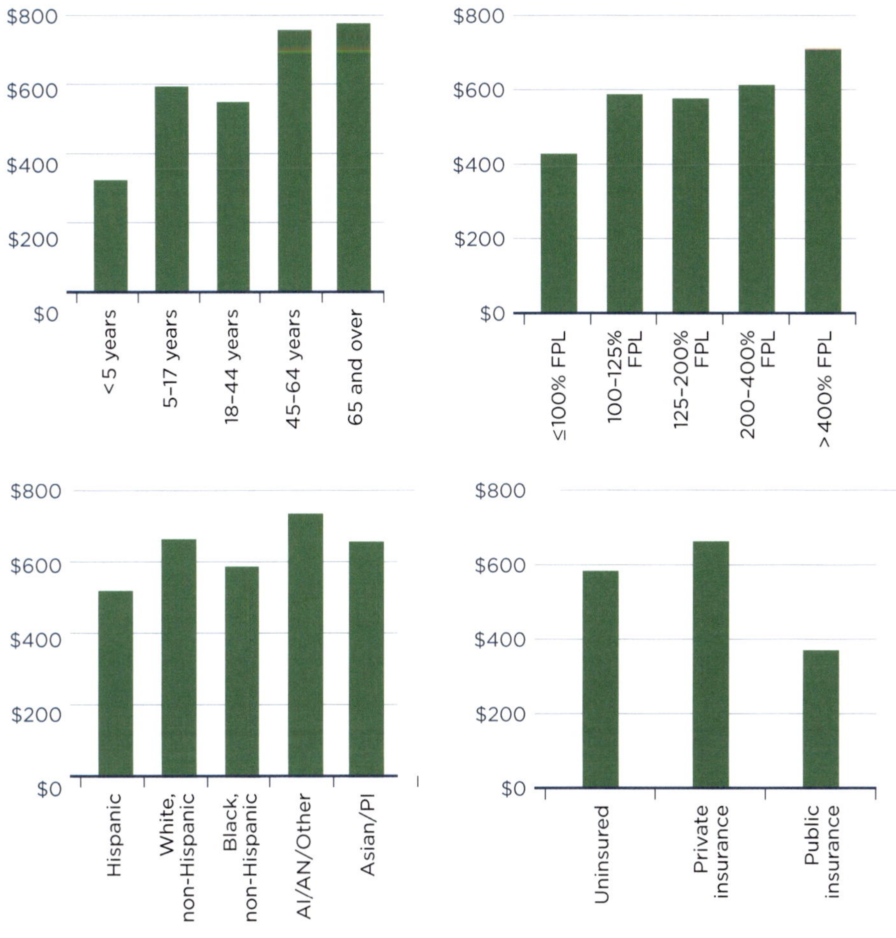

FIGURE 5-1
Mean annual dental expenses by age, income, race/ethnicity, and insurance status, United States, 2007.

NOTE: AI/AN = American Indians/Alaska Natives; FPL = federal poverty level; PI = Pacific Islander.
SOURCE: AHRQ, 2009.

incomes to pay for and use dental care. Finally, older adults (individuals 65 and over) had the highest average annual dental expenses at $776. By contrast, children and adolescents (individuals under age 18) had the lowest average annual dental expenses (AHRQ, 2009).

In 2007, the source of payments for dental care (e.g., private insurance, out-of-pocket, or public insurance) varied among individuals who had any

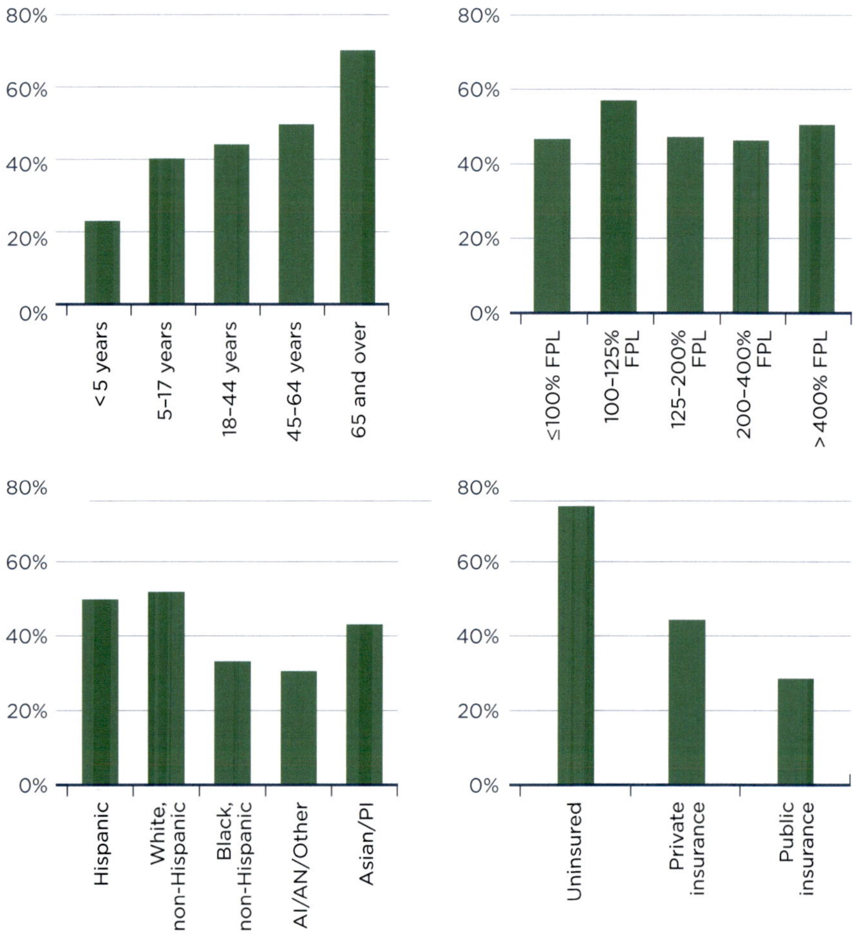

FIGURE 5-2
Percent of total annual dental expenses paid out of pocket by age, income, race/ethnicity, and insurance status, United States, 2007.

NOTE: AI/AN = American Indians/Alaska Natives; FPL = federal poverty level; PI = Pacific Islander.
SOURCE: AHRQ, 2009.

dental expenses. For example, the percentage of annual dental expenses paid out of pocket varied by age, race and ethnicity, income, and insurance status (see Figure 5-2). As would be expected, uninsured individuals pay the highest percentage—nearly three quarters—of their annual dental expenses out of pocket (74.7 percent) compared to individuals with private insurance and those with public insurance (44.3 percent and 28.5 percent, respectively) (AHRQ, 2009). Older adults (individuals 65 and over) had the highest percent of total annual dental expenses paid out of pocket than any other age group (70.3 percent). By contrast, children, who are more likely to have public insurance that includes dental coverage, had the lowest percent of total annual dental expenses paid out of pocket than any other age group (23 percent). Working age adults (individuals between 18 and 64 years of age), who are more likely to have employer-based dental coverage, had lower costs than older adults (AHRQ, 2009). The lack of dental coverage in Medicare and the lack of employee-based dental coverage translate into higher out-of-pocket dental expenses for older adults (Manski et al., 2010a).

OVERVIEW OF COVERAGE

Dental Coverage

There is strong evidence that dental coverage is positively tied to access to and utilization of oral health care (AHRQ, 2010; Decker, 2011; Sohn et al., 2007), although whether or not this relationship is causal is not clear. For example, it may be that those with greater demand for dental care are the ones most likely to purchase dental coverage. This suggests it is not clear if more coverage leads to greater use or greater demand leads to the purchase of dental coverage (and then greater use). The tie is clear, though: In 2007, 52 percent of adults with private dental coverage had at least one dental visit, compared to 31 percent of those without private dental coverage and 22 percent of uninsured individuals (Manski and Brown, 2010). Moreover, children who have dental coverage, through public programs (e.g., Medicaid or CHIP) or private insurance, use preventive care more routinely than their counterparts who lack coverage (Lewis et al., 2007). Studies using quasi-experimental designs to assess the impact of dental coverage on access and utilization indicate that, once children acquire coverage through a public program, they are significantly less likely to have unmet needs for dental care. For example, after enrolling in CHIP, unmet needs for oral health care decline among adolescents (Klein et al., 2007). Another study found that, after enrolling in CHIP, children with special health care needs had significantly improved access to a broad range of health care services, including dental care (Kenney, 2009). Overall, uninsured children are at least twice as likely as children with dental coverage to have unmet need for oral health care (Damiano et al., 2003; Feinberg et al., 2002; Fox et al., 2003; Kenney, 2007; Lave et al., 2002; McBroome et al., 2005; Mofidi et al., 2002; Szilagyi et al., 2004; Trenholm et al., 2005; Wang et al., 2007).

Millions of Americans lack dental coverage. Recent data from several sources underscore this deficiency among children, adults, and older adults:

- An estimated 130 million U.S. adults and children lack dental coverage (based on enrollment in private dental plans) (NADP, 2009).
- Over 40 percent adults ages 21–64 lack private dental coverage (see Figure 5-3) (Manski and Brown, 2010).
- Approximately 70 percent of adults age 65 and older, lack any kind of dental coverage—public or private (Manski and Brown, 2007).
- Over 22 percent of children ages 1–17 lack dental coverage (Liu et al., 2007).

What Do Dental Plans Cover?

The types of dental services covered by dental plans vary widely among private plans and between various public plans. Currently, there is no standard set of essential oral health benefits. For example, one plan may include "comprehensive" care such as routine diagnostic and preventive services, X-rays, restorative services, and oral surgery, while another may cover more limited services such as emergency care only. A recent survey of employer-sponsored health plans of the benefits typically covered by employers based on data from the National Compensation Survey provides an overview of employment-based dental benefits (see Box 5-1). Some of the variation in services covered is driven by employer and consumer choice. Dental benefits available to employees may be based upon their employers' selection of low-cost dental benefit packages or benefits packages that appeal to

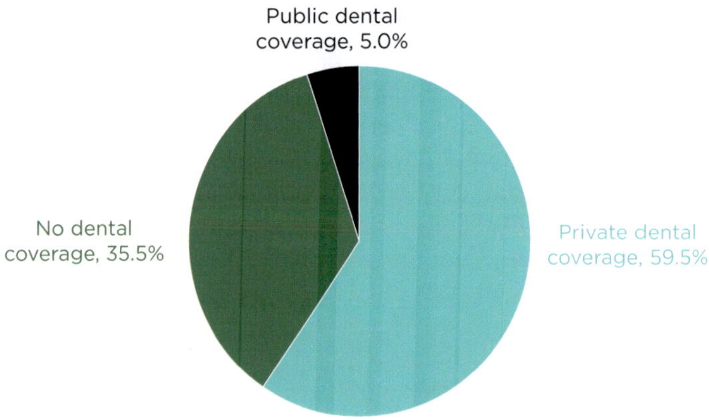

FIGURE 5-3
Percentage of adults 21–64 according to dental coverage status: U.S. civilian noninstitutionalized population, 2007.

SOURCE: Manski and Brown, 2010.

BOX 5-1
Summary of Employment-Based Dental Benefits

A recent report from the Department of Labor on selected medical benefits provided the following summary of employment-based dental benefits based on data from the National Compensation Survey (NCS):

> Plans typically grouped dental services into categories, such as preventive services (typically exams and cleanings), basic services (typically fillings, dental surgery, periodontal care, and endodontic care), major services (typically crowns and prosthetics), and orthodontia. Cost sharing for dental services typically involved an annual deductible—the median was $50 per person. After meeting the deductible, dental plans often paid a percent of covered services up to a maximum annual benefit. The median percent paid by the plan was 100 percent for preventive services, 80 percent for basic services, and 50 percent for major services and orthodontia. The median annual maximum was $1,500; a separate maximum applicable to orthodontic services also had a median value of $1,500.

SOURCE: BLS, 2011.

their higher paid workers. Alternatively, consumers may purchase or select employer-based coverage (when available) that provides a range of desired benefits and/or choice of providers. The dental benefits included in public plans are determined by federal law and/or state decisions. (A discussion of what is covered in public plans is included later in the chapter.) Each of the factors described above contribute to the tremendous variation in dental coverage.

How Is Dental Coverage Unique?

The usual premise for buying insurance is to cover unpredictable and rare events. This is the impetus behind purchasing health care, home, and car insurance. But this logic does not neatly fit most dental care. In general, dental care does not meet the criteria for casualty insurance that "the event or expense insured against (1) is relatively rare for the individual person but occurs at known rates for groups, (2) is very costly, and (3) cannot generally be controlled by the insured" (IOM, 1980). In fact, most people need or use oral health care at least annually.

Dental coverage is similar to health coverage in one notable way: the availability of a significant tax subsidy has led employers to offer dental coverage. Thus, most private dental coverage is employer provided, subsidized through the tax system. However, dental coverage typically requires higher percentage co-payments than health insurance.

The IOM report *Public Policy Options for Better Dental Health* (*Public Policy Options*) concluded that, despite the unique attributes of dental coverage, it is in the nation's best interest to cover dental services; the reasons provided by the committee over 30 years ago remain largely the same today:

- Use of oral health care is highly correlated with income, education, and occupational status.
- Effective preventive measures exist.
- The overall structure of dental benefit coverage does not adequately promote preventive services, often resulting in delayed treatment.

Finally, the Public Policy Options committee concluded that "well-designed public and private dental health insurance would be useful for achieving important objectives in dental health and that this advantage outweighs the inapplicability of some of the traditional insurance principles to dental care benefits." Specifically, the committee determined that dental coverage could, among other things, improve access to dental care delivery systems (IOM, 1980).

Variation in Coverage Rates by Race/Ethnicity

Dental coverage varies significantly by race and ethnicity (Flores and Tomany-Korman, 2008; Manski and Brown, 2007, 2008, 2010; Zuckerman et al., 2004). For example, data from the 2004 Household Component of the Medical Expenditure Panel Survey showed that among individuals of all ages, white non-Hispanics were more likely to have private dental coverage than black non-Hispanic and Hispanic individuals (who were more likely to have public dental coverage) (Manski and Brown, 2007). Data from the 2006 Health and Retirement Study showed that among older adults, non-Hispanic blacks were more likely to have dental coverage (56.8 percent) than non-Hispanic whites (46.7 percent) and Hispanics (42.4 percent) (Manski et al., 2010b).

PRIVATE SOURCES OF FINANCING

Dental care is financed primarily through private sources, including individual out-of-pocket payments and private coverage (see Table 5-1). For more than 50 years, these two sources have financed over 90 percent of all dental expenditures (CMS, 2010b). Americans spend billions of dollars out of pocket for dental services each year. In 2008, dental services accounted

TABLE 5-1
National Dental Expenditures, by Source of Funds, 2003–2009 (in $ billions)

		Private		Public		
Year	Total	Out-of-Pocket	Private Health Insurance	Medicare	Medicaid	Other Health Insurance Programs
2003	76.0	33.7	37.4	0.1	3.7	0.8
2004	81.8	36.0	40.5	0.1	4.0	0.9
2005	86.8	38.3	42.9	0.1	4.2	1.0
2006	91.4	40.3	45.1	0.1	4.4	1.1
2007	97.3	42.7	47.8	0.2	4.8	1.5
2008	102.3	44.9	49.1	0.2	5.8	1.7
2009	102.2	42.5	50.0	0.3	7.1	1.9

SOURCE: CMS, 2010b.

for 22 percent of all out-of-pocket health care expenditures, ranking second only to prescription drug expenditures (BLS, 2010a).

Variation in Coverage Rates by Employment and Income

Variations in dental coverage have been observed by employment status and income level. For example, data from the 2008 National Health Interview Survey showed that the percentage of individuals with private dental coverage increased as income levels increased (Bloom and Cohen, 2010). Similarly, higher-paid workers are also more likely to have access to and participate in stand-alone dental plans (Barsky, 2004; Ford, 2009). The availability of dental coverage through one's employer is associated with the size of the establishment; that is, the larger the number of employees overall, the greater the likelihood that stand-alone dental plans will be available to employees (Barsky, 2004; Ford, 2009). Employers can add a separate oral health product to their overall coverage package, but often they do not. In 2006, 56 percent of all employers offered health insurance but only 35 percent offered dental coverage (Manski and Cooper, 2010). Employees are more likely to be offered options for medical insurance than dental coverage, and a higher percentage of employees will take advantage of available dental benefits as compared with the percentage of employees who take advantage of available medical benefits (80 percent vs. 75 percent) (BLS, 2010b). As noted earlier, with the exception of coverage of

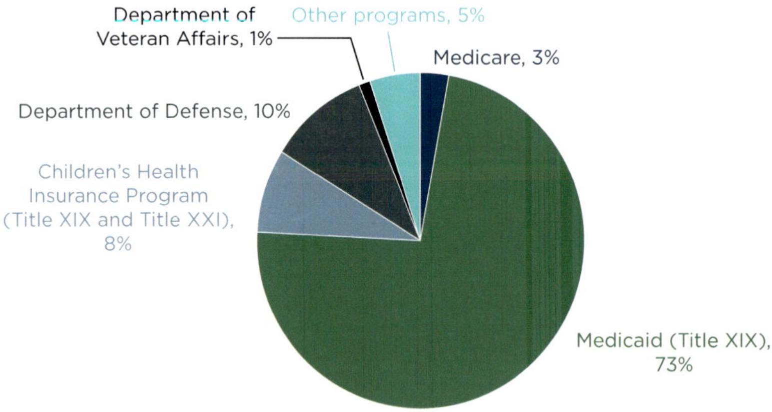

FIGURE 5-4
Public expenditures for dental services by program, 2009.

SOURCE: CMS, 2010b.

rare events, dental coverage differs from the typical insurance model; thus, employer-based dental coverage might be viewed as a fringe benefit that subsidizes oral health care utilization.

PUBLICLY SUBSIDIZED COVERAGE

Access to dental care depends on a variety of factors; however, chief among these is having a provider available and having the ability to pay for services (either through insurance, direct out-of-pocket payments, or subsidies) (Borchgrevink et al., 2008; Fisher and Mascarenhas, 2007; GAO, 2000; Hughes et al., 2005). In 2009, public subsidies or direct payments for dental services from public programs totaled $7.4 billion or less than 1 percent of national expenditures for dental services (CMS, 2010b). The overwhelming majority (73 percent) of these public expenditures for direct services or coverage came from Medicaid (CMS, 2010b) (Figure 5-4).

Medicaid and CHIP

Medicaid

Medicaid is a federal-state entitlement program for medical assistance to low-income children and pregnant women, persons over age 65, and those with disabilities who meet income and resource requirements; at the state's discretion, certain persons who are considered medically needy based on their high medical costs may also be covered. The vast majority of state Medicaid programs now purchase at least some medical care services through contracts with managed care plans (CMS, 2009).

Medicaid's Early and Periodic Screening, Diagnostic, and Treatment (EPSDT) service provides a comprehensive child health benefit, which requires states to fund well-child health care, diagnostic services, and medically necessary treatment services to Medicaid-eligible children ages birth to age 21 (CMS, 2005a). Under federal EPSDT law, states must cover any Medicaid-covered (i.e., allowed under the federal Medicaid statute) service that is necessary to prevent, correct, or ameliorate a child's physical health, which includes oral health (CMS, 2005b). Dental coverage is required for all Medicaid enrolled children under age 21 (CMS, 2011b). This is a comprehensive benefit, including preventive, diagnostic, and treatment services. At a minimum, these services must include relief of pain and infections, restoration of teeth, and maintenance of dental health. In contrast, states are not required to provide coverage for adults. For adults, states must only cover medical and surgical services furnished by a dentist to the extent those services can be performed under state law by either a doctor of medicine or a dentist. Beyond this, states' coverage of routine dental benefits for adults varies widely among the states, with a number of states limiting the benefit to emergency coverage (see Figure 5-5).

Medicaid coverage can improve access to medical and dental care; however, health status, age, race and ethnicity, gender, routine source of dental care, amount of reimbursement, and availability of providers all factor into the impact of coverage (Dasanayake et al., 2007; Edelstein and Chinn, 2009; Jablonski et al., 2005; Johnson et al., 2005; Kenney, 2009; Pourat and Finocchio, 2010; Rowley et al., 2006; Shiboski et al., 2005; Snyder, 2009). There are variations in the patterns of utilization for preventive, treatment, emergency, and specialty dental services associated with Medicaid populations compared to privately insured populations (Sweet et al., 2005).

At the same time, low provider participation in the Medicaid program has a direct and generally negative impact on access to oral health care for Medicaid beneficiaries (GAO, 2009, 2010; Lewis et al., 2009; Milgrom et al., 2010; Ramírez et al., 2011; Shortridge and Moore, 2009). For example, 74 percent of pediatricians cite the lack of dentists who accept Medicaid as a "moderate to severe barrier for 0–3-year-old Medicaid-insured patients to obtain dental care" (Lewis et al., 2009). In addition, a recent study in Illinois found that a child with public dental coverage (Medicaid/CHIP) was significantly less likely to obtain an appointment for an urgent oral injury than a child with the same injury with private dental coverage (Bisgaier et al., 2011). This effect was found even among Medicaid/CHIP-enrolled practices. Increases in Medicaid reimbursement, discussed later in this

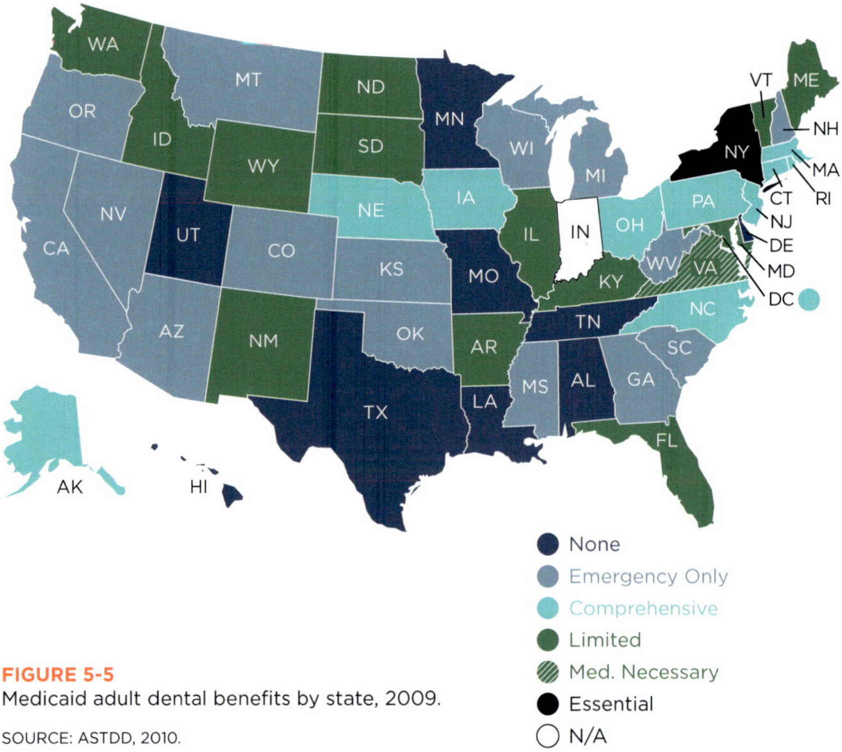

FIGURE 5-5
Medicaid adult dental benefits by state, 2009.

SOURCE: ASTDD, 2010.

chapter, have been shown by some studies to increase dentist participation (Griffin et al., 2007; Helgeson, 2005). Other approaches (e.g., training, administrative support, and quality improvement techniques) also have been shown to increase dentists' participation in Medicaid, particularly for children's services (Hughes et al., 2005). Multidimensional, strategically planned initiatives that include provider outreach, increased financing, and consumer education show particular promise (Greene-McIntyre et al., 2003; Kobayashi et al., 2005; Shirk, 2010; Taichman et al., 2009). As described in Chapter 3, state Medicaid programs are increasingly electing to reimburse primary medical care providers and dental hygienists for preventive oral health services, including the application of fluoride varnish, performing oral examinations, and providing anticipatory guidance (AAP, 2010; ADHA, 2010).

Children's Health Insurance Program (CHIP)

CHIP is a federal-state grant program that provides resources to states to expand health coverage to uninsured, low-income children up to age 19 and pregnant women. Unlike Medicaid, it is not an entitlement, but it does help states provide publicly subsidized health coverage to uninsured children in households earning up to 200 percent FPL (and with federal approval, well above that level). Following its enactment in 1997, millions of children received coverage for medical care and a portion of those were covered for dental care under CHIP (Rosenbach et al., 2003; VanLandeghem et al., 2003). CHIP plans either offer eligibility for children under Medicaid or create a separate children's health insurance approach managed by the state (and typically operated by private insurance companies). Non-Medicaid approaches must be equivalent to one of the so-called benchmark benefits packages (e.g., Federal Employees Health Benefits Program [FEHBP], Blue Cross/Blue Shield, or the state employee benefit plan). If CHIP is part of Medicaid, then benefits must be comparable, including EPSDT dental benefits.

The Children's Health Insurance Program Reauthorization Act (CHIPRA) enacted in February 2009 requires *all* states to provide dental coverage under CHIP, including "coverage of dental services necessary to prevent disease and promote oral health, restore oral structures to health and function, and treat emergency conditions."[1] States can meet this requirement in separate CHIP programs by providing dental coverage equivalent to one of three benchmark dental benefit packages: (1) the plan under FEHBP selected most frequently by employees seeking dependent coverage; (2) the state employee benefit plan selected most frequently by employees seeking dependent coverage; or (3) the commercial dental plan in the state that has the largest non-Medicaid enrollment of dependents (Paradise, 2008). In addition, states were given the option to offer a stand-alone or dental-only supplemental coverage to families whose children meet income eligibility requirements for CHIP and have private, employer-sponsored medical insurance but lack dental coverage.

CHIPRA also included provisions related to the dissemination of dental education materials, data reporting on dental access and quality, and requirements to post lists of participating dental professionals. For example, HHS's *Insure Kids Now* website was designed to provide families with more timely and accessible information about the participating providers in their communities and whether these providers are accepting new patients. However, a recent study by the Government Accountability Office

[1] *Children's Health Insurance Program Reauthorization Act of 2009*, Public Law 3, 111th Cong., 1st sess. (February 4, 2009).

(GAO) highlighted the significant deficiencies in the website's lists of dental professionals participating in Medicaid or CHIP including incomplete and inaccurate information (e.g., disconnected phone numbers, providers not accepting new patients, and providers no longer in practice) (GAO, 2010). In response to this report, HHS is taking steps to improve the *Insure Kids Now* website.

Factors That Influence Provider Participation in Medicaid and CHIP

According to the 2000 GAO report *Factors Contributing to Low Use of Dental Services by Low-Income Populations*, the primary reason individuals enrolled in Medicaid are unable to locate and use needed services is limited dentist participation in Medicaid (GAO, 2000). A recent report identified three main reasons given by dentists for not seeing more Medicaid patients: low reimbursement rates, administrative requirements, and patient-related issues (e.g., missed appointments) (Borchgrevink et al., 2008). The following sections provide a brief overview of how reimbursement rates and program-related administrative requirements influence provider participation in Medicaid. Patient-related issues are addressed in Chapter 4.

Low reimbursement rates Medicaid reimbursement rates are generally lower than dentists' usual and customary fees (GAO, 2000; Shirk, 2010). This is often cited as a disincentive to providers' willingness to participate in these publicly funded programs (Damiano et al., 1990; GAO, 2000; Lang and Weintraub, 1986; McKnight-Hanes et al., 1992; Venezie et al., 1997). For example, a recent state-by-state comparison of average retail fees and Medicaid reimbursement rates for oral evaluation revealed that, overall, Medicaid reimbursement rates were about 55 percent of the average retail fees ($18.00 vs. $33.00) (Shirk, 2010) (see Figure 5-6). While this comparison illustrates substantial variations by state, it should be noted that health care providers negotiate with insurers to determine discounts to retail fees. Since individuals without insurance have no one to negotiate such discounts on their behalf, they typically pay the full retail fee for services. Therefore, the only individuals who would be billed at the commercial rate would be the estimated 130 million U.S. adults and children who lack dental coverage. Furthermore, final negotiated rates depend on individual agreements; the larger the size of the insurer, the deeper discounts they may be able to negotiate. The impact of Medicaid reimbursement rates has also been observed in other health professions. For example, one study found a strong and significant correlation between low Medicaid reimbursement rates and low participation in Medicaid by pediatricians (Berman et al., 2002).

Before the recent economic downturn, a number of states had increased reimbursement rates for dentists in an effort to encourage broader participation of dentists in publicly funded programs and increase access to care. However, as states began to look for ways to address budgets shortfalls, many made cuts to dental reimbursement rates. In FY 2010, 13 states made cuts to dental rates, and seven more states adopted cuts to dental rates in FY 2011 (Smith et al., 2010).

Increases in reimbursement rates have shown promise in increasing dentists' participation in publicly funded programs (Borchgrevink et al., 2008; Eklund et al., 2003; Hughes et al., 2005; Mayer et al., 2000). A recent study found that both dentist participation in Medicaid and the number of Medicaid patients treated increased in states that implemented reimbursement rate increases (Borchgrevink et al., 2008). Moreover, the study found that dentists who were already enrolled in Medicaid began treating more Medicaid patients following the rate increases. Finally, in one state, both the number of providers and the geographic distribution of providers expanded following the increase in reimbursement rates. As a result, the average distance that children had to travel for care in the participating counties served decreased from 24.5 miles to 12.1 miles (Borchgrevink et al., 2008). (See the Innovations in Financing section later in this chapter for examples of enhanced Medicaid payment strategies.)

Efforts to improve access through financing strategies will necessarily be multifaceted and will be one component of broader efforts to improve access. For example, studies have demonstrated that increasing reimbursement rates alone is not sufficient in improving access to care. Without more comprehensive actions (including case management and streamlined enrollment and billing processes), barriers to oral health care persist (Borchgrevink et al., 2008).

Administrative requirements The administrative processes and requirements associated with Medicaid are frequently cited as a barrier to provider participation (ADA, 2004; GAO, 2000). In particular, dentists point to excessive paperwork, complex billing and preauthorization requirements, difficult eligibility-verification processes, slow payments, denials of submitted claims, and complicated provider enrollment as procedural obstacles to providing care to Medicaid patients (ADA, 2004; GAO, 2000; Greenberg et al., 2008). This corresponds with research in other health professions. For example, a nationally representative survey of U.S. physicians in direct patient care found that after inadequate reimbursement (84 percent of respondents), billing requirements and paperwork (70.4 percent of respondents) and delayed reimbursement (64.8 percent of respondents) were the most frequently reasons provided for limiting the number of Medicaid patients they see (Cunningham and May, 2006). Many states have taken measures to reduce administrative burdens as a strategy to improve provider participation in public programs. (See the Innovations in Financing section later in

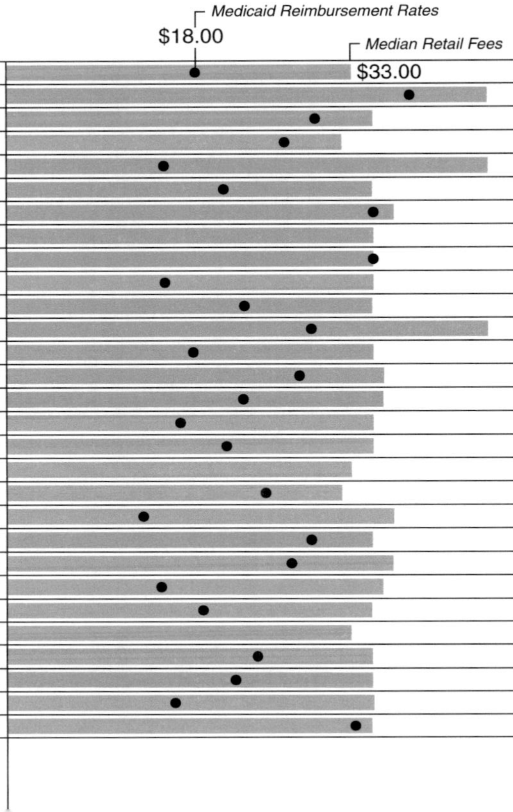

State	Median Retail Fees	Medicaid Reimbursement Rates
Alabama	$33.00	$18.00
Alaska	$46.00	$38.50
Arizona	$35.00	$29.50
Arkansas	$32.00	$26.60
California	$46.00	$15.00
Colorado	$35.00	$20.80
Connecticut	$37.00	$35.00
Delaware	$35.00	*
District of Columbia	$35.00	$35.00
Florida	$35.00	$15.00
Georgia	$35.00	$22.77
Hawaii	$46.00	$29.12
Idaho	$35.00	$17.76
Illinois	$36.00	$28.00
Indiana	$36.00	$22.58
Iowa	$35.00	$16.63
Kansas	$35.00	$21.00
Kentucky	$33.00	*
Louisiana	$32.00	$24.80
Maine	$37.00	$13.00
Maryland	$35.00	$29.08
Massachusetts	$37.00	$27.00
Michigan	$36.00	$14.89
Minnesota	$35.00	$18.70
Mississippi	$33.00	*
Missouri	$35.00	$24.00
Montana	$35.00	$21.89
Nebraska	$35.00	$16.00
Nevada	$35.00	$33.24

* No data recorded

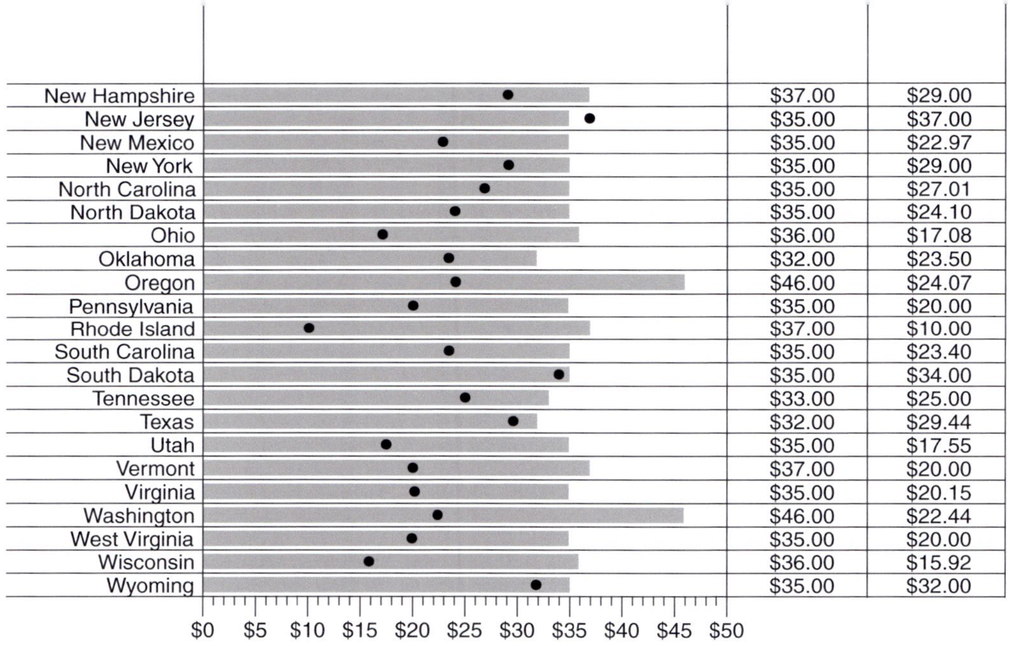

FIGURE 5-6
Median retail fees and Medicaid reimbursement rates for children's periodic oral evaluation, by state.

SOURCE: Used with permission by the National Health Policy Forum, from "Oral Health Checkup: Progress in Tough Fiscal Times?" figure 2 (Issue Brief No. 836, March 29, 2010).

this chapter for examples of how states are reducing administrative burdens associated with Medicaid.) These actions, in conjunction with rate increases and other supportive strategies (e.g., increased education and outreach to beneficiaries), can have a significant effect on increasing provider participation and patient utilization rates (Borchgrevink et al., 2008; GAO, 2009; Greenberg et al., 2008; Wysen et al., 2004).

Medicare

Medicare coverage is available to most Americans 65 and over,[2] regardless of income, and persons with disabilities. Medicare has several parts. Part A covers hospital and other institutional care for all who receive Social Security benefits, without a premium. Part B covers physician and certain other clinical services for those who elect to enroll and pay a premium. Most Medicare beneficiaries have both Part A and Part B coverage. In addition, Medicare Part D provides coverage for prescription drugs through private plans for those who wish to enroll.

The Medicare statute *explicitly excludes* coverage for what is generally known as dental care, specifically, "for services in connection with the care, treatment, filling, removal, or replacement of teeth or structures directly supporting the teeth."[3] Coverage is not determined by the value or the necessity of the dental care but by the type of service provided and the anatomical structure on which the procedure is performed. Medicare will not cover most dental care. For example, Medicare will not cover routine checkups, cleanings, fillings, or dentures.

The Centers for Medicare and Medicaid Services (CMS) has approved dental coverage in special situations that relate directly to medical needs. Currently, Medicare will pay for dental services that are an integral part either of a covered procedure (e.g., reconstruction of the jaw following accidental injury or removal of a facial tumor). Medicare also pays for extractions done in preparation for radiation treatment for diseases involving the jaw, which may be appropriate for patients with extensive periodontal disease and dental abscesses, but not for others who can be treated with less drastic interventions. Medicare will also reimburse for oral examinations, but not treatment, preceding kidney transplantation or heart valve replacement, under certain circumstances (i.e., such examination would be covered under Part A if performed by a dentist on the hospital's staff or under Part B if performed by a physician) (CMS, 2010a; IOM, 2000; Patton et al., 2001).

---

[2] Individuals who have not worked at all or have not worked enough to be eligible for Social Security are not eligible for Medicare.

[3] Section 1862(a)(12) of the U.S. Social Security Act.

As increasing numbers of baby boomers (individuals born between 1946 and 1964) become eligible for Medicare, considerable attention is being paid to how these aging adults will pay for and obtain oral health care (Ferguson et al., 2010; Manski et al., 2010a; Moeller et al., 2010). The relative size of this cohort—approximately 78 million in 2009—coupled with increases in longevity will create an unprecedented demand for oral health care for older adults.

ADDITIONAL SOURCES OF FEDERAL AND STATE FUNDING FOR ORAL HEALTH SERVICES, INFRASTRUCTURE, AND RESEARCH

Increasing access to oral health care is important, but improving oral health will require efforts that reach well beyond the dentist's office. Public health and community projects across the country are evidence of the important role of state and local health departments in promoting oral health, linking people to needed services, and developing population-based prevention programs. Such oral public health programs include efforts to reduce smoking, expand access to fluoridated water, and to educate the public about personal oral hygiene and prevention (ASTDD, 2011). Monitoring and surveillance are also key roles for oral public health. Table 5-2 provides an overview of additional public investments in oral health.

Maternal and Child Health Block Grant Program

Title V of the Social Security Act is a permanently authorized discretionary grant program that is viewed as a part of the oral health safety net for uninsured and underinsured women and children, including pregnant women and children with special health care needs.[4] Title V authorized the creation of the Maternal and Child Health (MCH) programs to promote and improve the health of all mothers and children. Title V operates as a federal-state partnership that requires a 75 percent match, that is, every $4 of federal money must be matched by $3 of state or local funds (HHS, 2008). Because oral health is an MCH priority area, Title V plays an important role in financing oral health care for vulnerable and underserved populations (see Box 5-2 for MCH Oral Health Goals). For example, in 2009, 32 states—or 63 percent—reported "oral health" as a priority need for preventive and primary care for pregnant women, mothers, infants, children, and children with special health care needs (HRSA, 2010). In addition, a recent survey of states found that Title V was the second most common source of funding for school-based health centers (SBHCs) for the 2004–2005 school year ($7.2 million) (Schlitt et al., 2008). As described

[4] United States Code, §701-710, subchapter V, chapter 7, Title 42.

TABLE 5-2
Federal and State Funding Sources for Oral Health Services, Infrastructure, and Research

Source	Appropriations, Grants, and Programs
Congress	Periodic federal legislation includes funding for oral health programs
State/local government	State-sponsored Dental Loan Repayment Programs; Community Support Grants; Funding for State Oral Health Sections, Bureaus, and Programs
Centers for Disease Control and Prevention (CDC)	State-based Oral Disease Prevention Programs Preventive Health and Health Services (PHHS) Block Grants Prevention Research Centers Program (PRCs)
National Center for Health Statistics (NCHS)	National Health Interview Survey (NHIS) and National Health and Nutrition Examination Survey (NHANES) include data on oral health status and access to services
Health Resources and Services Administration (HRSA)	
Maternal and Child Health Bureau (MCHB)	Maternal and Child Health Services Block Grants (Title V)
Bureau of Health Professions (BrHP)	National Health Service Corps (NHSC) Loan Repayment Program; Residency Training in General, Pediatric, and Public Health Dentistry; Dental Public Health Residency Training; and State Oral Health Workforce Grants
HIV/AIDS Bureau	Ryan White Comprehensive AIDS Resources Emergency (CARE) Act Funds; Community-Based Dental Partnership Program
Bureau of Primary Health Care (BPHC)	New Access Points Grants; Expanded Medical Capacity Grants; Service Expansion Grants
Office of Rural Health Policy (ORHP)	Rural Health Care Services Outreach Grants
Indian Health Service (IHS)	The Early Childhood Caries Initiative; Oral Health Promotion/Disease Prevention Awards

Centers for Medicare and Medicaid Services (CMS)	Medicaid reimbursement for: case management; services for children with special health care needs; school-based oral health services; selected administrative activities related to outreach, enrollment, and coordination of services; and referrals
U.S. Department of Agriculture (USDA)	Women, Infants, Children (WIC) Early Intervention for Oral Health Programs
Administration for Children and Families (ACF)	Head Start Oral Health Initiative

SOURCES: CDC, 2011a,b,c; Center for Oral Health, 2010; CMS, 2011a; HHS/ACF/OHS, 2011; HRSA, 2011d.

BOX 5-2
Maternal and Child Health Oral Health Goals

- Improve the health infrastructure and systems of care for all, especially underserved, vulnerable, and special needs population to ensure access to comprehensive, high-quality oral health services.
- Improve oral health status and outcomes (and their measurements) in seeking to eliminate health disparities.
- Improve the quality of oral health services (preventive and curative) for all, especially underserved, vulnerable, and special needs populations.
- Promote oral health through building public-private partnerships, including strengthening the dental public health infrastructure.

SOURCE: HHS, 2008.

in Chapter 4, SBHCs offer significant potential to increase access to oral health care among children.

The two major funding categories within the Title V MCH Block Grant program—formula grants and discretionary grants—and examples of oral health activities within both categories are described below.

Title V Block/Formula Grants

Title V Block/Formula Grants can be used to support direct health care services, enabling services (e.g., case management, transportation, outreach, and education), population-based services (e.g., surveillance), and infrastructure-building services (e.g., training and standards development). These broadly defined service areas and the design of the block grants inherently provide states with flexibility in how funds are used. For example, states that deem oral health as a priority have an existing source of annual funding from which to build. On the other hand, MCH block grants are a limited source of federal funds, and states may prioritize other critical maternal and child health issues over oral health. In 2010, Title V appropriations to states were $662 million, 85 percent—or $563 million—of which were set aside for formula block grants (HRSA, 2011a). However, the FY 2012 HRSA budget proposes over $6 million in overall cuts to the MCH block grants (HRSA, 2011d). HRSA maintains the Title V Information System website with "snapshots" of activities in the 59 states and jurisdictions that receive block grant funds from MCH (HRSA, 2011c). This website includes detailed annual reports from each state on programs and expenditures. However, oral health is not a line item on the budget and expenditure data forms and only some states include specific expenditures on oral health in their budget narratives. This makes estimating the exact amount spent on oral health care through MCH block grants difficult to determine. Data from the 2009 National Health Expenditure Accounts estimated that MCH spent 30 million dollars (11 million federal and 19 million state/local) on dental services (CMS, 2010b).

Title V Discretionary Grants

In addition to block grants, MCH supports oral health activities through Special Projects of Regional and National Significance (SPRANS) grants and Community Integrated Service Systems discretionary grants. These discretionary funds have been used to support a broad range of programs including school-based dental sealant programs, pediatric oral health leadership and leadership training programs, and infrastructure development within states and communities. The grants are intended to provide flexibility to states, communities, and institutions and promote innovation in addressing issues of timely importance that may not easily be accomplished through the formula block grants or through other federal/state programs. In 2010, the HRSA appropriation language included $4.9 million in SPRANS set aside as funds for oral health (HRSA, 2011a). However, the FY 2012 HRSA budget eliminated the SPRANS set-aside grants for oral health (HRSA, 2011d). HRSA maintains the Maternal and Child Health Bureau's Discretionary Grant Information System with program and performance measure data for these annual grants (HRSA, 2011b). For example, Iowa used Title V funding to develop a dental voucher program to increase access to oral health care for low-income, uninsured, and underinsured children. The program, which provides oral health screenings, examinations, and sealants to children in school-based settings, uses dental hygienists working under public health supervision. In 2005, the Iowa dental voucher program provided more than 25,000 services (e.g., screenings and fluoride varnish applications) and over 10,000 sealants (Association of Maternal and Child Health Programs, 2011).

THE PATIENT PROTECTION AND AFFORDABLE CARE ACT

The Patient Protection and Affordable Care Act (ACA) included numerous provisions to expand dental coverage, increase the number of oral health care professionals, and invest in oral health prevention and public health activities. Box 5-3 highlights key provisions of the ACA specifically related to dental coverage and the financing of oral health care. It also highlights selected provisions for oral public health initiatives, infrastruc-

BOX 5-3
Key Financing and Coverage Provisions for Oral Health Care in ACA

Dental coverage for children—Requires that all Qualified Health Plans offered under the Health Insurance Exchange provide coverage for an essential health benefits package, including oral care for children.

Stand-Alone Dental Plans—Allows stand-alone dental plans (i.e., those not offering medical and dental coverage) to participate in the Health Insurance Exchange.

Dental Coverage in Medicare Advantage—Requires Medicare Advantage Plans to use rebates to pay for dental coverage and other services.

MACPAC and Payments to Dental Professionals—Requires the Medicaid and CHIP Payment and Access Commission (MACPAC) to review and report to Congress on the process for updating payments to dental professionals, payment methodologies, and how the processes and methodologies relate to access and quality of care for Medicaid and CHIP beneficiaries.

Key Public Health, Infrastructure, and Research Provisions for Oral Health Care in ACA

Funding for Workforce Training—Establishes a separate appropriations line item for training of general, pediatric, and public health dentists and appropriates $30 million for FY 2010 to train the oral health workforce. Expands Title VII to create a "dental cluster" with a provision to support development of dental workforce training programs.

ture, and research grants that are likely to have an impact on access to oral health services for vulnerable and underserved populations. While these provisions may help expand access to care for vulnerable and underserved populations, it is unknown whether they will be fully funded.

INNOVATIONS IN FINANCING AND COVERAGE

The following sections provide descriptions of an array of financing and coverage innovations being used to improve access to oral health care. These examples include enhanced Medicaid payments, streamlined

Dental Faculty Loan Repayment Program—Establishes a dental faculty loan repayment program for faculty engaged in primary care dentistry, including general dentistry, pediatric dentistry, and public health dentistry.

Grants for Alternative Dental Health Care Providers Demonstration Projects—Authorizes grants to establish demonstration programs to "train or employ" alternative dental health care providers.

Funding for Oral Health Public Education Campaign—Requires a 5-year, evidence-based public education campaign to promote oral health, including a focus on early childhood caries, prevention, oral health of pregnant women, and oral health of at-risk populations.

Dental Caries Disease Management Grants—Establishes a grant program to demonstrate the effectiveness of research-based dental caries disease management.

Grants for School-based Dental Sealant Programs—Requires that all states, territories, and Indian tribes receive grants for school-based dental sealant programs.

Cooperative Agreements to Improve Oral Health Infrastructure—Requires the CDC to enter into cooperative agreements with states, territories, and Indian tribes to improve public health infrastructure related to oral health.

SOURCE: Children's Dental Health Project, 2010.

administrative processes, supportive activities, and integrating medical and oral health coverage. In some cases, these innovations are too new to have robust outcomes data for impact on access to care or oral health status, especially in the long term, and therefore the committee does not intend to imply it is recommending these approaches. In addition, these examples are not exhaustive of all of the strategies being used across the nation. Instead, they serve to illustrate the range of ideas and opportunities for improving how oral health care is financed and covered in order to improve access to care for vulnerable and underserved populations.

Enhanced Medicaid Payments

North Carolina Medicaid Waiver

North Carolina has developed a unique arrangement with the CMS to provide enhanced Medicaid payments to state-supported patient care facilities. These supplemental Medicaid payments have resulted in the development of a large network of 120 fixed and 16 mobile county-run dental clinics and an innovative clinical education model at a new School of Dental Medicine (SODM) at East Carolina University. As discussed in Chapter 3, this new clinical educational program is expected to significantly reduce dental access disparities in some of the poorest areas of the state.

In 1997 North Carolina obtained a CMS Medicaid waiver that allows enhanced payments to state-supported facilities that provide care to Medicaid patients. As a result:

1. Clinics bill fee-for-service for covered benefits provided to Medicaid-enrolled patients. On an annual basis, clinics determine the actual cost of providing services to Medicaid patients and submit the difference between actual costs and payments to the state Medicaid program.
2. The state pays the university 64 percent of the difference between actual and reimbursed costs. The money comes from CMS and reflects the fact that CMS pays 64 percent of Medicaid program costs in North Carolina.

As an example, assume the allowable cost for dental services is $2.0 million, and total reimbursement to the SODM under fee-for-service reimbursement is $1.75 million. Thus, the unreimbursed allowable amount is $250,000. Medicaid reimburses the unreimbursed costs to the extent of the federal Medicaid participation rate which is currently 64 percent. Accordingly, the school receives an additional settlement of $160,000. There is usually a 12-month period between submitting and receiving the additional funds (Bailit et al., 2010).

Minnesota Critical Access Dental Payment Program (CADPP)

In 2001, the Minnesota legislature established the Critical Access Dental Payment Program (CADPP) to offer increased reimbursement (through add-on payments) to providers that care for patients enrolled in the Minnesota Health Care Program (MHCP). MHCP provides health care coverage through three publicly funded health care programs: the Medical Assistance (MA) program, the General Assistance Medical Care (GAMC) program,

TABLE 5-3
Minnesota Fee-for-Service Payment to Charge Ratio, 2000–2006

	2000	2001	2002	2003	2004	2005	2006
CADPP providers	n/a	n/a	0.62	0.61	0.61	0.58	0.51
Non-CADPP providers	0.50	0.48	0.50	0.50	0.49	0.46	0.43

NOTE: n/a = not applicable.
SOURCE: Morales and Reisdorf, 2008.

and MinnesotaCare. While all three programs provide a dental benefit, only 44 percent of MA enrollees, 36 percent of GAMC enrollees, and 51 percent of MinnesotaCare enrollees visited a dentist in 2006 (Morales and Reisdorf, 2008).

A 2008 study of the program's impact on access showed that while a higher payment to charge ratio could be achieved with the CADPP designation in fee-for-service programs (see Table 5-3), providers continued to state that they could not afford to participate in the program.

The evaluation found that while the number of MHCP participants increased during the study period, the percent of continuously enrolled individuals receiving dental care remained stable while the rate of visits increased slightly. The researchers indicated a "growing concern for the creation of Medicaid dental mills" in which providers might deliver multiple procedures in order to maximize profitability. Overall, the researchers concluded that

> As measured by the overall number of enrollees obtaining dental services, the CADPP has demonstrated that add-on payment rates have not led to an increase in dental access for MHCP enrollees. Regardless of this finding, the program should continue to serve as a viable means of sustaining dental practices that see high volumes of MHCP enrollees and provide high quality evidence based care.

In addition, the researchers recommended further exploration into the effect of streamlining of administrative processes as well as payment rates.

Enhanced Medicaid Payments and Streamlined Administration

In 2000 the State of Michigan enrolled Medicaid-eligible children from 22 rural counties (increased to 59 counties in subsequent years) in a Delta Dental of Michigan plan called Healthy Kids Dental (HKD) (Eklund et al., 2003). Delta set fees (adjusted annually for inflation) for HKD children the same as for privately insured patients, used the same administrative processes for filing claims, and so forth, but did not charge patients any out-of-pocket expenses. In 5 years (2005), HKD utilization rates for those enrolled for 12 months increased to 53 percent, compared to the traditional Medicaid program (35 percent), but they were not as high as the privately insured (64 percent) (Eklund et al., 2003). The existing dental workforce was able to provide care to another 100,000 children (200,000 eligible).

Streamlined Administration and Supportive Activities

A recent CMS report features state-level efforts to improve the provision of Medicaid dental services through innovative practices (CMS, 2011a). For example, in Alabama, outreach to increase provider participation includes on-site assistance to dentists in completing Medicaid application forms; Maryland uses electronic funds transfer to improve the timeliness of reimbursement to providers; and Maryland and Virginia use a single contractor to administer their dental programs to reduce the paperwork providers and their office staff must complete; and Virginia reduced the prior authorizations needed for dental services (CMS, 2011a). The CMS report notes "states and providers interviewed say that these simplifications are extremely important to maintaining and increasing provider participation" (CMS, 2011a).

Integrating Medical and Oral Health Coverage

In Massachusetts, Blue Cross Blue Shield (BCBSMA) provides integrated medical and oral health coverage with the aim of improving overall health outcomes and removing cost barriers to oral health care among its vulnerable beneficiaries. Beneficiaries with diabetes, coronary artery disease (CAD), oral cancer, and women who are pregnant that have both medical and dental coverage are automatically enrolled in a program that provides "enhanced dental benefits." These individuals are eligible to receive additional services (such as cleanings or periodontal maintenance every 3 months) at no additional cost, based on their condition.

According to BCBSMA claims data, this approach has lowered medical costs among participants with diabetes and CAD. For example, BCBSMA claims data from 2007 showed that beneficiaries with CAD and diabetes who received periodontal services had lower overall monthly costs than those who received no dental care or preventive dental services alone (Lewando, 2010). BCBSMA claims data from 2009 showed that beneficiaries with CAD and diabetes who received dental prophylaxis and/or periodontal treatment had lower per-member-per-month medical costs than beneficiaries who did not receive treatment ($487 and $67, respectively) (Lewando, 2010). While this approach is not specifically designed to increase access, it is an example of an innovative cost-savings strategy targeted at vulnerable populations. Furthermore, it supports the committee's guiding principles that oral health care is an essential component of comprehensive health care and that oral health promotion and disease prevention are essential to any strategies aimed at improving access to care.

LIMITATIONS

As described in Chapter 1, the committee encountered considerable shortcomings in the research on expenditures and financing for oral health care during its review of the evidence. The committee made every effort to include the most up-to-date research published in peer-reviewed journals on these subjects. On the surface, it may appear that some of the references are dated. However, the committee determined that, in some cases, the strongest evidence on oral health financing and coverage was found in studies that have not been replicated in recent years. In other cases, newer data have been collected (through surveys such as NHANES and MEPS), but they have not been fully analyzed. Because the committee was not equipped to or charged with analyzing these data, it has cited the most current published analyses.

In addition to the lack of recent data in key areas, the committee was constrained by the somewhat limited analyses of data that exist on oral health coverage and financing. In general, the committee found few studies that provide detailed analyses of oral health financing by specific variables of interest or that analyzed complex relationships. For example, analyses of the different categories of dental coverage by subpopulations would provide a more complete picture of the impact of coverage on access and utilization and move beyond simple comparisons. In lieu of more detailed analyses, the committee relied on the strongest evidence available in the literature.

Finally, by reviewing and synthesizing the evidence, this chapter underscores the overall deficiencies in research on oral health financing. The committee hopes that this examination will help generate additional research questions and provide direction for future research.

FINDINGS AND CONCLUSIONS

The committee noted the following findings and conclusions:

- Financing for oral health care greatly influences where and whether individuals receive care.
- Per capita out-of-pocket spending for dental services is proportionally much greater than for medical services.
- Dental coverage is positively tied to access to and utilization of oral health care.

- Comprehensive dental benefits are federally required for all Medicaid-enrolled children, and all states are required to provide comparable dental coverage to children enrolled in CHIP.
- However, access to dental care continues to be a problem for children in Medicaid and CHIP.
- Medicaid benefits are not required for adults in every state, and among those states that offer dental coverage for adult Medicaid recipients, the benefits are typically limited to emergency coverage.
- Medicaid cannot properly address access to oral health services if it excludes oral health benefits.
- Low provider participation in the Medicaid program has a direct and generally negative impact on access to dental care for Medicaid beneficiaries.
- Medicare does not cover routine checkups, cleanings, fillings, or dentures for older adults.
- The federal government and states make considerable investments in dental coverage (e.g., Medicaid and CHIP), oral health services, infrastructure, and research. These investments, however, are insufficient in providing dental coverage and improving access to care for vulnerable and underserved populations.

REFERENCES

AAP (American Academy of Pediatrics). 2010. *Fluoride information by state.* http://www.aap.org/commpeds/dochs/oralhealth/fluoride.cfm (accessed March 15, 2011).

ADA (American Dental Association). 2004. *State and community models for improving access to dental care for the underserved—a white paper.* Chicago, IL.

ADHA (American Dental Hygienists' Association). 2010. States which directly reimburse dental hygienists for services under the Medicaid program. http://www.adha.org/governmental_affairs/downloads/medicaid.pdf (accessed March 12, 2011).

AHRQ (Agency for Healthcare Research and Quality). 2009. *Dental services—Mean and median expenses per person with expense and distribution of expenses by source of payment: United States, 2007.* http://www.meps.ahrq.gov/ (accessed March 15, 2011).

AHRQ. 2010. *2009 National healthcare disparities report.* Rockville, MD: U.S. Department of Health and Human Services.

Association of Maternal and Child Health Programs. 2011. *State profile: Iowa maternal and child health block grant 2011.* http://www.amchp.org/Advocacy/BLOCK-GRANT/2011PROFILES/Iowa.pdf (accessed March 16, 2011).

ASTDD (Association of State and Territorial Dental Directors). 2010. *Synopses of state dental public health programs: Data for FY 2008-2009.* http://www.astdd.org/docs/StateSynopsisReport2010SUMMARY.pdf (accessed April 5, 2011).

ASTDD. 2011. *Best practice approach reports.* http://www.astdd.org/best-practice-approach-reports (accessed March 17, 2011).

Bailit, H., J. D'Adamo, and T. Beazoglou. 2010 (unpublished). *Report to the Oral Health Access Committee: State case studies: Improving access to dental care for the underserved.*

Barsky, C. B. 2004. Incidence benefits measures in the national compensation survey. *Monthly Labor Review* 127(8):21-28.

Berman, S., J. Dolins, S. F. Tang, and B. Yudkowsky. 2002. Factors that influence the willingness of private primary care pediatricians to accept more Medicaid patients. *Pediatrics* 110(2 I):239-248.

Bisgaier, J., D. B. Cutts, B. L. Edelstein, and K. V. Rhodes. 2011. Disparities in child access to emergency care for acute oral injury. *Pediatrics*, doi:10.1542/peds.2011-0011.

Bloom, B., and R. A. Cohen. 2010. *Dental insurance for persons under age 65 years with private health insurance: United States, 2008*. Hyattsville, MD: National Center for Health Statistics.

BLS (Bureau of Labor Statistics). 2010a. *Consumer out-of-pocket health care expenditures in 2008*. http://www.bls.gov/opub/ted/2010/ted_20100325_data.htm (accessed January 9, 2011).

BLS. 2010b. *Employee benefits survey: Health care benefits, March 2010*. http://www.bls.gov/ncs/ebs/benefits/2010/benefits_health.htm (accessed December 28, 2010).

BLS. 2011. *Selected medical benefits: A report from the Department of Labor to the Department of Health and Human Services*. http://www.bls.gov/ncs/ebs/sp/selmedbensreport.pdf (accessed May 23, 2011).

Borchgrevink, A., A. Snyder, and S. Gehshan. 2008. *The effects of Medicaid reimbursement rates on access to dental care*. Washington, DC: National Academy for State Health Policy.

CDC (Centers for Disease Control and Prevention). 2011a. *Division of oral health state-based programs*. http://www.cdc.gov/oralhealth/state_programs.index.htm (accessed November 17, 2011).

CDC. 2011b. *Prevention research centers*. http://www.cdc.gov/prc (accessed November 17, 2011).

CDC. 2011c. *Preventive health and health services block grant funding by health program areas, fiscal year: 2010*. http://www.cdc.gov/phhsblockgrant/funding/blockgrant10.htm (accessed November 17, 2011).

Center for Oral Health. 2010. *WIC programs*. http://www.centerfororalhealth.org/programs/wic-programs (accessed January 31, 2011).

Children's Dental Health Project. 2010. *Oral health provisions in the Patient Protection and Affordable Care Act*. http://www.cdhp.org/system/files/FINAL%20HCR%20Senate%20Bill%20Summary%20-%203%2023%2010.pdf (accessed March 17, 2011).

CMS (Centers for Medicare and Medicaid Services). 2005a. *Early and periodic screening, diagnostic, and treatment benefit overview*. https://www.cms.gov/MedicaidEarlyPeriodicScrn/01_Overview.asp#TopOfPage (accessed March 16, 2011).

CMS. 2005b. *Early and periodic screening, diagnostic, and treatment benefits*. https://www.cms.gov/MedicaidEarlyPeriodicScrn/02_Benefits.asp#TopOfPage (accessed March 16, 2011).

CMS. 2009. *2009 Medicaid managed care enrollment report*. https://www.cms.gov/MedicaidDataSourcesGenInfo/04_MdManCrEnrllRep.asp (accessed March 16, 2011).

CMS. 2010a. *Medicare dental coverage: Overview*. http://www.cms.hhs.gov/MedicareDentalCoverage (accessed November 22, 2010).

CMS. 2010b. *National health expenditure accounts*. https://www.cms.gov/nationalhealthexpenddata/02_nationalhealthaccountshistorical.asp (accessed February 22, 2011).

CMS. 2010c. *National health expenditure projections 2009-2019*. https://www.cms.gov/NationalHealthExpendData/downloads/NHEProjections2009to2019.pdf (accessed February 22, 2011).

CMS. 2011a. *Innovative state practices for improving the provision of Medicaid dental services*. Baltimore, MD.

CMS. 2011b. *Overview Medicaid dental coverage*. https://www.cms.gov/MedicaidDentalCoverage/ (accessed March 16, 2011).

Cunningham, P. J., and J. H. May. 2006. *Medicaid patients increasingly concentrated among physicians.* Washington, DC: Center for Studying Health System Change.

Damiano, P. C., E. R. Brown, J. D. Johnson, and J. P. Scheetz. 1990. Factors affecting dentist participation in a state Medicaid program. *Journal of Dental Education* 54(11):638-643.

Damiano, P., J. Willard, E. Momany, and J. Chowdhury. 2003. The impact of the Iowa S-SCHIP program on access, health status, and family environment. *Ambulatory Pediatrics* 3:263-269.

Dasanayake, A. P., Y. Li, et al. 2007. Challenges faced by minority children in obtaining dental care. *Journal of Health Care for the Poor and Underserved* 18(4):779-788.

Decker, S. L. 2011. Medicaid payment levels to dentists and access to dental care among children and adolescents. *Journal of the American Medical Association* 306(2):187-193.

Edelstein, B. L., and C. H. Chinn. 2009. Update on disparities in oral health and access to dental care for America's children. *Academic Pediatrics* 9(6):415-419.

Eklund, S. A., J. L. Pittman, and S. J. Clark. 2003. Michigan Medicaid's healthy kids dental program: An assessment of the first 12 months. *Journal of the American Dental Association* 134(11):1509-1515.

Feinberg, E., K. Swartz, A. Zaslavsky, J. Gardner, and D. K. Walker. 2002. Family income and the impact of a Children's Health Insurance Program on reported need for health services and unmet health need. *Pediatrics* 109(2):E29.

Ferguson, D. A., B. J. Steinberg, and T. Schwien. 2010. Dental economics and the aging population. *Compendium of Continuing Education in Dentistry* 31(6):418-420, 422, 424-425.

Fisher, M. A., and A. K. Mascarenhas. 2007. Does Medicaid improve utilization of medical and dental services and health outcomes for Medicaid-eligible children in the United States? *Community Dentistry and Oral Epidemiology* 35(4):263-271.

Flores, G., and S. C. Tomany-Korman. 2008. Racial and ethnic disparities in medical and dental health, access to care, and use of services in U.S. children. *Pediatrics* 121(2): e286-e298.

Ford, J. L. 2009. *The new health participation and access data from the National Compensation Survey.* http://www.bls.gov/opub/cwc/cm20091022ar01p1.htm (accessed December 27, 2010).

Fox, M., J. Moore, R. Davis, and R. Heintzelman. 2003. Changes in reported health status and unmet need for children enrolling in the Kansas Children's Health Insurance Program. *American Journal of Public Health* 93(4):579-582.

GAO (Government Accountability Office). 2000. *Factors contributing to low use of dental services by low-income populations.* Washington, DC: U.S. General Accounting Office.

GAO. 2009. *State and federal actions have been taken to improve children's access to dental services, but gaps remain.* Washington, DC: U.S. Government Accountability Office.

GAO. 2010. *Efforts under way to improve children's access to dental services, but sustained attention needed to address ongoing concerns.* Washington, DC: U.S. Government Accountability Office.

Greenberg, B. J. S., J. V. Kumar, and H. Stevenson. 2008. Dental case management: Increasing access to oral health care for families and children with low incomes. *Journal of the American Dental Association* 139(8):1114-1121.

Greene-Mclntyre, M., M. Finch, and J. Searcy. 2003. Smile Alabama! Initiative: Interim results from a program to increase children's access to dental care. *Journal of Rural Health* 19(5):407-415.

Griffin, S. O., K. A. Jones, S. Lockwood, N. G. Mosca, and P. A. Honoré. 2007. Impact of increasing Medicaid dental reimbursement and implementing school sealant programs on sealant prevalence. *Journal of Public Health Management and Practice* 13(2):202-206.

Helgeson, M. J. 2005. The Minnesota oral health care solutions project: Implications for people with special needs. *CDA Journal* 33(8):641-649.

HHS (Department of Health and Human Services). 2008. State MCH-Medicaid coordination: A review of Title V and Title XIX interagency agreements (2nd ed). ftp://ftp.hrsa.gov/mchb/IAA/State_MCH_Medicaid_Coord.pdf (accessed April 5, 2011).

HHS/ACF (Administration for Children and Families)/OHS (Office of Head Start). 2011. *Head Start dental home initiative.* http://eclkc.ohs.acf.hhs.gov/hslc/tta-system/health/Health/Oral%20Health (accessed November 17, 2011). HRSA (Health Resources and Services Administration). 2010. *MCHB discretionary grant information system.* https://perfdata.hrsa.gov/mchb/mchreports/search/program/prgsch02_result.asp (accessed March 31, 2011).

HRSA (Health Resources and Services Administration). 2011a. *Fiscal year 2011 justification of estimates for appropriations committees.* http://www.hrsa.gov/about/budgetjustification/budgetjustification11.pdf (accessed April 5, 2011).

HRSA. 2011b. *Maternal and Child Health Bureau discretionary grant information system reports.* https://perfdata.hrsa.gov/MCHB/DGISReports/default.aspx (accessed March 17, 2011).

HRSA. 2011c. *Maternal and Child Health Bureau: TVIS snapshots.* https://perfdata.hrsa.gov/mchb/TVISReports/Snapshot/SnapShotMenu.aspx (accessed March 17, 2011).

HRSA. 2011d. *Fiscal year 2011 justification of estimates for appropriations committees.* http://www.hrsa.gov/about/budget/budgetjustification2012.pdf (accessed May 11, 2011).

Hughes, R. J., P. C. Damiano, M. J. Kanellis, R. Kuthy, and R. Slayton. 2005. Dentists' participation and children's use of services in the Indiana dental Medicaid program and SCHIP: Assessing the impact of increased fees and administrative changes. *Journal of the American Dental Association* 136(4):517-523.

IOM (Institute of Medicine). 1980. *Public policy options for better dental health.* Washington, DC: National Academy Press.

IOM. 2000. *Extending Medicare coverage for preventive and other services.* Washington, DC: National Academy Press.

Jablonski, R. A., C. L. Munro, M. J. Grap, and R. K. Elswick. 2005. The role of biobehavioral, environmental, and social forces on oral health disparities in frail and functionally dependent nursing home elders. *Biological Research for Nursing* 7(1):75-82.

Johnson, J. T., E. G. Turner, K. F. Novak, and A. L. Kaplan. 2005. Factors associated with comprehensive dental care following an initial emergency dental visit. *Journal of Dentistry for Children* 72(2):78-80.

Kenney, G. 2007. The impacts of the State Children's Health Insurance Program on children who enroll: Findings from ten states. *Health Services Research* 42(4):1520-1543.

Kenney, M. K. 2009. Oral health care in CSHCN: State Medicaid policy considerations. *Pediatrics* 124(Supp. 4):S384-S391.

Klein, J. D., L. P. Shone, P. G. Szilagyi, A. Bajorska, K. Wilson, and A. W. Dick. 2007. Impact of the state children's health insurance program on adolescents in New York. *Pediatrics* 119(4):e885-e892.

Kobayashi, M., D. Chi, S. E. Coldwell, P. Domoto, and P. Milgrom. 2005. The effectiveness and estimated costs of the access to baby and child dentistry program in Washington state. *Journal of the American Dental Association* 136(9):1257-1263.

Lang, W. P., and J. A. Weintraub. 1986. Comparison of Medicaid and non-Medicaid dental providers. *Journal of Public Health Dentistry* 46(4):207-211.

Lave, J. R., C. R. Keane, C. J. Lin, and E. M. Ricci. 2002. The impact of dental benefits on the utilization of dental services by low-income children in western Pennsylvania. *Pediatric Dentistry* 24(3):234-240.

Lewando, R. 2010. *Periodontal disease and chronic diseases: Emerging science and programs: BCBSMA Total Health Solutions*. Presentation to the National Oral Health Conference, April 27, 2010. http://www.nationaloralhealthconference.com/docs/presentations/2010/Robert%20Lewando%20-%20Periodontal%20Disease.pdf (accessed May 12, 2011).

Lewis, C., W. Mouradian, R. Slayton, and A. Williams. 2007. Dental insurance and its impact on preventative dental care visits for U.S. children. *Journal of the American Dental Association* 138(3):369-380.

Lewis, C. W., S. Boulter, M. A. Keels, D. M. Krol, W. E. Mouradian, K. G. O'Connor, and R. B. Quinonez. 2009. Oral health and pediatricians: Results of a national survey. *Academic Pediatrics* 9(6):457-461.

Liu, J., J. C. Probst, A. B. Martin, J.-Y. Wang, and C. F. Salinas. 2007. Disparities in dental insurance coverage and dental care among U.S. children: The National Survey of Children's Health. *Pediatrics* 119(Supp. 1):S12-S21.

Manski, R. J., and E. Brown. 2007. *Dental use, expenses, private dental coverage, and changes, 1996 and 2004*. Rockville, MD: Agency for Healthcare Research and Quality.

Manski, R. J., and E. Brown. 2008. *Dental coverage of children and young adults under age 21, United States, 1996 and 2006. Statistical brief #221*. Rockville, MD: Agency for Healthcare Research and Quality.

Manski, R. J., and E. Brown. 2010. *Dental coverage of adults ages 21-64, United States, 1997 and 2007*. Rockville, MD: Agency for Healthcare Research and Quality.

Manski, R. J., and P. F. Cooper. 2010. Characteristics of employers offering dental coverage in the united states. *Journal of the American Dental Association* 141(6):700-711.

Manski, R. J., J. Moeller, H. Chen, P. A. St. Clair, J. Schimmel, L. Magder, and J. V. Pepper. 2010a. Dental care expenditures and retirement. *Journal of Public Health Dentistry* 70(2):148-155.

Manski, R. J., J. Moeller, J. Schimmel, P. A. St. Clair, H. Chen, L. Magder, and J. V. Pepper. 2010b. Dental care coverage and retirement. *Journal of Public Health Dentistry* 70(1):1-12.

Mayer, M. L., S. C. Stearns, E. C. Norton, and R. G. Rozier. 2000. The effects of Medicaid expansions and reimbursement increases on dentists' participation. *Inquiry* 37(1):33-44.

McBroome, K., P. C. Damiano, and J. C. Willard. 2005. Impact of the Iowa S-SCHIP program on access to dental care for adolescents. *Pediatric Dentistry* 27(1):47-53.

McKnight-Hanes, C., D. R. Myers, and J. C. Dushku. 1992. Method of payment for children's dental services by practice type and geographic location. *Pediatric Dentistry* 14(5):338-341.

Milgrom, P., R. S.-Y. Lee, C. E. Huebner, and D. A. Conrad. 2010. Medicaid reforms in Oregon and suboptimal utilization of dental care by women of childbearing age. *Journal of the American Dental Association* 141(6):688-695.

Moeller, J. F., H. Chen, and R. J. Manski. 2010. Investing in preventive dental care for the Medicare population: A preliminary analysis. *American Journal of Public Health* 100(11):2262-2269.

Mofidi, M., R. Slifkin, V. Freeman, and P. Silberman. 2002. The impact of a state children's health insurance program on access to dental care. *Journal of the American Dental Association* 133(6):707-714.

Morales, M. and C. Reisdorf. 2008. *Minnesota health care programs: Critical Access Dental Program—results and recommendations*. St. Paul, MN: Minnesota Department of Human Services.

NADP (National Association of Dental Plans). 2009. *Dental benefits improve access to dental care*. http://www.nadp.org/Libraries/HCR_Documents/nadphcr-dentalbenefitsimproveaccesstocare-3-28-09.sflb.ashx (accessed January 10, 2011).

Paradise, J. 2008. *Dental coverage and care for low-income children: The role of Medicaid and SCHIP.* Washington, DC: Kaiser Family Foundation.

Patton, L. L., B. A. White, and M. J. Field. 2001. Extending Medicare coverage to medically necessary dental care. *Journal of the American Dental Association* 132(9):1294-1299.

Pourat, N., and L. Finocchio. 2010. Racial and ethnic disparities in dental care for publicly insured children. *Health Affairs* 29(7):1356-1363.

Ramírez, M., K. P. Ahluwalia, and J. A. Teresi. 2011. Correlates of dental visits among community-residing Latino elders: A public health alert. *Gerodontology* 28(1):12-18.

Rohde, F. 2010. *Dental expenditures in the 10 largest states, 2007.* Rockville, MD: Agency for Healthcare Research and Quality.

Rosenbach, M., M. Ellwood, C. Irvin, C. Young, W. Conroy, B. Quinn, and M. Kell. 2003. *Implementation of the state children's health insurance program: Synthesis of state evaluations.* Washington, DC: Mathematica Policy Research Inc.

Rowley, S. T., B. Sheller, B. J. Williams, and L. Mancl. 2006. Utilization of a hospital for treatment of pediatric dental emergencies. *Pediatric Dentistry* 28(1):10-17.

Schlitt, J. J., L. J. Juszczak, and N. H. Eichner. 2008. Current status of state policies that support school-based health centers. *Public Health Reports* 123(6):731-738.

Shiboski, C. H., M. Cohen, K. Weber, A. Shansky, K. Malvin, and R. M. Greenblatt. 2005. Factors associated with use of dental services among HIV-infected and high-risk uninfected women. *Journal of the American Dental Association* 136(9):1242-1255.

Shirk, C. 2010. *Oral health checkup: Progress in tough fiscal times?* Washington, DC: National Health Policy Forum.

Shortridge, E. F., and J. R. Moore. 2009. Use of emergency departments for conditions related to poor oral healthcare: Implications for rural and low-resource urban areas for three states. *Journal of Public Health Management and Practice* 15(3):238-245.

Smith, V., K. Gifford, E. Ellis, R. Rudowitz, and L. Snyder. 2010. *Hoping for economic recovery, preparing for health reform: A look at Medicaid spending, coverage and policy trends.* Washington, DC: Kaiser Family Foundation.

Snowden, C. B., T. R. Miller, A. F. Jensen, and B. A. Lawrence. 2003. Costs of medically treated craniofacial conditions. *Public Health Reports* 118(1):10-17.

Snyder, A. 2009. *Increasing access to dental care in Medicaid: Targeted programs for four populations.* Washington, DC: National Association for State Health Policy.

Sohn, W., A. Ismail, A. Amaya, and J. Lepkowski. 2007. Determinants of dental care visits among low-income African-American children. *Journal of the American Dental Association* 138(3):309-318.

Sweet, M., P. Damiamo, E. Rivera, R. Kuthy, and K. Heller. 2005. A comparison of dental services received by Medicaid and privately insured adult populations. *Journal of the American Dental Association* 136(1):93-100.

Szilagyi, P. G., A. W. Dick, J. D. Klein, L. P. Shone, J. Zwanziger, and T. McInerny. 2004. Improved access and quality of care after enrollment in the New York State Children's Health Insurance Program (SCHIP). *Pediatrics* 113(5):e395-e404.

Taichman, L. S., W. Sohn, S. Lim, S. Eklund, and A. Ismail. 2009. Assessing patterns of restorative and preventive care among children enrolled in Medicaid, by type of dental care provider. *Journal of the American Dental Association* 140(7):886-894.

Trenholm, C., E. Howell, D. Hughes, and S. Orzol. 2005. The Santa Clara County Healthy Kids Program: Impacts on children's medical, dental, and vision care. *Mathematica Policy Research Report,* http://www.mathematica-mpr.com/publications/PDFs/santaclara.pdf (accessed May 10, 2011).

VanLandeghem, K., J. Bronstein, and C. Brach. 2003. *Children's dental care access in Medicaid: The role of medical care use and dentist participation.* Rockville, MD: Agency for Healthcare Research and Quality.

Venezie, R., W. Vann Jr., S. Cashion, and R. Rozier. 1997. Pediatric and general dentists' participation in the North Carolina Medicaid program: Trends from 1986 to 1992. *Pediatric Dentistry* 19(2):114-117.

Wang, H., E. C. Norton, and R. G. Rozier. 2007. Effects of the State Children's Health Insurance Program on access to dental care and use of dental services. *Health Services Research* 42(4):1544-1563.

Wysen, K. H., P. M. Hennessy, M. I. Lieberman, T. E. Garland, and S. M. Johnson. 2004. Kids get care: Integrating preventive dental and medical care using a public health case management model. *Journal of Dental Education* 68(5):522-530.

Zuckerman, S., J. Haley, Y. Roubideaux, and M. Lillie-Blanton. 2004. Health service access, use, and insurance coverage among American Indians/Alaska Natives and whites: What role does the Indian Health Service play? *American Journal of Public Health* 94(1):53-59.

6

A Vision for the Delivery of Oral Health Care to Vulnerable and Underserved Populations

The committee's ultimate goals in this report are to synthesize current issues related to accessing oral health care, to examine strengths and deficiencies in the delivery system that responds to these issues, and to provide a vision for improving the delivery of oral health care to underserved and vulnerable populations across the life cycle.

The committee faced several challenges in addressing these goals because (1) vulnerable and underserved populations in the United States are numerous and heterogeneous; (2) as such, these populations have a broad range of unmet needs and face diverse barriers to access; (3) oral health care for vulnerable and underserved populations is delivered in myriad settings and through varied institutional structures, with limited common goals and no coherent, organizing system; (4) there is no agreed-upon set of essential oral health services with which to evaluate the success of efforts designed to improve access; and (5) there is a lack of agreement on how to expand the capacity of the oral health workforce to meet the needs of underserved and vulnerable populations, and this issue is politically charged.

Recognizing the challenges described above, the committee drew upon the existing literature to formulate a number of key findings and conclusions that are highlighted in the preceding chapters. In this final chapter, the findings are consolidated into four overall conclusions. These conclusions in turn serve as the foundation for the committee's vision for improving the delivery of oral health care to underserved and vulnerable populations across the life cycle. This chapter presents the committee's vision and 10 specific recommendations—directed to both public and private entities—for improving access to oral health care.

Numerous coordinated and sustained actions will be needed to implement the committee's recommendations and to achieve its vision. Therefore, the committee identifies important actions that various stakeholders can take and identifies the relevant policy levers that are most likely to produce both short-term and long-term change (see later in this chapter for a summary of key implementation strategies by actor).

OVERALL CONCLUSIONS

After reviewing the evidence, the committee concluded the following:

1. *Improving access to oral health care is a critical and necessary first step to improving oral health outcomes and reducing disparities.*
2. *The continued separation of oral health care from overall health care contributes to limited access to oral health care for many Americans.*
3. *Sources of financing for oral health care for vulnerable and underserved populations are limited and tenuous.*
4. *Improving access to oral health care will necessarily require multiple solutions that use an array of providers in a variety of settings.*

The committee's overall conclusions reflect the need for action to address issues of access to oral health care. If the current approaches to oral health education, financing, and regulation continue unchanged, equitable access to oral health care cannot be achieved. However, this report should not be perceived as simply a call for more spending. Investing additional money in a delivery system that is poorly designed to meet the oral health care needs of the nation's underserved and vulnerable populations would produce limited results and would be fiscally irresponsible. Rather, the report calls for transformation through targeted investments in programs and policies that are most likely to yield the greatest impact.

A VISION FOR IMPROVING ACCESS TO ORAL HEALTH CARE

While the majority of the U.S. population is able to routinely obtain oral health care in traditional dental practice settings, millions of Americans have unmet oral health needs due, in part, to major barriers in access to care. This is especially true for the nation's vulnerable and underserved populations. The committee's review of the evidence, as presented in this report, makes a compelling case for action. Failure to address the challenges that millions of Americans face in accessing oral health care will exacerbate the disproportionate burden of oral diseases experienced by vulnerable and underserved populations. Therefore, the committee provides a vision of

BOX 6-1
Vision for Oral Health Care in the United States

Everyone has access to quality oral health care across the life cycle.

To be successful with underserved and vulnerable populations, an evidence-based oral health system will

1. **Eliminate barriers that contribute to oral health disparities;**
2. **Prioritize disease prevention and health promotion;**
3. **Provide oral health services in a variety of settings;**
4. **Rely on a diverse and expanded array of providers competent, compensated, and authorized to provide evidence-based care;**
5. **Include collaborative and multidisciplinary teams working across the health care system; and**
6. **Foster continuous improvement and innovation.**

how public and private providers should address the delivery of oral health care to underserved and vulnerable populations (see Box 6-1).

The committee's vision is both aspirational and achievable. That is, there are immediate steps that can be taken to improve access to oral health care, while other goals focus beyond what is attainable exclusively in the near term. These goals will only be realized by sustained and concerted efforts over time. The committee's recommendations, therefore, spell out what is achievable at present as well as what our nation should aspire to.

RECOMMENDATIONS

The committee arrived at set of 10 recommendations. If acted upon in a coordinated and comprehensive manner, these recommendations will improve access to oral health care for underserved and vulnerable populations.

Integrating Oral Health Care into Overall Health Care

The committee's vision calls for an array of providers to participate in the delivery of oral health care. This strategy will help groups that are unable to obtain oral health services in traditional dental practice settings to receive care from the range of health care professionals that they encounter more routinely. For populations that rarely visit dentists, nondental health care professionals may be in the best position to provide oral health education, screening, and prevention. Young children, for example, visit pediatricians and family physicians earlier and more frequently than they visit dentists (Dela Cruz et al., 2004). With proper training, these primary care providers are well situated to educate parents about how to prevent oral disease, assess risk for oral disease, screen for early childhood caries, and deliver preventive services (e.g., fluoride varnish). Similarly, older adults living in institutions receive much of their routine care from nurses and nursing assistants who can also screen for dental disease, provide routine oral health care (e.g., toothbrushing and denture care), and promote preventive care.

Ensuring that nondental health care professionals are properly trained to take a role in delivering quality oral health care will be crucial. Defining a multidisciplinary, core set of oral health competencies is the first step in training nondental health care professionals to provide oral health care. These competencies would describe essential skills that health care professionals need in order to provide quality oral health care upon completing their training. The overall aim of a minimum core set is to establish base standards across the health professions and to reduce the burden on each profession to develop their own competencies for oral health. Individual professions, however, may choose to build upon the core set to reflect their specific expertise and interaction with individuals and within communities.

The core set of oral health competencies for nondental health care professionals needs to be developed with input from a variety of stakeholders to ensure that they are appropriately broad and, therefore, applicable to many health professions. The competencies also need to reflect the collective expertise and experience of dental professionals and their nondental health care professional counterparts to ensure that the competencies prepare professionals to provide care that meets appropriate standards of quality (i.e., care that is safe, timely, effective, efficient, equitable, and patient-centered). Therefore, the committee recommends

> **RECOMMENDATION 1a: The Healthcare Resources and Services Administration (HRSA) should convene key stakeholders from both the public and private sectors to develop a core set of oral health competencies for health care professionals.**

At minimum, the core competencies need to prepare graduates to

- Recognize risk for oral disease through competent oral examinations,
- Provide basic oral health information,
- Integrate oral health information with diet and lifestyle counseling, and
- Make and track referrals to oral health care professionals.

Fortunately, there are models that can serve as a basis for developing a core set of oral health competencies for nondental health care professionals. For example, as discussed in Chapter 3, the University of Washington developed and implemented curriculum to train medical students about oral health that has subsequently been endorsed by the American Association of Medical Colleges (Mouradian et al., 2005). The curriculum includes competencies in five general areas: oral public health, dental caries, periodontal disease, oral cancer, and oral-systemic interactions. Similar sets of competencies have been developed or proposed for other disciplines (e.g., geriatrics and physician assistants [PAs]) and health issues (e.g., family violence) (Danielsen et al., 2006; Knox and Spivak, 2005; Partnership for Health in Aging, 2008).

Once a core set of competencies has been developed, it will need to be adopted by health professional schools and incorporated into the curriculum. The committee concludes the best way to incorporate the oral health competencies into health professional education is for accrediting and certification bodies to require them for accreditation and maintenance of certification. Therefore, the committee recommends

RECOMMENDATION 1b: Following the development of a core set of oral health competencies for nondental health care professionals

- **Accrediting bodies for undergraduate and graduate-level nondental health care professional education programs should integrate these core competencies into their requirements for accreditation; and**
- **All certification and maintenance of certification for health care professionals should include demonstration of competence in oral health care as a criterion.**

Finally, HRSA can play an important role in supporting the adoption of oral health core competencies into nondental health professional education programs. To that end, the committee suggests the following strategies:

- HRSA can strengthen the integration of oral health core competencies into nondental health professional education programs by requiring that Title VII–funded programs include interprofessional education on oral health.
- HRSA can support curriculum development and dissemination efforts for nondental health professional education programs.

Creating Optimal Laws and Regulations

The committee's vision underscores the need to eliminate barriers to accessing oral health care. Due to their powerful influence on oral health practice, the committee identified the variety of regulations and policies that determine *how* care is provided—and more importantly *by whom*—as a key area of focus for efforts to eliminate barriers.

Despite the existence of national accreditation standards on education and training of oral health professionals, regulations defining supervision levels and scopes of practice vary widely by state. For example, a recent review of dental hygiene practice acts revealed great variability among states regarding required levels of supervision by settings of care, type of service, and other special requirements (e.g., minimum hours/years of clinical experience or possession of professional liability insurance) (ADHA, 2011). In some instances, dental hygienists are permitted to provide some services in public health settings under the general supervision of a dentist, but in the same state, are not permitted to provide the same services in private dental offices without direct supervision (ADHA, 2011; HRSA, 2004). Furthermore, seven states require that a dentist be present when a hygienist applies dental sealants (ADHA, 2011). As a result of overly restrictive regulation, states may miss critical opportunities to serve greater numbers of individuals in need of care.

Some states seek to meet the growing public needs by altering their scope of practice and supervision regulations to allow a broader range of oral health care professionals to see patients without a dentist's direct supervision. For example, California's Health Workforce Pilot Project includes a process to evaluate new workforce models prior to adoption of new professions or expanded scope of practice for existing professions. The registered dental hygienist in alternative practice license in California, which allows dental hygienists to practice in certain community settings without a dentist's direct supervision, was a result of this process. California also has a current project evaluating the placement of Interim Therapeutic Restorations by Dental Hygienists and Dental Assistants under general supervision in community settings. The majority of state laws, however, lag behind in this regard. As a result, the services that oral health care professionals are able to provide vary significantly and decision making regarding such regulations are often unrelated to competence, education and training, or the safety of those services.

Previous IOM reports have supported the idea of expanding scope of practice in alignment with professional competencies (IOM, 2001, 2008, 2010). For example, the report *Crossing the Quality Chasm: A New Health System for the 21st Century* noted that, "scope of practice acts and other workforce regulations need to allow for innovation in the use of all types of clinicians to meet patient needs in the most effective and efficient way possible" (IOM, 2001). More recently, the report *The Future of Nursing: Leading Change, Advancing Health* recommended that scope-of-practice barriers be removed to enable advanced nurse practitioners "to practice to the full extent of their training and education" (IOM, 2010). Building from these reports and the evidence from other professions, the committee determined that amending existing state laws, including practice acts, will set the stage to increase access to basic oral health care. Therefore, the committee recommends

RECOMMENDATION 2: State legislatures should amend existing state laws, including practice acts, to optimize access to oral health care.
At minimum, state dental practice acts should

- **Allow allied dental professionals to practice to the full extent of their education and training;**
- **Allow allied dental professionals to work in a variety of settings under evidence-supported supervision levels; and**
- **Allow technology-supported remote collaboration and supervision.**

This recommendation will enable an array of health care professionals to work in community settings, change supervision requirements to levels supported by evidence, and allow the use of telehealth technologies to reach underserved populations with care that is as effective as that delivered in person. By allowing an array of health care professionals to address basic oral health needs, dentists will be able to dedicate themselves to providing more complex care and treating more patients with complex needs.

Because amendments to state practice acts provide an important opportunity to expand access to oral health care, it is incumbent upon the states to adopt effective reforms. States can be supported in these efforts with strong evidence and clear guidance. This committee, therefore, proposes the following as strategies for implementation and dissemination:

- In the short term, the Centers for Medicare and Medicaid Services (CMS) can support states by disseminating rules and policies that promote Medicaid and Children's Health Insurance Program (CHIP) beneficiaries' access to appropriate care, and ensuring that its rules and polices reflect the practice abilities of current and new types of licensed providers.
- In the long term, the Office of the Assistant Secretary for Planning and Evaluation can help ensure that state practice acts are structured to optimize access to oral health care by examining and reporting on the impact of state practice acts on oral health care delivery to vulnerable and underserved populations. These reports would need to be conducted and published periodically to support sustained attention to increasing access.

Private foundations and organizations that focus on state policy can also play an important role in supporting efforts to eliminate unnecessary regulatory and policy barriers to oral health care. Therefore, the committee suggests the following as specific examples of activities for such organizations:

- Foundations, professional organizations, and public policy organizations are ideally suited to conduct and disseminate an initial review of state practice acts with a focus on access to services.
- Foundations, professional organizations, and public policy organizations can support states by issuing "best practices" briefs to highlight what each state is doing and what impact it is having on access.

Improving Dental Education and Training

The committee's vision supports changes to dental education and training that will ensure that current and future generations of dental professionals can deliver quality care to diverse populations, in a variety of settings, using a variety of service-delivery mechanisms, and across the life cycle. Greater emphasis will need to be placed on increasing the diversity of the workforce, including in the areas of race and ethnicity, as well as geographic distribution. The creation of such an improved and responsive education system can play a key role in eliminating barriers to oral health care.

Training a Diverse and Experienced Workforce

The 2004 Institute of Medicine (IOM) report *In the Nation's Compelling Interest* emphasized the importance of ensuring greater diversity among health care professionals as it "is associated with improved access to care for racial and ethnic minority patients, greater patient choice and satisfaction, better patient–provider communication, and better educational experiences for *all* students while in training" (IOM, 2004). Similarly, the ADA's *Future of Dentistry* report concluded that, "Dental schools have a responsibility to recruit and retain underrepresented minority students and faculty and for training students to be culturally competent in dealing with various populations" (ADA, 2001). Several innovative strategies have been used across the country to achieve these aims. For example, as discussed in Chapter 3, bridge and pipeline programs are two strategies used to address the imbalance between the numbers of minorities in the oral health professions and those in the general population. While evidence indicates that strategies undertaken by dental pipeline programs show promise, they have made only modest gains in national enrollment among underrepresented minority students to date (Brunson et al., 2010).

In addition to efforts to increase the diversity of dental professional students, oral health curricula need to be updated to ensure that future dental professionals have substantial practical experiences in a variety of settings (e.g., Federally Qualified Health Centers [FQHCs], nursing homes, local health departments). Skills needed to work in these settings and with these populations include the ability to work in interprofessional teams with general health, education, and social service professionals; the ability to work in dental professional teams; and the ability to use new service-delivery mechanisms such as telehealth technologies for supervision, consultation, and collaboration. Providing students with clinical exposure in community-based settings increases the likelihood that students may return to such settings in their future careers and improves their comfort level with caring for vulnerable and underserved populations. The ADA recognized the importance of clinical experience in community settings in its *Future of Dentistry* report, that stated: "Dental schools should develop programs in which students, residents, and faculty provide care for members of the underserved populations in community clinics and practices" (ADA, 2001). And more recently, the ADA reaffirmed this position on community-based education programs in its new *Accreditation Standards for Dental Education Programs*. The new standards state that: "Dental education programs must make available opportunities and encourage students to engage in service learning experiences and/or community-based learning experiences" (ADA, 2010).

Finally, schools will require more faculty members with experience and expertise in caring for vulnerable and underserved populations to adequately prepare students to work with these groups. Therefore, the committee recommends

RECOMMENDATION 3: Dental professional education programs should

- **Increase recruitment and support for enrollment of students from underrepresented minority, lower-income, and rural populations;**
- **Require all students to participate in community-based education rotations with opportunities to work with interdisciplinary teams; and**
- **Recruit and retain faculty with experience and expertise in caring for underserved and vulnerable populations.**

To support Recommendation 3, the committee further recommends

RECOMMENDATION 4: HRSA should dedicate Title VII funding to

- **Support the development, implementation, and maintenance of substantial community-based education rotations, and**

- **Increase funding for recruitment and scholarships for underrepresented minorities, lower-income, and rural populations to attend dental professional schools.**

Continuation and scaling up of proven strategies will help prepare and ultimately promote a greater desire among future oral health care professionals to provide care to underserved and vulnerable populations. HRSA can play an important role in supporting this important shift in dental education and training. The committee, therefore, suggests that

- HRSA can help dental professional schools meet the requirement for all students to participate in substantial rotations in community-based settings by dedicating Title VII funding to support the development and implementation of these programs.
- Furthermore, HRSA could provide additional funding to disseminate model practices.

Private foundations have been at the forefront of efforts to increase enrollment of students from underrepresented minority, lower-income, and rural populations, and they can continue to play an important role. The committee, therefore, suggests that

- Private foundations and professional organizations can strengthen the efforts of dental professional education by funding bridge programs that recruit high school students from underrepresented minority, lower-income, and rural populations for predental college education.
- Private foundations and professional organizations can also fund the development of innovative educational models to prepare students to work in diverse settings and with new delivery mechanisms.

Promoting Advanced Practical Experience

As discussed throughout this report, underserved and vulnerable populations have both distinct and heterogeneous needs. Therefore, all oral health care professionals need to be sufficiently educated and trained to care for a broad range of individuals and populations. This is especially critical for dentists who will be called upon to provide specialized care and treat patients with the most complex needs. However, as discussed in Chapter 3, upon completion of dental school, students may have had few opportunities to integrate their skills and knowledge with practical hands-on experience and may not feel adequately prepared for independent practice. To address this problem, the committee maintains that more dental students need to pursue postgraduate residency training so they are prepared to work with all populations.

Moreover, the evidence reviewed in Chapter 3 demonstrates that additional training is needed to better prepare oral health care professionals to care for underserved and vulnerable populations. Postgraduate dental education is seen as an opportunity to address these needs. Dentists who have completed general dentistry residency programs report feeling more comfortable caring for underserved patients and patients with complex needs, and they deliver care for those patients more often, even after completing residency. Residencies in dentistry are also an important source of care for the underserved. Therefore, the committee recommends

RECOMMENDATION 5: HRSA should dedicate Title VII funding to support and expand opportunities for dental residencies in community-based settings.

Subsequently, state legislatures should require a minimum of 1 year of dental residency before a dentist can be licensed to practice.

This recommendation is not new; it was included in the 1995 IOM report, *Dental Education at the Crossroads* (*Crossroads*), where the committee found that

> A year of postgraduate or advanced education in general dentistry would allow students to gain speed and confidence in procedures, broaden their patient management skills to cover more complex problems, and mature in the nontechnical aspects of patient care. (IOM, 1995)

To be optimally effective in preparing dentists to care for underserved and vulnerable populations, it will be necessary for dental residencies to include clinical experiences with young children, individuals with special health care needs, and older adults.

It should be noted that the authoring committee of *Crossroads* recommended creating more opportunities for residencies rather than require them (IOM, 1995). This current committee recommends the same as a short-term goal. To be maximally effective in addressing issues of access, the committee recommends that these residency opportunities should take place in settings where services are most needed. To that end, the committee has identified "community-based settings" as logical partners for dental residencies. Further, as *Crossroads* noted, "financial pressures on hospitals have resulted in a modest decline in the number of hospital-based general dentistry programs, and uncertainties over future funding for graduate medical education may have some spillover effects on dentistry" (IOM, 1995). This committee, therefore, recommends a continuous source of existing funding—Title VII of the Public Health Services Act—be directed to support dental residencies.

Given the strength of the evidence supporting the value of at least 1 year of practical training in community settings, the committee recommends that state legislatures should ultimately *require* a minimum of 1 year of dental residency before a dentist can be licensed to practice. This recommendation was also included in the ADA report *The Future of Dentistry* that stated: "When economically and logistically feasible, a Postgraduate Year One (PGY-1) year should be a requirement for all dental graduates" (ADA, 2001). Because this recommendation will involve, among other actions, the need for each state to revise its statutes to make postgraduate education a requirement for licensure, the committee proposes that this recommendation be implemented as a long-term goal.

This committee suggests the following as strategies for implementation:

- HRSA can support care for underserved and vulnerable populations where they live, work, and learn (i.e., schools, FQHCs, nursing homes) by designating the types of clinical experiences and settings that would qualify for dental residencies.
- The public and private sectors can support efforts to identify and address barriers to having all states make postgraduate education a requirement for licensure.
- Hospitals and dental schools can increase the number of formal relationships with community-based care settings (such as FQHCs, nursing homes, state and local health departments, and prisons) for dental residency programs.

Reducing Financial and Administrative Barriers

Evidence cited throughout this report demonstrates that oral health is integral to overall health and that dental coverage is a major determinant of access to and utilization of oral health care. Reducing financial and administrative barriers to oral health care are among the most significant actions that can be taken to achieve the committee's vision.

Expanding Dental Coverage

Despite its importance, millions of Americans lack dental coverage. As discussed in Chapter 5, recent data from several sources underscore this deficiency among children, adults, and older adults.

All states are required to provide comprehensive dental benefits (including preventive, diagnostic, and treatment services) for all Medicaid-enrolled children, and all states are required to provide comparable dental coverage to children enrolled in CHIP. In contrast, states are not required to provide Medicaid benefits for adults. Among those states that offer dental coverage for adult Medicaid recipients, the benefits are typically limited to emergency coverage. Furthermore, the enactment of the Patient Protection and Affordable Care Act (ACA) is not likely to change the structure of oral health coverage—particularly for adults. For example, the ACA charges the Secretary of Health and Human Services with defining essential health benefits. While the Act specifies that oral health benefits for children must be included as essential, it does not make the same stipulation for adults. As a result, among adults, publicly funded programs reinforce an artificial separation of oral health from overall health.

The committee concludes that (1) publicly funded programs should not separate oral health from overall health, and (2) because publicly funded programs are the primary source of coverage for underserved and vulnerable populations, Medicaid cannot properly address the issue of access if oral health services are excluded from Medicaid benefits. However, in the absence of a comprehensive cost–benefit analysis and in a climate of significantly limited resources, the committee lacks the necessary evidence base to recommend that all states be required to cover essential dental benefits for all Medicaid beneficiaries. Nevertheless, the committee firmly concludes that this is a critical and necessary action worth building toward.

Therefore, the committee recommends

RECOMMENDATION 6: The Centers for Medicare and Medicaid Services (CMS) should fund and evaluate state-based demonstration projects that cover essential oral health benefits for Medicaid beneficiaries.

State-based demonstration projects will help establish a basis for sound policy and fiscal decision making both for participating states and for future federal and state action. Recognizing the different challenges faced by individual states, the committee suggests that CMS build flexibility into and encourage innovation in the demonstrations. For example, states may choose to focus on providing oral health benefits to specific populations (e.g., "high-risk" enrollees with underlying health problems who are most likely to have associated general health care consequences and costs from poor oral health) or to examine the effects of providing benefits to populations across the board. Providing flexibility to the states will help to surface a variety of promising strategies. Finally, strategies for state-based demonstration projects can be informed by data from states that currently have adult dental benefits as well as the experience of states that have eliminated or reduced adult dental benefits for budgetary reasons.

In addition, the committee suggests the following as strategies for implementation:

- CMS can ensure that Medicaid beneficiaries receive the appropriate level of care by appointing and convening a committee of key stakeholders to establish an essential dental benefits package for Medicaid.
- CMS can provide technical assistance and oversight to state-based demonstration projects including guidance on program design elements that address the specialized needs of targeted beneficiaries and consultation on program evaluation and monitoring systems.
- CMS can develop a report at the culmination of the demonstration projects to review, translate, and disseminate evidence and guidance to all states.
- Private foundations can partner with CMS and participating states to support outreach for state-based demonstration projects including campaigns to raise awareness of changes in state oral health benefits available and to promote the use of newly covered services.

Adjusting Payments and Streamlining Administrative Processes

Financing also has a profound influence on providers' practice patterns. For example, as discussed in Chapter 5, low reimbursement by third-party payers and public programs, such as Medicaid and CHIP, is often cited as a disincentive to providers' willingness to participate in these publicly funded programs. Increases in reimbursement rate have shown promise in increasing dentists' participation in publicly funded programs.

However, efforts to improve access through financing strategies will necessarily be multifaceted and will be one component of broader efforts to improve access. For example, studies have demonstrated that increasing reimbursement rates alone is not sufficient in improving access to care. Without more comprehensive actions (including case management and streamlined enrollment and billing processes), barriers to oral health care access persist. To that end, many states have taken measures to reduce administrative burdens associated with poor participation in publicly funded programs. These actions, in conjunction with rate increases and other supportive strategies (e.g., increased education and outreach to beneficiaries), can have a greater impact on increasing provider participation and patient utilization rates (Borchgrevink et al., 2008; GAO, 2009; Greenberg et al., 2008; Wysen et al., 2004). Therefore, the committee recommends

RECOMMENDATION 7: To increase provider participation in publicly funded programs, states should

- Set Medicaid and CHIP reimbursement rates so that beneficiaries have equitable access to essential oral health services, as required by law;
- Provide case-management services; and
- Streamline administrative processes.

In light of current economic circumstances and perennial demands on tight state budgets, states will need additional support to carry out this recommendation. Therefore, the committee suggests the following as strategies:

- Congress can support state efforts by providing enhanced federal matching funds to help offset the additional expense to the states.
- To be most effective, Congress can require that an enhanced match be tied to efforts by states to streamline administrative procedures related to provider and patient participation in Medicaid.
- CMS can ensure that Medicaid beneficiaries have equitable access to essential oral health services by appointing and convening a committee of key stakeholders to establish an essential dental benefits package for Medicaid.

There is a precedent for this type of enhanced federal match, most recently in the Patient Protection and Affordable Care Act (ACA).[1] For example, the regular Medicaid matching rate—which ranges from 50 percent to 76 percent—is designed to provide additional federal support to states with lower per capita incomes. Under the ACA, the federal matching rate will increase to cover of the cost of additional newly eligible Medicaid beneficiaries (those added under the Medicaid expansion to 133 percent of the federal poverty level [FPL]).

As noted previously in this report, simply increasing reimbursement rates, in the absence of other actions, will not be sufficient in improving access to care. Therefore, the committee proposes the following strategies to enhance the recommendations:

- CMS can support state efforts to streamline administrative processes by issuing guidance to state Medicaid officers on strategies to reduce administrative burdens associated with provider participation in Medicaid.

---

[1] *Patient Protection and Affordable Care Act*, Public Law 148, 111th Cong., 2nd sess. (March 23, 2010).

- States can use Maternal and Child Health Services Block Grant (Title V) funds to evaluate and assess their case-management services to to determine the most effective strategies to improve access to oral health care.
- Professional organizations and patient advocacy organizations can work with their constituencies to help identify populations in need of case management and the specific administrative barriers serving these populations.

Promoting Research

Over the course of this study, the committee encountered considerable gaps in the evidence base regarding important aspects of oral health and the delivery of oral health care to vulnerable and underserved populations. For example, little is known about the best ways to care for the distinct segments of the American public that are not well served by the traditional oral health care system. To this end, there are a number of programs currently under way designed to deliver oral health care to underserved and vulnerable populations through innovations in use of the workforce and in alternative settings of care. Additional research on the effectiveness of these (and other) strategies toward improving access to oral health care will provide the evidence needed to make policy decisions. It will also foster the continuous improvement and innovation in the delivery of oral health care that the committee calls for in its vision.

First, as discussed earlier, research is needed on how to best include nondental health care professionals in oral health care. In addition, within the dental professions, several new models seek to develop new types of dental professionals, or expand the role of existing dental professionals. For example, as discussed in Chapter 3, evaluations of the dental health aide therapist program in Alaska to date point to the quality and acceptability of dental therapists in providing care to remote populations. These findings are similar to evaluations of dental therapist programs in other countries where these professionals have a long history of serving as members of the dental team. However, evaluations to date have also been limited owing to the small number of dental therapists in Alaska, and it is not yet possible to determine the broader implications of this and similar programs designed to improve access to oral health care in the United States. More research is needed to establish a sufficient evidence base to support broader dissemination of these programs. Research is also needed to evaluate newer methods and technologies for providing oral health care to underserved and vulnerable populations. For example, as discussed in Chapter 4, the use of telehealth technologies is emerging as a strategy to provide dental services in underserved communities where significant barriers to receiving care in a traditional dental office setting exist.

As described in Chapter 4, a range of strategies has been developed to deliver oral health care to vulnerable and underserved populations in a variety of settings outside the traditional dental practice setting. Some of these efforts build on the capacity of existing community services (e.g., dental professionals partnering with the Special Supplemental Nutrition Program for Women, Infants, and Children [WIC]); others broaden the kinds of services provided at sites in the community (e.g., school-based health centers, mobile vans and other mobile equipment, and state and local health departments); still others are entirely new settings of care (e.g., retail dental clinics). While individual programs have been evaluated in terms of acceptability and effectiveness, less is known about which settings of care are most effective for reaching underserved and vulnerable populations. Therefore, more research is needed to determine the best strategies for reaching these populations in general as well as strategies for addressing the needs of specific subpopulations (e.g., individuals with special health care needs or older adults).

In addition, as discussed in Chapter 2, quality improvement efforts in oral health are hampered by a deficiency in the collection, analysis, and use of data related to important aspects of oral health. For example, a review of current National Quality Forum–endorsed measures finds no measures related to oral health (NQF, 2010). Further, the annual AHRQ National Healthcare Quality Report and the National Healthcare Disparities Report currently include only information about access to dental services, and not about the state of quality in oral health care (AHRQ, 2010). The lack of quality measures and the absence of a universally accepted and used set of diagnosis codes among dentists make it difficult to assess the quality of specific services and procedures and limits the conclusions that can be drawn regarding their relationship to longer-term oral health outcomes. While concerns have been raised for the quality of care provided by dental professionals that are not dentists, there is little ability to assess the technical competence, practice procedures, and quality of care and outcomes of care provided by *any* dental professionals, which makes comparison of care rendered by different types of professionals even more challenging.

Finally, as alluded to earlier, little has been done to investigate better methods of financing and regulation that might lead to improvements in dental coverage, access to oral health care, and, again, improvements in oral health status. Therefore, the committee recommends

RECOMMENDATION 8: Congress, the Department of Health and Human Services (HHS), federal agencies, and private foundations should increase funding for oral health research and evaluation related to underserved and vulnerable populations, including

- **New methods and technologies (e.g., nontraditional settings, non-dental professionals, new provider types, and telehealth);**
- **Measures of access, quality, and outcomes; and**
- **Payment and regulatory systems.**

Given the need for further research, the committee concludes that a variety of stakeholders will need to take additional actions to support this recommendation, including

- Federal agencies can increase funding for programs that successfully provide education and preventive and treatment services to vulnerable and underserved populations such as Head Start, the WIC program, and school-based health centers.
- HRSA can support the research agenda by providing funding for oral health demonstration projects that use a new delivery system—including new workforce models—that will successfully provide education, prevention, and treatment services to underserved populations through Head Start, WIC, and school-based health centers.

Expanding Capacity

Achieving the committee's vision for oral health care will require that there are adequate resources available to meet the oral health needs of the public. As described throughout this report, these needs are great, and they are growing. For example, the ACA requires health plans offered on state health insurance exchanges to offer pediatric oral health benefits. The ACA, thus, will increase the number of children with oral health benefits. As more children receive coverage, there will be a need for increased capacity of the oral health delivery system.

Supporting State Oral Health Programs

State oral health programs are essential to effectively direct resources and monitor the impact of oral health efforts. One important function of state oral health programs is their ability to monitor and analyze the burden of oral health diseases, conditions, and personal behaviors over time. This information is critical to judicious planning, implementation, and evaluation of dental public health services. A recent examination of progress in children's oral health since the surgeon general's report on oral health concluded

> The importance of surveillance and the dental public health infrastructure, including the dental public health workforce, cannot be overemphasized.

> Data are essential for establishing baselines and evaluating programs, policies, and trends. (Mouradian et al., 2009)

While there is little evidence regarding the specific impact and effectiveness of oral health surveillance (Beltrán-Aguilar et al., 2003; Tomar and Reeves, 2009), there is strong evidence from other fields (e.g., communicable diseases and occupational health) to support the effectiveness and importance of surveillance activities (IOM, 2002). For example, HIV/AIDS surveillance efforts were critical to understanding the number and characteristics of individuals affected by the epidemic (Gostin et al., 1997). Ultimately, these data helped guide targeted resource allocation for prevention and treatment programs (Fleming et al., 2000).

The impact of other functions of state oral health programs (e.g., planning and supporting community water fluoridation, dental sealant programs, fluoride varnish programs, dental screening programs, and oral health programs specifically for pregnant women) as well as relevant state characteristics (e.g., provision of Medicaid adult dental benefits, counties without dentists and/or Medicaid dentists, and overall demographic information) are documented in the annual Association of State and Territorial Dental Directors (ASTDD) *Synopses of State Dental Public Health Programs* (ASTDD, 2010). According to the ASTDD,

> With expanded infrastructure and capacity, state oral health programs are better able to monitor oral health status, address high-risk populations, increase population-based prevention activities, and extend resources to local health agencies and communities in order to implement oral health strategies. (ASTDD, 2000)

Despite the positive impact of state oral health programs, funding for state and local dental public health services continues to be limited. In FY 2010, the Centers for Disease Control and Prevention (CDC) provided $6.8 million to just 19 state oral health programs to support evidence-based prevention programs (e.g., community water fluoridation and school-based sealant programs), surveillance of oral disease burden, and to develop plans to improve oral health and address disparities.

Recognizing the critical role of state-based programs, the committee recommends

> **RECOMMENDATION 9: The Centers for Disease Control and Prevention (CDC) and the Maternal and Child Health Bureau (MCHB) should collaborate with states to ensure that each state has the infrastructure and support necessary to perform core dental public health functions (e.g., assessment, policy development, and assurance).**

The committee proposes the following strategies to support the implementation of this recommendation:

- The CDC can continue to increase the number of states that receive cooperative agreement funding for dental public health programs.
- The MCHB can support an oral health component under Title V through block grants (formulary grants to states), discretionary funds, and/or "set asides" (a percentage of funds) for oral health.
- Congress can fund the *Oral Healthcare Prevention Education Campaign* authorized by the Patient Protection and Affordable Care Act (ACA) [Public Law 111-148, Title IV, Sec. 4102] which calls for a national public education campaign focused on oral health and disease prevention targeted towards vulnerable and underserved populations.
- Private foundations can partner with public agencies to develop, implement, and evaluate public education and oral health literacy campaigns.

Capitalizing on Federally Qualified Health Centers

FQHCs play an important role in increasing access to oral health care for vulnerable and underserved populations. For example, FQHCs are required to provide certain services—including preventive, but not comprehensive, dental services—either in the clinic or by referral. The FQHC program is growing steadily. In 2009, HRSA funded 1,131 FQHCs, which are located in all 50 states, the District of Columbia, and Puerto Rico (HRSA, 2011). That is an increase from 914 FQHCs in 2004. Funding for FQHCs is also increasing. The American Recovery and Rehabilitation Act[2] includes $2 billion for FQHCs (HHS, 2010), and the health care reform bills include $11 billion for a Community Health Centers Trust Fund that will allow FQHCs to expand access and make capital improvements, and also appropriate $1.5 billion to a new National Health Service Corps Trust Fund.[3,4] In 2009, over 3.4 million patients used dental services in the health center system (HRSA, 2011). Still, the number of patients whose oral health needs are served by the health center system has been only a small fraction of the underserved population (Bailit et al., 2006). Even with the expected health center expansion, the health center dental system will be inadequate to meet the demand for oral health services. Support and reform

---

[2] *American Recovery and Reinvestment Act of 2009*, Public Law 5, 111th Cong., 1st sess. (February 17, 2009).

[3] *Health Care and Education Reconciliation Act of 2010*, Public Law 152, 111th Cong., 2nd sess. (March 30, 2010).

[4] *Patient Protection and Affordable Care Act*, Public Law 148, 111th Cong., 2nd sess. (March 23, 2010).

of the health center oral health delivery system will be needed to realize the potential of this vital national resource.

Based on these findings, the committee concludes that with adequate support, FQHCs are well positioned to significantly expand the delivery of oral health care to vulnerable and underserved populations. Furthermore, because FQHCs employ both dental and nondental health professionals, clinics can engage additional members the health care team in providing basic oral health care to the populations they serve. The committee, therefore, recommends

RECOMMENDATION 10: To expand the capacity of FQHCs to deliver essential oral health services, HRSA should

- **Support the use of a variety of oral health care professionals;**
- **Enhance financial incentives to attract and retain more oral health care professionals;**
- **Provide guidance to implement best practices in management, operation, and efficiency; and**
- **Assist FQHCs in all states to operate programs outside their physical facilities and take advantage of new systems to improve the oral health of the population they serve.**

The committee believes that the following strategies will be needed to support the implementation of this recommendation:

- Public-private partnerships can supplement loan repayment programs for oral health care professionals who are willing to serve a designated amount of time in medically underserved areas.
- HRSA can support dissemination and implementation of this recommendation by identifying FQHC "best practices" to highlight what states and/or individual clinics are doing and what impact these efforts are having on access.
- HRSA can support the demonstration and dissemination of models that extend the reach of FQHCs by operating programs outside their physical facilities and that use new delivery models and techniques.
- Other nonprofit community health centers can take the steps outlined in this recommendation to increase the delivery of essential oral health services to greater numbers of vulnerable and underserved individuals.

Box 6-2 provides a summary of the committee's suggestions for a variety of ways in which the implementation of the preceding recommendations may be supported.

BOX 6-2
Summary of Key Implementation Strategies for the Committee's Recommendations

Health Resources and Services Administration (HRSA)

- Require that Title VII–funded programs include interprofessional education on oral health to promote the integration of oral health core competencies in nondental health professional education programs.
- Support curriculum development and dissemination efforts for nondental health professional education programs.
- Dedicate Title VII funding to support the development and implementation of required substantial rotations in community-based settings at dental professional schools. Additional funding could be provided to disseminate model practices.
- Support care for underserved and vulnerable populations where they live, work, and learn by designating the types of clinical experiences and settings that would qualify for dental residencies.
- Provide funding for oral health demonstration projects that use a new delivery system—including new workforce models—that will successfully provide education, prevention, and treatment services to underserved populations through Head Start, WIC, and school-based health centers.
- Identify FQHC "best practices" to highlight what states and/or individual clinics are doing and what impact it is having on access.
- Support demonstration and dissemination of models that extend the reach of FQHCs by operating programs outside their physical facilities and that use new delivery models and techniques.

The Centers for Medicare and Medicaid Services (CMS)

- Disseminate rules and policies that promote Medicaid and CHIP beneficiaries' access to appropriate care, and ensure that rules and polices reflect the practice abilities of current and new types of licensed providers.
- Ensure that Medicaid beneficiaries receive the appropriate level of care and equitable access to care by appointing and convening a committee of key stakeholders to establish an essential dental benefits package for Medicaid.
- Ensure that Medicaid beneficiaries receive the services for which they are eligible by issuing guidance to states on how to reach populations that are covered but do not receive the care.
- Require states periodically to submit plans on how to increase Medicaid visit rates, and provide technical assistance on how to help them improve.
- Issue guidance to state Medicaid officers on strategies to reduce administrative burdens associated with provider participation in Medicaid.

The Office of the Assistant Secretary for Planning and Evaluation (ASPE)

- Examine and report on the impact of state practice acts on oral health care delivery to vulnerable and underserved populations. These reports will need to be conducted and published every 5 years to support sustained attention to optimizing access.

Congress

- Provide enhanced federal matching funds to the states to help offset the additional expense of increasing Medicaid reimbursement rates to cover the cost of providing oral health care. To be most effective, Congress can require that an enhanced match be tied to efforts by states to streamline administrative procedures related to provider and patient participation in Medicaid.
- Fund the *Oral Healthcare Prevention Education Campaign* authorized by the Patient Protection and Affordable Care Act (ACA) [Public Law 111-148, Title IV, Sec. 4102] which calls for a national public education campaign focused on oral health and disease prevention targeted towards vulnerable and underserved populations.

Dental Professional Schools and Teaching Hospitals

- Establish formal relationships with community-based care settings (such as FQHCs, nursing homes, state and local health departments and prisons) for dental residency programs.

Foundations and Organizations

Conduct and disseminate an initial review of state practice acts with a focus on access to services.

- Issue "best practices" briefs to highlight what each state is doing and what impact it is having on access.
- Work with constituencies to help identify populations in need of case management and the specific administrative barriers serving vulnerable and underserved populations.
- Fund bridge programs that recruit high school students from underrepresented minority, lower-income, and rural populations for predental college education.
- Fund programs and public campaigns to raise awareness that oral health care is a Medicaid benefit that people need to use.
- Partner with public agencies to develop, implement, and evaluate public education and oral health literacy campaigns.

CLOSING THOUGHTS

The release of this report coincides with a transformative moment in the nation's health care system. Efforts are under way to ensure that all Americans have access to affordable health coverage. In the midst of these changes, the distinct deficits faced by vulnerable and underserved populations deserve particular attention. As the nation struggles to address the larger systemic issues of access to health care, greater effort will be needed to ensure that oral health is included in this conversation. The enduring separation of oral health care from overall health care has marginalized issues related to oral health. As a result, oral health coverage has not been a primary focus of health reform.

Further complicating matters is that these issues emerge at a time of significant economic challenges. For example, as states look for ways to address budgets shortfalls, many are eliminating their already limited coverage of oral health services. This strategy was even highlighted in a February 2011 letter to states providing guidance on potential cost-savings in Medicaid programs in which the secretary of HHS reminded governors that "while some benefits, such as hospital and physician services, are required to be provided by State Medicaid programs, many services, such as prescription drugs, dental services, and speech therapy, are optional" (HHS, 2011).

Finally, there will be a sharp increase in the demands on the oral health delivery system by children and the growing numbers of retirees. For one, the ACA will increase coverage for oral health benefits for children. Even more significant, as increasing numbers of baby boomers (those born between 1946 and 1964) become eligible for Medicare, considerable attention will need to be paid to how these aging adults will pay for and obtain oral health care. The relative size of this cohort—approximately 78 million—coupled with increases in longevity will create an unprecedented demand for oral health care for older adults.

In light of the above issues, it is the committee's strong intent that this report calls into sharp focus the challenges that millions of Americans face in accessing oral health care. The recommendations in this report provide a roadmap for creating an integrated delivery system that provides quality oral health care to vulnerable and underserved people where they live, work, and learn through changes to education, financing, and regulation of oral health services. Failure to act now virtually guarantees that the nation's inadequate and inequitable access to oral health care will persist with far-reaching individual and societal consequences.

REFERENCES

ADA (American Dental Association). 2001. *Future of dentistry*. Chicago, IL: American Dental Association.

ADA. 2010. *Standards for dental education programs*. http://www.ada.org/115.aspx (accessed November 5, 2010).

ADHA (American Dental Hygienists' Association). 2011. *Direct access states chart*. http://www.adha.org/governmental_affairs/downloads/direct_access.pdf (accessed May 18, 2011).

AHRQ (Agency for Healthcare Research and Quality). 2010. *National Healthcare Quality & Disparities Reports: NHQDRnet*. http://nhqrnet.ahrq.gov/nhqrdr/jsp/nhqrdr.jsp (accessed November 29, 2010).

ASTDD (Association of State and Territorial Dental Directors). 2000. *Building infrastructure and capacity in state and territorial oral health programs*. Sparks, NV: Association of State and Territorial Dental Directors.

ASTDD. 2010. *Synopses of state dental public health programs: Data for FY 2008-2009*.

Bailit, H., T. Beazoglou, N. Demby, J. McFarland, P. Robinson, and R. Weaver. 2006. Dental safety net: Current capacity and potential for expansion. *Journal of the American Dental Association* 137(6):807-815.

Beltrán-Aguilar, E., M. M. Dolores, S. A. Lockwood, G. Rozier, and S. L. Tomar. 2003. Oral health surveillance: Past, present, and future challenges. *Journal of Public Health Dentistry* 63(3):141-149.

Borchgrevink, A., A. Snyder, and S. Gehshan. 2008. *The effects of Medicaid reimbursement rates on access to dental care*. Washington, DC: National Academy for State Health Policy.

Brunson, W. D., D. L. Jackson, J. C. Sinkford, and R. W. Valachovic. 2010. Components of effective outreach and recruitment programs for underrepresented minority and low-income dental students. *Journal of Dental Education* 74(Supp. 10):S74-S86.

Danielsen, R., J. Dillenberg, and C. Bay. 2006. Oral health competencies for physician assistants and nurse practitioners. *Journal of Physician Assistant Education* 17(4):12-16.

Dela Cruz, G. G., R. G. Rozier, and G. Slade. 2004. Dental screening and referral of young children by pediatric primary care providers. *Pediatrics* 114(5).

Fleming, P. L., P. M. Wortley, J. M. Karon, K. M. DeCock, and R. S. Janssen. 2000. Tracking the HIV epidemic: Current issues, future challenges. *American Journal of Public Health* 90(7):1037-1041.

GAO (Government Accountability Office). 2009. *State and federal actions have been taken to improve children's access to dental services, but gaps remain*. Washington, DC: U.S. Government Accountability Office.

Gostin, L. O., J. W. Ward, and A. Cornelius Baker. 1997. National HIV case reporting for the United States a defining moment in the history of the epidemic. *New England Journal of Medicine* 337(16):1162-1167.

Greenberg, B. J. S., J. V. Kumar, and H. Stevenson. 2008. Dental case management: Increasing access to oral health care for families and children with low incomes. *Journal of the American Dental Association* 139(8):1114-1121.

HHS (U.S. Department of Health and Human Services). 2010. *Recovery Act (ARRA): Community health centers*. http://www.hhs.gov/recovery/hrsa/healthcentergrants.html (accessed February 3, 2010).

HHS. 2011. Sebelius outlines state flexibility and federal support available for Medicaid. http://www.hhs.gov/news/press/2011pres/01/20110203c.html (accessed February 24, 2011).

HRSA (Healthcare Resources and Services Administration). 2004. *The professional practice environment of dental hygienists in the fifty states and the District of Columbia, 2001.* Rockville, MD: Department of Health and Human Services.

HRSA. 2011. *Health centers: 2009 at-a-glance.* http://www.hrsa.gov/data-statistics/health-center-data/NationalData/2009/2009datasnapshot.html (accessed March 1, 2011).

IOM (Institute of Medicine). 1995. *Dental education at the crossroads: Challenges and change.* Washington, DC: National Academy Press.

IOM. 2001. *Crossing the quality chasm: A new health system for the 21st century.* Washington, DC: National Academy Press.

IOM. 2002. *The future of the public's health in the 21st century.* Washington, DC: The National Academies Press.

IOM. 2004. *In the nation's compelling interest: Ensuring diversity in the health-care workforce.* Washington, DC: The National Academies Press.

IOM. 2008. *Retooling for an aging America: Building the health care workforce.* Washington, DC: The National Academies Press.

IOM. 2010. *The future of nursing: Leading change, advancing health.* Washington, DC: The National Academies Press.

Knox, L. M., and H. Spivak. 2005. What health professionals should know: Core competencies for effective practice in youth violence prevention. *American Journal of Preventive Medicine* 29(5 Supp. 2):191-199.

Mouradian, W. E., A. Reeves, S. Kim, R. Evans, D. Schaad, S. G. Marshall, and R. Slayton. 2005. An oral health curriculum for medical students at the University of Washington. *Academic Medicine* 80(5):434-442.

Mouradian, W. E., R. L. Slayton, W. R. Maas, D. V. Kleinman, H. Slavkin, D. DePaola, C. Evans Jr., and J. Wilentz. 2009. Progress in children's oral health since the surgeon general's report on oral health. *Academic Pediatrics* 9(6):374-379.

NQF (National Quality Forum). 2010. *NQF-endorsed standards.* http://www.qualityforum.org/Measures_List.aspx (accessed November 29, 2010).

Partnership for Health in Aging. 2008. *Multidisciplinary competencies in the care of older adults at the completion of the entry-level health professional degree.* http://www.americangeriatrics.org/files/documents/health_care_pros/PHA_Multidisc_Competencies.pdf (accessed December 7, 2010).

Tomar, S. L., and A. F. Reeves. 2009. Changes in the oral health of U.S. children and adolescents and dental public health infrastructure since the release of the Healthy People 2010 objectives. *Academic Pediatrics* 9(6):388-395.

Wysen, K. H., P. M. Hennessy, M. I. Lieberman, T. E. Garland, and S. M. Johnson. 2004. Kids get care: Integrating preventive dental and medical care using a public health case management model. *Journal of Dental Education* 68(5):522-530.

Appendix A

Acronyms

AAP	American Academy of Pediatrics
AAPA	American Academy of Physician Assistants
AAPD	American Academy of Pediatric Dentistry
ABCD	Access to Baby and Child Dentistry
ACA	Patient Protection and Affordable Care Act
ACF	Administration for Children and Families
ACGME	Accreditation Council for Graduate Medical Education
ADA	American Dental Association
ADHA	American Dental Hygienists' Association
ADHP	advanced dental hygiene practitioner
ADT	Minnesota advanced dental therapist
AGD	Academy of General Dentistry
AHRQ	Agency for Healthcare Research and Quality
AI/AN	American Indians and Alaska Natives
APHA	American Public Health Association
ARC-PA	Accreditation Review Commission on Education for the Physician Assistant
ASTDD	Association of State and Territorial Dental Directors
BCBSMA	Blue Cross Blue Shield of Massachusetts
BLS	Bureau of Labor Statistics
CAD	coronary artery disease
CADPP	Critical Access Dental Payment Program
CDA	certified dental assistant

CDC	Centers for Disease Control and Prevention
CDHC	community dental health coordinator
CDT	certified dental technician
CHC	community health center
CHIP	Children's Health Insurance Program
CHIPRA	Children's Health Insurance Program Reauthorization Act
CMS	Centers for Medicare and Medicaid Services
CODA	Commission on Dental Accreditation
DHAT	dental health aide therapist
DDS	Doctor of Dental Surgery
DGME	direct Graduate Medical Education
DMD	Doctor of Dental Medicine
DT	Minnesota dental therapist
ECC	early childhood caries
ED	(hospital) emergency department
EFDA	expanded function dental assistant
EPSDT	Early and Periodic Screening, Diagnostic, and Treatment
FEHBP	Federal Employees Health Benefits Program
FPL	federal poverty level
FQHC	Federally Qualified Health Center
FTC	Federal Trade Commission
GAMC	General Assistance Medical Care
GAO	U.S. Government Accountability Office
GME	Graduate Medical Education
HHS	U.S. Department of Health and Human Services
HIPAA	Health Insurance Portability and Accountability Act
HKD	Healthy Kids Dental
HPSA	Health Professional Shortage Area
HRSA	Health Resources and Services Administration
IHS	Indian Health Service
IME	indirect medical education
IOM	Institute of Medicine
LHD	local health department
LTC	long-term care

MCH	Maternal and Child Health
MCHB	Maternal and Child Health Bureau
MEPS	Medical Expenditure Panel Survey
MHCP	Minnesota Health Care Program
MOM	Missions of Mercy
NCHS	National Center for Health Statistics
NHANES	National Health and Nutrition Examination Survey
NHIS	National Health Interview Survey
NHSC	National Health Service Corps
NIDCR	National Institute of Dental and Craniofacial Research
NIH	National Institutes of Health
NOHSS	National Oral Health Surveillance System
NP	nurse practitioner
NRC	National Research Council
OHS	Office of Head Start
OIG	Office of the Inspector General
PA	physician assistant
PGY-1	Postgraduate Year One
RDHAP	registered dental hygienist in alternative practice
SBHC	school-based health center
SHCN	special health care needs
SNODENT	Systematized Nomenclature of Dentistry
SODM	School of Dental Medicine at East Carolina University
SPRANS	Special Projects of Regional and National Significance
STFM	Society of Teachers in Family Medicine
URM	underrepresented minority
USDA	U.S. Department of Agriculture
USPHS	U.S. Public Health Service
USPSTF	U.S. Preventive Services Task Force
VA	U.S. Department of Veterans Affairs
WDOH	Washington Department of Health
WDSHS	Washington Department of Social and Health Services
WHO	World Health Organization
WIC	Special Supplemental Nutrition Program for Women, Infants, and Children

Appendix B

Commissioned Papers

Lessons from Medicine: Opportunities and Constraints for Oral Disease Management
Author: Burton L. Edelstein

The Oral Health Workforce in the United States
Authors: Margaret Langelier
Tracey Continelli
David Armstrong
Jean Moore

State Case Studies: Improving Access to Dental Care for the Underserved
Authors: Howard Bailit
John D'Adamo
Tryfon Beazoglou

NOTE: All commissioned papers have been placed into this project's public access file.

Appendix C

Workshop Agendas

MARCH 4, 2010

National Academy of Sciences Building
2100 C Street, NW, Washington, DC 20418

11:45 AM	**Welcome**
	Frederick P. Rivara, Committee Chair, University of Washington
12:00 PM	**Remarks from Study Sponsors and Discussion** *Marcia Brand, Health Resources and Services Administration* *Len Finocchio, California HealthCare Foundation*
1:00	**Lunch**
1:40	**Position Statements—Professional Societies** *David Halpern, Academy of General Dentistry* *James Crall, American Academy of Pediatric Dentistry* *Ron Tankersley, American Dental Association* *Ann Battrell, American Dental Hygienists' Association*
2:30	**The Status of Children's Oral Health** *Bruce Dye, Centers for Disease Control and Prevention*
	Women and Oral Health *Renee Samelson, Albany Medical College*

3:15 **Federally Qualified Health Centers**
Gina Capra, Health Resources and Services Administration

3:45 **Missions of Mercy Project—Creating Partnerships in the Community**
Terry Dickinson, Virginia Dental Association

Oral Health in the Emergency Room
Robert Shesser, George Washington University

4:30 **Open Public Comment Period**

5:00 **Concluding Remarks and Adjourn Open Session**

JULY 27, 2010

Sir Francis Drake Hotel
450 Powell Street, San Francisco, CA

9:00 AM **Welcome and Opening Remarks**
Frederick P. Rivara, Committee Chair

9:05 **Oral Health Within Overall Health Care Trends**
Edward O'Neil, University of California, San Francisco

9:30 **Navigating the System—the Patient's Perspective**
Laurie Norris, Pew Center on the States

9:50 **Caring for Underserved and Vulnerable Populations—I**

Implementation and Dissemination of Oral Prevention Services in Well Child Care at Group Health: Key Learnings
David Grossman, GroupHealth Cooperative

Retail Dental Clinics
Mary Kate Scott, Scott & Company, Inc.

Michigan Healthy Kids Dental Program
Woosung Sohn, University of Michigan

10:55	Break
11:20	Caring for Underserved and Vulnerable Populations—II
	An Overview of Health Centers *John McFarland, Salud Family Health Center and National Network for Oral Health Access*
	Solving Oral Health Access: A Regionalized, Integrated, and Rural Dental System *Greg Nycz, Family Health Center of Marshfield, Inc.*
	Nursing Homes and Mobile Clinics *Greg Folse, private practice*
	School-Based Health Care *Larry Hill, CincySmiles Foundation*
12:45 PM	Lunch
1:45	Supporting Oral Health Providers
	Expertise and Technical Assistance in Health Centers *Steven P. Geiermann, American Dental Association*
	Supporting Ohio's Dental Care Safety Net: Grants and Accessible Information *Mark Siegal, Ohio State Department of Health*
	Practice Management *Jesley Ruff, American Dental Partners*
2:45	Break
3:05	Perspectives on Access Issues
	Rural Issues *Jessica Van Arsdale, Humboldt State University*
	Social Determinants of Oral Health *Peter Milgrom, University of Washington*

	Management of Health Service Through Outcome-Based Statistics *Michael Griffiths, Institutional Dental Care*
4:05	**Discussants** *Louise T. Veselicky* *Kristen Simmons* *Bob Russell*
4:45	**Public Comment**
5:00	**Adjourn**

Appendix D

Summary of *Advancing Oral Health in America:* A Report of the IOM Committee on an Oral Health Initiative

In February 2010, with support from the Health Resources and Services Administration (HRSA), the Institute of Medicine (IOM) formed the Committee on an Oral Health Initiative to assess the current oral health care system and to advise the Department of Health and Human Services (HHS) on actions that should be taken for an HHS oral health initiative (see Box D-1). This study was conducted at the same time that the IOM's Committee on Oral Health Access to Services study was under way. While

BOX D-1
The Committee on an Oral Health Initiative Statement of Task

The IOM Board on Health Care Services, in collaboration with the Board on Children, Youth, and Families, will undertake a study to

- Assess the current oral health care system for the entire U.S. population;
- Examine preventive oral care interventions, their use and promotion;
- Explore ways of improving health literacy for oral health;
- Review elements of a potential HHS oral health initiative, including possible or current regulations, statutes, programs, research, data, financing, and policy; and
- Recommend strategic actions for HHS agencies and, if relevant and important, other actors, as well as ways to evaluate this initiative.

the two studies had related statements of task, the two projects had separate committees, meetings, and report review processes. The two committees were not made aware of the other's conclusions or recommendations.

The IOM Committee on an Oral Health Initiative's report, *Advancing Oral Health in America*, released in April 2011, summarizes the state of oral health today, underscores the important oral-systemic connection, describes the current role of HHS, and provides lessons learned from previous related efforts. The committee made seven recommendations in six key areas, including establishing and evaluating an oral health initiative; focusing on prevention; improving oral health literacy; enhancing the delivery of oral health care; expanding research; and measuring progress. Finally, the committee identified three key areas needed to ensure success: strong leadership, sustained interest, and the involvement of multiple stakeholders. This appendix provides an overview of the report, *Advancing Oral Health in America*. Full text of the report can be found online at http://www.iom.edu/oralhealthinitiative.

ORGANIZING PRINCIPLES FOR AN HHS ORAL HEALTH INITIATIVE

The Committee on an Oral Health Initiative developed a set of organizing principles based on the areas in greatest need of attention as well as approaches that have the most potential for creating improvements:

1. Establish high-level accountability.
2. Emphasize disease prevention and oral health promotion.
3. Improve oral health literacy and cultural competence.
4. Reduce oral health disparities.
5. Explore new models for payment and delivery of care.
6. Enhance the role of nondental health care professionals.[1]
7. Expand oral health research, and improve data collection.
8. Promote collaboration among private and public stakeholders.
9. Measure progress toward short-term and long-term goals and objectives.
10. Advance the goals and objectives of *Healthy People 2020*.

RECOMMENDATIONS

Based on these principles, the Committee on an Oral Health Initiative recommended several approaches that HHS could take to help improve the

[1] *Nondental health care professionals* includes, but is not limited to, nurses, pharmacists, physician assistants, and physicians.

oral health of the nation. The committee referred to this set of recommendations as the New Oral Health Initiative (NOHI), to distinguish it from and build upon HHS' existing Oral Health Initiative.

RECOMMENDATION 1: The secretary of HHS should give the leader(s) of the New Oral Health Initiative (NOHI) the authority and resources needed to successfully integrate oral health into the planning, programming, policies, and research that occur across all HHS programs and agencies:

- Each agency within HHS that has a role in oral health should provide an annual plan for how it will integrate oral health into existing programs within the first year.
- Each agency should identify specific opportunities for public–private partnerships and collaborating with other agencies inside and outside HHS.
- The leader(s) of the NOHI should coordinate, review, and implement these plans.
- The leaders(s) of the NOHI should incorporate patient and consumer input into the design and implementation of the NOHI.

RECOMMENDATION 2: All relevant HHS agencies should promote and monitor the use of evidence-based preventive services in oral health (both clinical and community based) and counseling across the life span by

- Consulting with the U.S. Preventive Services Task Force and the Task Force on Community Preventive Services to give priority to evidentiary reviews of preventive services in oral health;
- Ensuring that HHS-administered health care systems (e.g., Federally Qualified Health Centers, Indian Health Service) provide recommended preventive services and counseling to improve oral health;
- Providing guidance and assistance to state and local health systems to implement these same approaches; and
- Communicating with other federally administered health care systems to share best practices.

RECOMMENDATION 3: All relevant HHS agencies should undertake oral health literacy and education efforts aimed at individuals, communities, and health care professionals. These efforts should include, but not be limited to,

- Community-wide public education on the causes and implications of oral diseases and the effectiveness of preventive interventions;

- o Focus areas should include
    - The infectious nature of dental caries,
    - The effectiveness of fluorides and sealants,
    - The role of diet and nutrition in oral health, and
    - How oral diseases affect other health conditions.
- Community-wide guidance on how to access oral health care; and
  - o Focus areas should include using and promoting websites such as the National Oral Health Clearinghouse and www.healthcare.gov.
- Professional education on best practices in patient–provider communication skills that result in improved oral health behaviors.
  - o Focus areas should include how to communicate to an increasingly diverse population about prevention of oral cancers, dental caries, and periodontal disease.

RECOMMENDATION 4: HHS should invest in workforce innovations to improve oral health that focus on

- Core competency development, education, and training, to allow for the use of all health care professionals in oral health care;
- Interprofessional, team-based approaches to the prevention and treatment of oral diseases;
- Best use of new and existing oral health care professionals; and
- Increasing the diversity and improving the cultural competence of the workforce providing oral health care.

RECOMMENDATION 5: CMS should explore new delivery and payment models for Medicare, Medicaid, and CHIP to improve access, quality, and coverage of oral health care across the life span.

RECOMMENDATION 6: HHS should place a high priority on efforts to improve open, actionable, and timely information to advance science and improve oral health through research by

- Leveraging resources for research to promote a more robust evidence base specific to oral health care, including but not limited to
  - o oral health disparities, and
  - o best practices in oral health care and oral health behavior change;
- Working across HHS agencies, in collaboration with other federal departments (e.g., Department of Defense, Veterans Administration) involved in the collection of oral health data, to integrate,

standardize, and promote public availability of relevant databases; and

- Promoting the creation and implementation of new, useful, and appropriate measures of quality oral health care practices, cost and efficiency, and oral health outcomes.

RECOMMENDATION 7: To evaluate the NOHI, the leader(s) of the NOHI should convene an annual public meeting of the agency heads to report on the progress of the NOHI, including

- Progress of each agency in reaching goals;
- New innovations and data;
- Dissemination of best practices and data into the community; and
- Improvement in health outcomes of populations served by HHS programs, especially as they relate to Healthy People 2020 goals and specific objectives.

HHS should provide a forum for public response and comment and make the final proceedings of each meeting available to the public.

The recommendations in *Advancing Oral Health in America* highlight the vital role that HHS can play in improving oral health and oral health care in the United States. The committee concluded that an HHS oral health initiative could be successful if it had clearly articulated goals, effective coordination, and adequate funding. The committee stressed that three key areas were needed to successfully maintain oral health as a priority issue for HHS: strong leadership, sustained interest, and the involvement of multiple stakeholders.

Appendix F

Committee and Staff Biographies

Frederick P. Rivara, M.D., M.P.H. (*Chair*), is currently the Seattle Children's Guild Endowed Chair in Pediatrics and Professor of Pediatrics at the University of Washington School of Medicine, Adjunct Professor of Epidemiology in the University of Washington School of Public Health, Vice-Chair of the Department of Pediatrics, and Head of the Division of General Pediatrics. He is Editor of *Archives of Pediatrics and Adolescent Medicine*. Dr. Rivara's current research interests include prevention of intimate partner violence, reducing alcohol-related trauma, determining the long-term outcome of children with traumatic brain injury, and studying the effectiveness of trauma systems in the care of pediatric and adult trauma patients. He served as founding director of the Harborview Injury and Research Center in Seattle for 13 years, founding president of the International Society for Child and Adolescent Injury Prevention, and his contributions to the field have spanned 30 years. He has received numerous honors including the Charles C. Shepard Science Award from the Centers for Disease Control and Prevention, the American Public Health Association, Injury Control and Emergency Health Services Section Distinguished Career Award, and the American Academy of Pediatrics, Section on Injury and Poison Prevention, Physician Achievement Award. He is a member of the Institute of Medicine. Dr. Rivara received his medical degree from the University of Pennsylvania School of Medicine.

Paul C. Erwin, M.D., Dr.P.H., is Professor and Chair of the Department of Public Health at the University of Tennessee in Knoxville. Prior to this appointment he served as the Regional Director, East Tennessee Region, in the Tennessee Department of Health for 12 years. Dr. Erwin received a B.S. from the University of the South (Sewanee, Tennessee); an M.D. from the University of Alabama in Birmingham; an M.P.H. in International Health at the Johns Hopkins University School of Hygiene and Public Health; and a Dr.P.H. at UNC/Chapel Hill. Dr. Erwin was a Fellow in International Health at the Aga Khan University in Karachi, Pakistan. He also served as a Scholar of the CDC/University of California Public Health Leadership Institute, 1995. Currently, Dr. Erwin is board certified in Internal Medicine and Public Health/General Preventive Medicine and is a Fellow of the American College of Preventive Medicine. He is also a board member of the Tennessee Institute of Public Health, 2007–present, and the Public Health Foundation, 2009–present. Since 2007, he has been a member of the Scientific Advisory Committee for United Health Foundation's *America's Health Rankings* report and the Research and Evaluation Committee of the Public Health Accreditation Board. Dr. Erwin's public health-related research and publications have been in the areas of public health systems and services research, health inequities/poverty and health, and infectious/communicable diseases.

Caswell A. Evans, Jr., D.D.S., M.P.H., is currently the Associate Dean for Prevention and Public Health Sciences at the University of Illinois, Chicago College of Dentistry. He served as the Executive Editor and Project Director of *Oral Health in America: A Report of the U.S. Surgeon General.* For 12 years, Dr. Evans served as Director of Public Health Programs and Services for the Los Angeles County Department of Health Services. He also served as Adjunct Professor for the School of Public Health and the School of Dentistry at the University of California, Los Angeles; Visiting Professor of Dentistry at Columbia University School of Dental and Oral Surgery; and Distinguished Minority Visiting Professor at the Boston University Health Sciences Center. He is a member of the Institute of Medicine. Dr. Evans is a Past President of the American Public Health Association, the American Association of Public Health Dentistry, and the American Board of Dental Public Health. He was the first recipient of the Beverlee A. Myers Award for Excellence in Public Health, conferred by the California State Department of Health Services. He was also honored with the Champion of Prevention Award from the Centers for Disease Control and Prevention.

Theodore G. Ganiats, M.D., is professor of Department of Family and Preventive Medicine at the University of California, San Diego School of Medicine, and Executive Director of the UCSD Health Services Research Center. He has been a member or chair of over 40 national guideline and quality/performance panels spanning multiple disciplines. His research interests involve outcomes research, focusing on quality-of-life assessment and cost-effectiveness analysis. He is a member of the Society for Medical

Decision Making, Academy Health, the American Public Health Association, and the International Society for Quality of Life Research. Dr. Ganiats is a member of the IOM, Section 8 for Family Medicine, Emergency Medicine, and Physical Medicine. He received his medical degree from the University of California, San Diego.

Shelly Gehshan, M.P.P., is the director of the Pew Children's Dental Campaign. Prior to joining Pew, she spent nearly 20 years working for state policy makers on a range of issues affecting low-income women and children, such as oral health, behavioral health, reproductive health, service delivery, and health care financing through Medicaid and SCHIP. From 2005 to 2008, Ms. Gehshan served as a senior program director at the National Academy for State Health Policy (NASHP) in Washington, DC. She developed NASHP's extensive portfolio of work in the area of oral health and directed projects on health care reform, Medicaid, behavioral health, and juvenile justice. Before joining NASHP, Ms. Gehshan spent 9 years as a program director for the National Conference of State Legislatures. At NCSL, she served as managing director and senior policy analyst for the Forum for State Health Policy Leadership, which provides training, policy analyses, and technical assistance for legislators and legislative staff. Ms. Gehshan spent 6 years as deputy director of the Southern Governors' Association's Infant Mortality Project, where she worked with governors and state legislators to expand access to prenatal care for low-income women. Ms. Gehshan has also served as the vice-chair of the board of directors for the Children's Dental Health Project. She has a master's degree in public policy from the Goldman School of Public Policy at the University of California, Berkeley.

Kathy Voigt Geurink, R.D.H., B.S., M.A., is a Clinical Associate Professor in the Department of Dental Hygiene, School of Health Professions, University of Texas Health Science Center. She has been recognized with various awards for her impact on the field of dental hygiene and in advancing the role of the dental hygienist in public health. Her textbook, *Community Oral Health Practice*, is widely used in dental hygiene programs nationwide. She serves as a consultant on the ASTDD School and Adolescent Oral Health Committee working with experts from around the country to advocate and support efforts to improve the oral health of children and adolescents. She has worked throughout her career with Head Start in addressing access to care for pregnant women, children, and families through the development of programs including oral health education, disease prevention, and referrals to dental homes. She also coordinates an ASTDD Committee on Healthy Aging to support assessment, policy development and assurance efforts in states. In 2011, she received the ASTDD

Distinguished Service Award for service to ASTDD and community oral health programs.

Paul Glassman, D.D.S., M.A., M.B.A., is professor of Dental Practice and Director of Community Oral Health at the Arthur A. Dugoni School of Dentistry at the University of the Pacific. He is a former president of the Special Care Dentistry Association, a national organization dedicated to improving oral health for people with special needs and older adults. He is director of the Pacific Center for Special Care and director of the California Statewide Task Force on Oral Health for People with Disabilities and Aging Californians. His research focuses on developing community-based systems for improving oral health for underserved populations; dentistry for patients with special needs, medical disabilities, and dental fear; and geriatric dentistry. He received his dental degree from the University of California, San Francisco.

David M. Krol, M.D., M.P.H., a general pediatrician, is Team Director and Senior Program Officer, Human Capital for the Robert Wood Johnson Foundation. Prior to joining the Foundation, Dr. Krol was an Associate Professor and Chair of the Department of Pediatrics at the University of Toledo College of Medicine. He is a leader in children's oral health advocacy and policy with a focus on the interface between primary care pediatrics and dentistry. Dr. Krol has published in scientific journals such as *Pediatrics*, *Advances in Pediatrics*, *Pediatrics in Review*, and others on topics such as children's oral health and health workforce policy. He partnered with the Children's Dental Health Project in his role as recipient of a Soros Advocacy Fellowship for Physicians. He was a RWJ Clinical Scholar and Bush Fellow in Child Development and Social Policy at Yale University. He was selected as a Pediatric Leader of the 21st Century by the American Academy of Pediatrics. Dr. Krol received his medical degree from the Yale School of Medicine and his M.P.H. from Columbia University, Mailman School of Public Health.

Jane Perkins, J.D., M.P.H., is the Legal Director for National Health Law Program. She focuses on Medicaid, particularly the Early and Periodic Screening, Diagnostic, and Treatment (EPSDT) program and discrimination in the delivery of health care. She engages in litigation and policy advocacy on these topics, manages NHeLP's litigation docket, and has written manuals, fact sheets, and numerous articles on Medicaid, civil rights, and federal court access. She also provides legal assistance and training to consumer advocates and health care consumers. Ms. Perkins is the co-author of *Toward a Healthy Future: Medicaid Early and Periodic Screening, Diagnostic and Treatment Services for Poor Children and Youth*, a Medicaid EPSDT resource manual. She was a 1997 recipient of the Reginald Heber Smith Award from the National Legal Aid and Defender Association for dedicated service and outstanding achievement as an indigent defense attorney. In 2009, Ms. Perkins received the Defender of Justice award from the North Carolina Justice Center. She earned her M.P.H. from the University of California, Berkeley, in 1982; her J.D. from the University of North Carolina, Chapel Hill, in 1981; and her B.A. from Davidson College in 1978.

Margaret A. Potter, M.S., J.D., is at the University of Pittsburgh holding positions in the Graduate School of Public Health as Associate Dean & Director of the Center for Public Health Practice and Associate Professor of Health Policy & Management. Her research interests include access to health services, public health systems including workforce development and financing, and public health law and policy. She has chaired national work groups on academic public health practice, focusing on the translation of scholarship to policy and practice. She is immediate past-chair of the board of directors of the Public Health Foundation. She earned a Master of Science degree in biomedical information systems from the Illinois Institute of Technology and a Juris Doctor degree from the Rutgers-Newark School of Law.

Renee Samelson, M.D., M.P.H., FACOG, is currently Associate Professor of Obstetrics and Gynecology at Albany Medical College and is a member of the Division of Maternal Fetal Medicine. She is board certified in Obstetrics and Gynecology and Preventive Medicine/Public Health with subspecialty board certification in Maternal-Fetal Medicine. Her high-risk obstetrical practice includes management of medical problems including diabetes and hypertension, obstetrical complications, prepregnancy consultations, prenatal diagnosis and treatment including evaluation of congenital anomalies, and first trimester screening. In 2006, Samelson was the co-editor of *Oral Health Care During Pregnancy and Early Childhood Clinical Practice Guidelines*. This document was the result of the work of an expert panel convened by the New York State Department of Health to develop recommendations for health care professionals in educating women about oral health and improving the overall health of women and children. Dr. Samelson had participated in multiple committees of the NIH Pediatric Aids Clinical Trial Group and was the Albany obstetrical principal investigator in several HIV perinatal trials. She continues to serve as a consultant to the NYS AIDS Institute.

Phyllis W. Sharps, Ph.D., RN, CNE, FAAN, is professor at Johns Hopkins University School of Nursing and the Associate Dean for Community and Global Programs. Her research and expertise focuses on addressing maternal child health disparities for vulnerable populations. She is currently Principal Investigator of a major NIH-funded test of a home visiting intervention for pregnant women to help end violence in their lives and prevent consequent trauma-related mental and physical health outcomes for both women and their infants. The intervention builds on her years of clinical practice and research including her work to develop, provide, and test a prenatal intervention to prevent low birth weight and other maternal child health problems in inner-city Baltimore and Washington, DC. She provides leadership in interdisciplinary research efforts and policy initiatives that are culturally appropriate, real-world based, and that address health iniquities. She received her Ph.D. from the University of Maryland School of Nursing, Baltimore.

Linda H. Southward, Ph.D., ACSW, is a Research Fellow at the Social Science Research Center of Mississippi State University. She was a leader in establishing the Child Care, Health, and Early Education Research Consortium (CHEER) of the American Academy of Pediatrics. She has led several surveys of children care directors' perspectives of a variety of early care and education issues, enabling investigation of systemic and pervasive child care research issues, including children's oral health status. She has also led a project on children's oral health with the Mississippi chapter of the American Academy of Pediatrics and has served as Principal Investigator in a 5-year AHRQ-funded study to determine to feasibility of developing an intervention to reduce dental caries of preschool children in 12 Mississippi Delta counties. Currently, Dr. Southward is leading a 5-year RWJ-funded study to evaluate the effectiveness of the Mississippi Healthy Student Act of 2007 in the areas of health education, physical education, and nutritional practices among Mississippi's public schools, students, parents, and policy makers in addressing childhood overweight and obesity in Mississippi. In addition, she coordinates the MS KIDS COUNT program. She earned a Ph.D. in Social Work from the University of Alabama.

Maria Rosa Watson, D.D.S., M.S., Dr.PH., is Board Diplomate of the American Board of Dental Public Health, a licensed Dentist in the District of Columbia, and has a Dr.PH from the Department of Epidemiology, Johns Hopkins University School of Public Health. From 1994 to 2002 she served on the faculty of the Department of Pediatric Dentistry at the University of Maryland Dental School. She has received NIH funding in the areas of community-based participatory research and health literacy. She is currently co-investigator of a NIH/NIMH Intervention and Practice Research Infrastructure Program (IP-RISP) grant, "Improving Health Services for Low-Income Latinos in Primary Care," of the Boston University and NIH-funded study "Partnering with Community Health Centers to Prevent

Early Childhood Caries," and of a project to develop a research agenda from the community perspective. She has served as independent evaluator to a University of South Florida-CDC grant focused on using CBPR in the implementation of a peer-led chronic illness self-management program, and to an oral health pilot program to increase access to dental care for adult Montgomery County residents, which now has been expanded to serve uninsured children. She received her B.S. and D.D.S. from the Peruvian University Cayetano Heredia, a M.S. in Pediatric Dentistry and an M.P.H. from the University of Michigan, followed by postgraduate residency training in dental public health with the U.S. Department of Veterans Affairs.

Barbara Wolfe, Ph.D., is Professor of Economics, Population Health Sciences, and Public Affairs and Faculty Affiliate at the Institute for Research on Poverty at the University of Wisconsin-Madison. Her research focuses broadly on poverty and health issues. Current projects examine the effect of expansions in public health insurance on health care coverage and labor force outcomes; the role of income on health using a natural experiment and using evidence from brain scans; whether housing voucher programs lead to higher earnings, higher-quality child care, and less reliance on other public assistance programs; and the increasing selectivity of high-quality universities. Recent work addresses the effects of welfare reform; economics of disability; ties among income, wealth, and health; racial disparities in health; and intergenerational determinants of success in young adults. She is a member of the IOM, Section 11 for social sciences, humanities, and law, and previously served as vice-chair of the Board on Children, Youth and Families. Her recent articles have appeared in the *Journal of Public Economics, Journal of Human Resources*, *International Journal of Health Care Finance and Economics*, *Journal of Policy Analysis and Management*, *Economy Inquiry*, *Journal of Health Economics*, and *Demography*. She received her doctorate in Economics from the University of Pennsylvania.

INSTITUTE OF MEDICINE STAFF

Tracy A. Harris, D.P.M., M.P.H., is a Senior Program Officer with the Institute of Medicine's (IOM's) Board on Health Care Services. Dr. Harris was trained in podiatric medicine and surgery and spent several years in private practice. In 1999, she was awarded a Congressional Fellowship with the American Association for the Advancement of Science and spent 1 year working in the U.S. Senate. Dr. Harris joined the IOM in 2004. Her most recent work has focused on aging and the health care workforce. She was the study director for the 2008 report *Retooling for an Aging America: Building the Health Care Workforce*. In 2009, she staffed a National Academies-wide initiative on the "Grand Challenges of an Aging Society" and directed a workshop on the oral health care workforce. Dr. Harris is the study director for this current report, the recently released report *Advancing Oral Health in America*, and director of a workshop on the allied health workforce. Dr. Harris has a doctor of podiatric medicine degree from Temple University and a master of public health degree with a concentration in health policy from The George Washington University.

Patti Simon, M.P.H., is a Senior Program Officer with the Institute of Medicine's (IOM's) Board on Children, Youth, and Families. In addition to her work on this current report, Ms. Simon served as the program officer for the recently released report *Child and Adolescent Health and Health Care Quality: Measuring What Matters*. Prior to joining the IOM in 2009, Ms. Simon worked in the Department of Health Policy at The George Washington University, where she managed a national program focused on health disparities and the social determinants of health. She holds an M.P.H. with a concentration in health education and health promotion from the University of Texas School of Public Health.

Meg Barry, J.D., M.P.H., is an Associate Program Officer on the Board on Health Care Services. She joined the IOM in 2009. She has worked on two studies related to oral health, and recently began working on a study of geographic variation in health care spending and promotion of high value care. Before joining the IOM, she worked on health care regulatory matters at a national law firm and reauthorization of the State Children's Health Insurance Program at the New America Foundation. Previously, she worked as a research scientist at Northwestern University. She is a graduate of the University of Michigan Law School and School of Public Health.

Wendy E. Keenan is a program associate for the Board on Children, Youth, and Families. She helps organize planning meetings and workshops that cover current issues related to children, youth, and families, and provides administrative and research support to the Board's various program committees. Ms. Keenan has been on the National Academies' staff for 10 years and has worked on studies for both the IOM and NRC. As a senior program assistant, she worked with the NRC's Board on Behavioral, Cognitive, and Sensory Sciences. Prior to joining the National Academies, she taught English as a second language for Washington, DC, public schools. She received a B.A. in sociology from The Pennsylvania State University and took graduate courses in liberal studies at Georgetown University.

Amy Asheroff joined the IOM in 2009 as a senior program assistant for the Board on Health Care Services and the Board on Children, Youth, and Families. She works on several projects: the Committee on an Oral Health

Initiative, Committee on Oral Health Access to Services, Committee on the Mental Health Workforce for Geriatric Populations, and a workshop on the allied health workforce. Prior to joining the IOM, she served a year of service in a safety net medical clinic in northwest Washington, DC, through AmeriCorps. She graduated from the University of California, Berkeley, with a bachelor's degree in the History of Art and Italian.

Rosemary Chalk is director of the Board on Children, Youth, and Families, a joint effort of the IOM and NRC. She is a policy analyst who has been a study director at the National Academies since 1987. She has directed or served as a senior staff member for more than a dozen IOM and NRC studies, including studies on vaccine finance, the public health infrastructure for immunization, family violence, child abuse and neglect, research ethics and misconduct in science, and education finance. From 2000 to 2003, Ms. Chalk directed a research project on the development of child well-being indicators for the child welfare system at Child Trends in Washington, DC. She previously served as a consultant for science and society research projects at the Harvard School of Public Health and was an Exxon research fellow in the Program on Science, Technology, and Society at the Massachusetts Institute of Technology. She was program head of the Committee on Scientific Freedom and Responsibility of the American Association for the Advancement of Science from 1976 to 1986. She holds a B.A. in foreign affairs from the University of Cincinnati.